Computer-Aided Drug Design

Computer-Aided Drug Design

Methods and Applications

edited by

THOMAS J. PERUN

Abbott Laboratories
Abbott Park, Illinois

C. L. PROPST

Affiliated Scientific, Inc.
Ingleside, Illinois

MARCEL DEKKER, INC.   New York and Basel

Library of Congress Cataloging-in-Publication Data

Computer-aided drug design : methods and applications / edited by Thomas J.
  Perun, C. L. Propst.
        p.   cm.
    Includes bibliographies and index.
    ISBN 0-8247-8037-X (alk. paper)
    1. Drugs--Design--Data processing. 2. Computer-aided design. I. Perun,
  Thomas J. II. Propst, C. L. (Catherine Lamb)
    [DNLM: 1. Chemistry, Pharmaceutical. 2. Computers. 3. Models, Molecu-
  lar.   QV 744 C738]
  RS420.C66   1989
  615'.19'00285--dc19
  DNLM/DLC
  for Library of Congress   88-37186
                                                                    CIP

The computer-generated figure on the cover is a previously unpublished renin
model derived from the crystal structure of porcine pepsin with a potent inhibitor in the active site. (Courtesy of Dr. Charles Hutchins, Abbott Laboratories.)

This book is printed on acid-free paper.

MARCEL DEKKER, INC.
270 Madison Avenue, New York, New York 10016

Current printing (last digit):
10 9 8 7 6 5 4 3 2 1

PRINTED IN THE UNITED STATES OF AMERICA

In Memory of
Eliza Mayo Mills Propst
and
John Thomas Perun

Preface

The development of new drugs has been responsible for decreasing human morbidity and mortality more than any other scientific endeavor in our lifetime. These products have dramatically improved the quality of life across all age ranges and socioeconomic groups. Moreover, modern drugs are a highly cost-effective form of treatment. They can prevent illness or, when illness occurs, speed recovery, reduce hospital stays, and decrease the need for surgery.

Drugs can be discovered in a number of ways. Sometimes they are found by accident. Most frequently, they are developed as part of an organized effort to discover new ways to treat specific diseases. With the general acceptance of the molecular basis of disease has come the realization that the disease process can be understood at the chemical level, and consequently the disease can be interrupted chemically. This has led to the mechanistic approach for the development of drugs to treat diseases.

The mechanistic approach to drug discovery begins with knowledge of the disease process itself. It also requires that one know about the chemical structures of the interacting molecules. Since substrates, ligands, or drugs that mimic them (effectors) and their enzymes or receptors (targets) interact via a lock-and-key type mechanism, knowledge of their three-dimensional structures is of critical importance. Once these are known, scientists can begin to design new chemical entities (NCEs) to influence the targets which are involved in the disease process.

Because of the vast amount of information involved in determining the three-dimensional structures of the effector and its target, and in the use of this information for the design of new medicinal agents, computers have been a major requirement for this process. Consequently this approach to new drug design has frequently been called "computer-aided drug design" (CADD). Such a designation, however, loses sight of the fact that the computer functions as a tool in the drug design process. CADD is critically dependent on the physical techniques of crystallization and spectroscopy to provide the practical parameters for its calculations, and on the wisdom of the medicinal scientists to interpret and utilize its output data.

This book has been written to provide an overview of the process of mechanistic, computer-aided drug design. To accomplish this, the book has been divided into two sections: "Methods" and "Applications." It is intended to be of use to students who plan to enter the field of drug design and to individuals who are currently involved with drug research but may not be fully familiar with the approaches used in CADD. Since this is a very rapidly moving field, some of the theoretical sections present concepts that are at the forefront of this technology; consequently this book should also be of use to scientists who are intimately involved with CADD.

The process of mechanistic design of new drugs is only in its infancy. This is because the knowledge base about both disease processes and the structures and interactions of molecules is still developing. This in no way prevents the use of this technology in discovering new pharmaceuticals. Rather it challenges the creativity of the scientist to supplement current knowledge with ingenuity. The Applications section of the book has been added as a complement to the Methods section in order to demonstrate how scientists are currently coping with the available knowledge base and at the same time successfully developing new drugs.

Thomas J. Perun
C. L. Propst

Contributors

Donald J. Abraham   Department of Medicinal Chemistry, Medical College of Virginia, Virginia Commonwealth University, Richmond, Virginia

Giorgio Bolis*   Computer-Assisted Molecular Design, Abbott Laboratories, Abbott Park, Illinois

Stanley K. Burt   Sandoz Research Institute, East Hanover, New Jersey

Stephen W. Fesik   NMR Research, Abbott Laboratories, Abbott Park, Illinois

Jonathan Greer   Computer-Assisted Molecular Design, Abbott Laboratories, Abbott Park, Illinois

Arnold T. Hagler   Department of Biophysics, The Agouron Institute, La Jolla, California, and Biosym Technologies, Inc., San Diego, California

David G. Hangauer   Department of Exploratory Chemistry, Merck Sharp & Dohme Research Laboratories, Rahway, New Jersey

Andreas Haupt   Institute of Organic Chemistry, J. W. Goethe University, Frankfurt, Federal Republic of Germany

---

Present affiliation: Computer Aided Molecular Design Department, Farmitalia Carlo Erba, Milan, Italy.

Victor J. Hruby   Department of Chemistry, University of Arizona, Tucson, Arizona

Horst Kessler   Institute of Organic Chemistry, J. W. Goethe University, Frankfurt, Federal Republic of Germany

Lee F. Kuyper   Wellcome Research Laboratories, Research Triangle Park, North Carolina

Donald Mackay   Department of Biophysics, The Agouron Institute, La Jolla, California, and Biosym Technologies, Inc., San Diego, California

Dexter B. Northrop   School of Pharmacy, University of Wisconsin—Madison, Madison, Wisconsin

T. J. O'Donnell*   Computer-Assisted Molecular Design, Abbott Laboratories, Abbott Park, Illinois

Thomas J. Perun   Pharmaceutical Discovery Division, Abbott Laboratories, Abbott Park, Illinois

B. Montgomery Pettitt   Department of Chemistry, University of Houston, Houston, Texas

C. L. Propst   Affiliated Scientific, Inc., Ingleside, Illinois

Daniel H. Rich   School of Pharmacy, University of Wisconsin—Madison, Madison, Wisconsin

Thomas J. Smith   Department of Biological Sciences, Purdue University, West Lafayette, Indiana

Martin Will   Institute of Organic Chemistry, J. W. Goethe University, Frankfurt, Federal Republic of Germany

---

Present affiliation: Scientific Graphics and Computing, O'Donnell Associates, Chicago, Illinois.

Contents

APPLICATIONS

Computer-Aided Drug Design

1
Introduction to Computer-Aided Drug Design

C. L. Propst
Affiliated Scientific, Inc., Ingleside, Illinois

Thomas J. Perun
Abbott Laboratories, Abbott Park, Illinois

I. INTRODUCTION

Although the phrase computer-aided drug design may seem to imply that drug discovery lies in the hands of the computational scientists who are able to manipulate molecules on their computer screens, the drug design process is actually a complex and interactive one, involving scientists from many disciplines working together to provide many types of information. This book has been written to show how the modern computational and experimental techniques that have been developed in recent years can be used together to provide structural information about the biologically active molecules that are involved in disease processes and in modulating disease processes.

II. HOW DRUGS ARE DISCOVERED

Occasionally new drugs are found by accident. More frequently they are developed as part of an organized effort to discover new ways to treat specific diseases. The discovery of new pharmaceutical agents has gone through an evolution over the years and has been adding new technologies to this increasingly complex process (1).

A. Screening for New Drugs

The traditional way to discover new drugs has been to screen a large number of synthetic chemical compounds or natural products for desirable effects. Although this approach for the development of new pharmaceutical agents has been successful in the past, it is not an ideal one for a number of reasons.

The biggest drawback to the screening process is the requirement for an appropriate screening procedure. Although drugs are ultimately developed in the clinic, it is usually inappropriate to put chemicals of unknown efficacy directly into humans. Consequently, other systems have to be developed. Normally a battery of screens is used to select potential new drug candidates, with activity in initial, rough screens feeding compounds into later, more sophisticated screens. Initial screens are often in vitro tests for some fundamental activity, such as the ability to kill bacteria in solution. Ultimately, however, more sophisticated in vivo screens are needed. This second level of screening is normally carried out using animal model systems for the disease.

Screens have inherent limitations (2). Primary screens are used for large numbers of chemicals to choose which compounds should be further tested with more sophisticated tests. If the primary screen does not select for an appropriate activity, however, an active structure will appear to be inactive and will not be discovered. Secondary screening in animal model systems has additional problems, such as: (1) the animal model may not accurately reflect the human disease; (2) the chemical may be extensively metabolized to a different compound in the animal before it reaches its target; (3) the chemical may not be absorbed or distributed as it is in humans. In each of these cases, the active structure potentially will not be identified.

Another serious problem with the screening process is that, because of its random nature, it is inherently repetitious and time-consuming just to find a chemical with the desired activity. Furthermore, chemical compounds discovered by this approach commonly do not have optimal structures for modulating the biological process. This in turn may require administration of larger quantities of the drug and increase the risk of unwanted side effects.

The major advantage of screening is the large amount of information that is *not* needed to carry out the process. One does not need to know the structure of the drug being sought. Nor does one need to know the structure of the target upon which the drug will act. Most importantly, one does not need to know about the underlying mechanism of the disease process itself.

B. Modifications for Improvements

Once an active (lead) compound has been identified and its chemical structure determined, it is usually possible to improve on this activity and/or to reduce side effects by making modifications to the basic chemical structure. Modifications to improve performance are often carried out using chemical or bioformentative means to make changes in the lead structure or its intermediates. Alternatively, for some natural products, the gene itself may be engineered so that the producer organism synthesizes the modified compound directly.

The process of developing drugs via modification of active lead compounds requires that the structure of the compound be known. One still does not need to know the structure of the target on which the drug works. Likewise, no information about the underlying disease process is required.

As with screening, the process of modification is often based on a primarily trial-and-error approach. Because more information is known, however, this process can be carried out with much greater probability of success than a purely random process. A prime example of the power of this approach is in the antiinfective area where modifications of the original first-generation cephalosporins have led to second- and now third generation offspring with substantially improved characteristics (3).

The limitations of this process are inherent to the fact that one is using a single lead compound as the basis for further drug design. Improvements are likely; however, no major breakthrough in developing new chemical entities (NCEs) is probable. Furthermore, if the original lead compound fails to generate a desirable drug, one must start the process over again by finding a new lead molecule.

C. Mechanism-Based Drug Design

As still more information becomes available about the biological basis of a disease, it is possible to begin to design drugs using a mechanistic approach to the disease process. When the disease process is understood at the molecular level and the target molecule(s) are defined, drugs can be designed specifically to interact with the target molecule in such a way as to disrupt the disease (1–6).

Clearly a mechanistic approach to drug design requires a great deal of knowledge. Furthermore, processing this knowledge in such a way that a scientist can use the knowledge to develop a new drug is a formidable task. Nonetheless, it is clear that the major breakthroughs in drug design in the future are most likely to come via the use of this approach. Because of the massive amount of information that must be harnessed to develop drugs by this technique, it is in this area where computer-aided drug design will have its greatest impact. This will be discussed further in Section III.

D. Combining Techniques

In discussing the various techniques for finding new drugs, it is important to remember that drug discovery is both a cumulative and a reiterative process. Potential drugs developed by modifying a lead structure are certain to be sent through selective screening processes to confirm activity and select for the best candidate to go on for further development. Likewise, drugs developed mechanistically will likely be both screened and later modified in order to produce the best candidate drug. Figure 1 presents schematically some of the various interactions that can occur in the discovery of a new drug.

Furthermore, every new chemical entity that affects the disease process—whether found by accident, screening, modification, or mechanistic design—provides useful information for developing still better compounds. This is true whether the chemical has positive or negative effects on the disease process. Each new chemical increases the data base of information about the disease-target-drug interaction. This in turn is the basis for rational drug design.

III. THE BASICS OF MECHANISTIC DRUG DESIGN

Most diseases affecting man have been identified by their clinical manifestations. Thus we are familiar with medical conditions such as hypertension, cancer, infections, etc. Modern biological techniques now have enabled

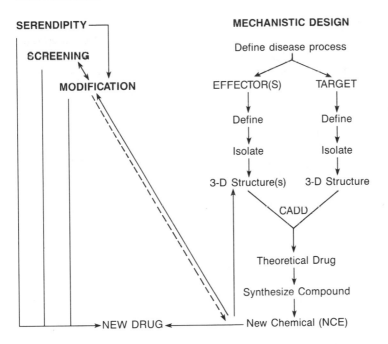

Figure 1 Flow diagram of some of the potential interactions that can occur in the process of discovering a new chemical entity. Modification has the potential to produce improvements in structures but is unlikely to discover a new chemical entity (dashed line).

researchers to study such diseases at the molecular level and to identify the processes or molecules responsible for producing the clinical effects.

A. Defining the Disease Process

The first step in the mechanistic design of drugs to treat diseases is to determine the biochemical basis of the disease process. Ideally, one would know the various steps involved in the physiological pathway that carries out the normal function. In addition, one would know the exact step(s) in the pathway that are altered in the diseased state. Knowledge about the regulation of the pathway is also important. Finally, one would know the three-dimensional structures of the molecules involved in the process.

Once the biochemical basis of the disease is understood, one can select a target for modulating the disease process. These targets are often macromolecules such as enzymes, receptors, or nucleic acids, and are discussed further in the next section. In the normal condition the interaction of targets with their effector molecules produces a necessary physiologic function. Although most diseases have not been so fully characterized that all the above information is available, in many instances sufficient information is available to design a rational approach to block or reverse the disease process.

B. Defining the Target

There are potentially many ways in which biochemical pathways could become abnormal and result in disease. Therefore, knowledge of the molecular basis of the disease is important in order to select a target at which to disrupt the process. Targets for mechanistic drug design usually fall into three categories: enzymes, receptors, and nucleic acids.

1.   Enzymes as Targets

Enzymes are frequently the target of choice for disruption of a disease. If a disease is the result of the overproduction of a certain compound, then one or more of the enzymes involved in its synthesis can often be inhibited, resulting in a decrease in production of the compound and disruption of the disease process. This is the theoretical basis behind the design of both the angiotensin-converting enzyme inhibitors (Chapter 7) and the renin inhibitors (Chapter 8). Inhibition of either of these enzymes, which are in the same biochemical pathway, decreases the production of angiotensin II and consequently reduces blood pressure. In other instances specific enzymes may be required for pathogenic microorganisms or cancerous cells to live and grow, thereby causing disease. Inhibition of such enzymes would prevent the growth of these microbes or cells and hence reverse the disease. Such is the case with the enzyme dihydrofolate reductase which is described in Chapter 9.

   Enzymes are usually the targets of choice because they are relatively small, aqueous-soluble proteins that often can be isolated for study. When enough of the enzyme is difficult to obtain from its natural source, genetic engineering techniques are frequently utilized to provide material for conducting x-ray crystallography, NMR spectroscopy, and enzyme kinetic studies. Ultimately the data obtained by these techniques allow one to determine the three-dimensional structures of the enzyme molecule in its active conformation. These structures provide a starting point for the design of new effector molecules (i.e., drugs) by computer graphics and molecular modeling techniques.

2.   Receptors as Targets

Sometimes a disease can be modulated by blocking the action of an effector at its cellular receptor. A classic example of this is the well-known inhibition of the gastric histamine-2 receptor by the drug cimetidine which decreases acid secretion in the stomach and reduces ulcer formation (7). Unlike enzymes, which often circulate in the body and can be isolated and studied outside their biological environment, cellular receptors consist of proteins imbedded in a surface membrane. Consequently these targets are difficult to isolate, and thus it is difficult to determine their structures. Nonetheless, molecular biological techniques are beginning to produce these macromolecules in larger amounts. Structural information will soon be available for many of them, using the same experimental techniques used for determining enzyme structures.

Receptors that are easily isolated are the most amenable to rational design of effectors. An illustrative use of this concept is in the three-dimensional structural determination of rhinoviruses, which then can serve as a receptor-type target for the design of antiviral drugs. Chapter 10 describes compounds that can bind to and block the uncoating of the target rhinovirus, thereby potentially preventing diseases such as the common cold. Chapters 11 and 12 deal with more conventional receptors and show the difficulties of working with these targets as well as the techniques used to compensate for the difficulties.

3. Nucleic Acids as Targets

Diseases can also potentially be blocked by preventing the synthesis of undesirable proteins at the nucleic acid level. This strategy has frequently been employed in the antimicrobial and antitumor areas, where DNA-blocking drugs are used to prevent the synthesis of critical proteins. Since the microorganisms or tumor cells cannot grow and/or replicate, the disease process is effectively blocked. Examples include the use of the DNA-intercalating drug adriamycin to treat certain forms of cancer (8).

Although nucleic acids are legitimate targets for computer-aided drug design, for exemplary reasons this book deals only with protein targets. Nevertheless the principles derived from the use of protein targets are, for the most part, also applicable to the nucleic acids.

C. Defining the Effector

Effector molecules are compounds that can occupy an active site of a target molecule. As used in this context, they can be substrates, natural effectors that regulate the target in positive or negative ways, or drugs. Effector molecules and their targets interact with each other via a lock-and-key type of mechanism, in which the target enzyme or receptor is the lock and the effector is the key (9). Implicit in this concept is that the two fit together in a physically complementary fashion. Therefore, it should be possible to determine the shape of the mutual contact surface of either by knowing the three-dimensional conformation of the active portion of one.

In reality, the relationship between effector and target is more complex. The natural effector molecule fits into the active site of the enzyme or the binding site of the receptor in a manner that maximizes the complementarity of the two molecules (10). In addition, this complementarity not only is recognized as a function of shape, but also includes the interaction of charged regions, hydrogen bonding, hydrophilic interactions, etc. (see Chapters 2, 3). Because the interactions between the effector and its target are so complex, the best information for designing drugs is obtained when one can determine the three-dimensional structure of both the target and effector molecules. However, since effector molecules are often much smaller and more readily available than their targets (see previous section), they are usually more amenable to structural analyses. Again the information obtained from experimental techniques provides the spatial coordinates that are utilized in the computerized analysis of the effector's structure.

D. Designing New Drugs to Effect Targets

To make a good drug, a compound should exhibit a number of useful characteristics. In addition to producing the desired effect, it should be sufficiently potent that large amounts do not have to be administered. It should have low toxicity and minimal side effects. Drugs that have to be given for chronic conditions should have considerable residence time in the body (half-life) so that continuous administration is not needed. Oral administration of a drug is the preferred route in order to encourage patient compliance.

In the normal condition, natural effectors interact with their targets to carry out a needed physiological function. The natural effector for a target thus often represents an optimal structure for the complex formed. These natural molecules are not often used as drugs, however, for a number of reasons. The body generally has the ability to produce these effectors whenever they are needed to modulate a biological process. Once they have fulfilled their function, they are rapidly removed via metabolic and elimination mechanisms. Natural effectors also generally are not orally active. The metabolic instability built into the molecule to facilitate natural inactivation often allows it to be degraded by enzymes in the gastrointestinal tract. Even when natural effectors survive this process, they typically do not have the properties necessary to pass through the gastrointestinal mucosa. Additionally, endogenous effectors frequently interact with similar targets in a variety of systems. Thus, they tend to cause substantial unrelated side effects under conditions of high-level or long-term administration.

On the other hand, natural effector molecules are often used as the starting point for the development of new drugs, since they generally have selectivity and potency for the desired target. By careful manipulation of the native structure, one can frequently retain the binding characteristics of the effector while designing in other desirable characteristics. Examples of drug design with natural effectors as the starting point include the use of the structure of luteinizing hormone-releasing hormone in the design of LHRH receptor agonists such as the anticancer drug leuprolide (11) and the use of the structure of the enkephalins in the design of opioid receptor agonists as potential analgesics (Chapter 11).

There are other sources for complementary structures for enzyme and receptor targets, which can also be used as a starting point, or to provide additional structural information, for designing new drugs. If the natural effector is unavailable, similar effectors from a different host may be used— e.g., the structure of equine angiotensinogen was used in the development of early human renin inhibitors (Chapter 8 and ref. 12). Natural products, particularly those obtained from microbes, often provide novel structures that are potent effectors. For example, pepstatin, a natural product produced by an actinomycete, is a potent inhibitor of aspartic proteinases and therefore was useful in the design of renin inhibitors (Chapter 8). Likewise, antamanide, a substance found in mushrooms, has been useful in the study of hepatocellular receptors (Chapter 12).

Synthetic compounds with only a vague resemblance to the effector may also have regions of complementarity and provide useful information. For example, trimethoprim, a unique synthetic compound with little resemblance to folic acid, is an excellent inhibitor of bacterial dihydrofolate reductase and was an important lead structure in the design of inhibitors of DHFR enzymes (Chapter 9). In each case the goal of the drug designer, when modifying the natural or other effectors, is to remove those characteristics that confer instability and poor absorption and to add features that improve potency while providing greater specificity.

E. Overcoming Obstacles in Mechanistic Drug Design

It is easiest to design new drugs when one has a full understanding of the disease process and reliable structural information about the target and its effectors. Unfortunately, such complete information is not often available.

In the design of a new drug, structural information about the target molecule is frequently unavailable. Enzymes are the target of choice because they are generally smaller and not attached to other structures and thus are often easier to isolate and characterize. Even when enzymes are selected as targets, however, there can be problems obtaining structural information. Sometimes it is difficult to isolate or produce sufficient quantities of the target enzyme to study it directly. Human enzymes are especially difficult to obtain in large quantities. When this happens, one can often take advantage of the fact that many enzymes belong to families with a high degree of homology in their amino acid sequence. Thus enzymes with similar functions often retain similar structural features and catalytic sites. It is therefore possible to model an enzyme with an unknown structure by using the structural information from a known enzyme. Sometimes one can use the "same" enzyme from a different species as a model. A good example is the use of various dihydro-folate reductase enzymes from different species to define the structure and specificity of the target enzyme (Chapter 9). Alternatively, enzymes of the same class or sharing similar properties can be used. Such is the case with the use of both carboxypeptidase A and thermolysin as models for human angiotensin-converting enzyme, which is described by Hangauer in Chapter 7. Likewise aspartic proteinases from fungal and mammalian sources have been used to model the human renin enzyme (Chapter 8).

Receptor molecules make still more difficult targets, because they are much larger and frequently membrane-associated. In many cases, the receptor has never been isolated in pure form, and little about its chemical and structural characteristics is known. In these cases all the information available about the effector-receptor complex comes from the effector's structure alone (see Section III. C). Accurate structural information about the complex is made more difficult when the effector molecule is a flexible one with many possible conformations in solution. In such a case, attempts are made to constrain the structure of the effector through cyclization or other chemical modifications. These more rigid structures then become useful probes for the macromolecular receptor and are often able to select for specific receptor subtypes. Good examples of this technique are described in the chapters by Hruby and Pettitt (Chapter 11) and by Kessler, Haupt, and Will (Chapter 12), which deal with the opioid and hepatocellular receptors, respectively.

Finally, it should be reiterated that mechanistic drug design is based on knowledge. Since the data base that supports that knowledge is still developing, and is growing at a very rapid rate, it is important for medicinal scientists both to be receptive to new information and to be creative with its use. It is to be anticipated that important new data for the design of drugs will become available from scientific disciplines that by tradition are widely divergent, including clinical medicine, pharmacology, microbiology, mole-cular biology, enzymology, biochemistry, medicinal chemistry, and physical chemistry. With the current state of knowledge, success in designing new drugs depends on the ability to overcome obstacles, which in turn is dependent on the scope and the ingenuity of the medicinal scientists involved in the process.

IV. IMPORTANT TECHNIQUES FOR DRUG DESIGN

To obtain the structural information about molecules necessary for mechanistic design of drugs, a variety of chemical, physical, and theoretical techniques must be used. Different techniques provide complementary types of information, which together can be used to determine how molecules interact.

A. X-Ray Crystallography

X-ray crystallography is often the starting point for gathering information for mechanistic drug design. This technology has the potential to determine total structural information about a molecule. Furthermore it provides the critically important coordinates needed for the handling of data by computer modeling systems.

To carry out an x-ray crystallographic analysis, material of very high purity is needed. This material must be carefully crystallized to yield crystals of a suitably high quality for study. Small molecules can generally be crystallized using standard chemical techniques. Macromolecules such as proteins, however, require specialized techniques to produce suitable crystals. Even with suitable crystals, the solution of a macromolecular structure is much more difficult than for a small molecule. The larger number of atoms in a macromolecule makes it hard to attain the high degree of resolution needed. Furthermore, the instrumentation required is complex, and the data analysis and refinement take substantial computer time. Finally, because x-ray crystallography must be carried out with molecules in the solid phase, the three-dimensional structure obtained may differ from the molecule in its biologically active state.

Nevertheless, this technology is very important for determining the structure of the drug (effector), the structure of the drug's target, and the interaction of the two. The methodology behind the use of this technology in new drug discovery is described in Chapter 4. An application of this technology is detailed in the x-ray work of Abraham and Perutz on hemoglobin and its implications for antisickling drugs, which is also described in Chapter 4. Additional examples of the use of x-ray crystallography can be found throughout the Applications section of the text. An especially illustrative application is shown in Chapter 10 which describes how this technology is being applied to the search for antiviral drugs. Here Smith describes how x-ray crystallography has been used first to determine the structure of the infectious virus (the target) and later the structure of drug candidates and their interaction with the virus.

B. NMR Spectroscopy

As previously mentioned, the major limitations of x-ray crystallography are the necessity to obtain good crystals and the fact that three-dimensional data obtained with crystals may not reflect the molecular structure under biological conditions that involve molecules in solution. The best technique for determining structural information on molecules in solution is nuclear magnetic resonance (NMR) spectroscopy. NMR uses much softer radiation which can examine molecules in the more mobile liquid phase, so the three-dimensional information obtained may be more representative of the molecule in its biological environment. Another advantage of NMR is its ability to examine small molecule-macromolecule complexes, such as an enzyme inhibitor in the active site of the enzyme. Such information can be obtained by x-ray crystallography only after cocrystallization or crystal "soaking" techniques. In addition, NMR can often be used to gather structural information more rapidly than x-ray crystallography.

The disadvantage of NMR is that the data obtained are not as precise or complete as those from an x-ray structure determination. There is also a limit on the size of molecule that can be studied with present equipment. Modern high-field NMR spectrometers have recently been developed that can obtain data on smaller samples and, by the use of two-dimensional techniques, are able to obtain more precise information about macromolecules.

The mechanics of NMR spectroscopy in new drug design are detailed by Fesik in Chapter 5. Additional discussions and examples of the application of this technology in designing pharmaceuticals are seen in Chapter 11, which reviews the design of conformationally constrained opioid peptides.

C. Computerized Molecular Modeling

One of the most important advances in mechanistic drug design has been the recent development of computerized molecular modeling. Computerized modeling can provide scientists with five major types of information that are important for mechanistic design of drugs: (1) the three-dimensional structure of a molecule; (2) the chemical and physical characteristics of a molecule; (3) comparison of the structure of one molecule with other different molecules; (4) visualization of complexes formed between different molecules; and (5) predictions about how related new molecules might look.

Model building has been used for many years to approximate structures of biomolecules. The advent of computer techniques, however, has enabled this to be accomplished with greater speed and precision and has allowed the incorporation of information not previously available into the modeling process. Modern computer graphic techniques have enabled the three-dimensional visualization of structures on specialized computer terminals. It has made possible the manipulation of these structures in real time to allow visualization of different parts of the molecule, to change the orientation of specific functions while holding others constant, and to look at different feasible conformations.

Molecular modeling can also present the scientist with a visualization of specific characteristics of a molecule that influence its interactions with other molecules. Examples include structures that show the van der Waals radii of atoms, the electrostatic potential of molecules, the solvent accessible surface of molecules, the contour of electron density, etc.

Molecular modeling also has the ability to compare the structure of one molecule with related molecules to determine areas of similarity and difference. This comparison can include charged regions and other chemical characteristics as well as gross structural features. In addition, it can visualize in three dimensions how two different molecules—e.g., a drug and its target enzyme—can fit together.

Finally, this technology has the potential power to design theoretical new molecules to satisfy predetermined shapes. An example would be "finding" a new structure that mimics the shape of an active compound and is therefore able to occupy the active site of an enzyme.

This powerful new methodology is described in detail by O'Donnell in Chapter 2. Although all chapters in the Applications section of this book use this technology, the power of this methodology in new drug discovery is especially evident in the chapters by Bolis and Greer (Chapter 8), describing the development of a new class of cardiovascular drugs (the renin inhibitors), and by Kuyper (Chapter 9), describing work on the enzyme dihydrofolate reductase.

D. Other Important Considerations

It has long been realized that biological molecules can exist in a variety of different conformations and, depending on the energetics of the molecules and the environmental conditions, will shift among these conformations. The initial application of molecular modeling to design drugs generally begins with the use of rigid constructs for structures and their targets. This concept of molecular behavior is often satisfactory for answering simple questions, such as whether a drug will fit into the active site of the target. As the questions about molecular interactions become more complex, however, the concept of molecules in different dynamic energetic states and configurations becomes much more important. Sophisticated questions such as what is the most favorable position for a drug in its target's active site require more information, based on additional physical parameters, than simply answering the question, will a molecule fit into a given space.

The flexibility of molecular conformations, both in single molecules and in molecules interacting with each other, is an important and challenging concept in drug design. One of the major potentials of computer-aided drug design is the development of completely new effector compounds for targets. To date, however, this has been very difficult. A significant reason is our lack of knowledge about the factors that govern conformational states and flexibility. Two chapters in this book deal extensively with the theoretical aspects of drug design and the complex concepts surrounding molecular interactions. Chapter 3, by Burt and Hagler, discusses in detail molecular mechanics and molecular dynamics as applied to new drug design. Chapter 6 by Rich and Northrop, details the importance of enzyme kinetics in the design of new drugs.

Both of these chapters present concepts that are at the forefront of mechanistic drug design. These concepts and the problems they attempt to understand and handle are important, since it is in these areas that breakthroughs are still needed to realize the real potential of computer-aided drug design in predicting new chemical structures that will interact with the desired targets.

V. CONCLUSIONS AND FUTURE PERSPECTIVES

The process of drug discovery and development is a long and difficult one, and the costs of developing new therapeutic agents are increasing rapidly (13). Today it takes approximately 10 years and $100 million to bring a new drug to market (14,15). In spite of the tremendous costs involved, the payoff is also high, both in dollars and in the improvements made in preventing and controlling human diseases. The emphasis now is not just on finding new ways to treat human diseases, but also on improving the quality of life of people in general. The use of new computer-based drug design techniques has the ability to accomplish both of these goals and to improve the efficiency of the process as well, thus reducing costs.

Mechanism-based drug design tackles medical problems directly. It provides an opportunity to discover entirely new lead compounds not possible using other techniques for drug development. Thus it offers the potential for treating diseases that are not currently controllable by existing drugs.

Similarly, these new techniques in drug design can improve the lead optimization process. By understanding the physical interaction of a drug and its receptor, one has the means to improve on the potency and selectivity of a drug and thereby reduce its undesirable interactions with other physiological processes in the body. We are already seeing improvements in the quality of life of patients receiving these newer drugs, which have greater potency and fewer side effects. An example is the emerging use of angiotensin-converting enzyme inhibitors as first-line antihypertensive agents (16).

Finally, since the traditional lead optimization process typically requires the synthesis of hundreds or even thousands of new compounds, it is a time-consuming and labor-intensive process. The use of newer computer-based techniques in combination with techniques that have been successful in the past provides a means to greatly reduce the number of new compounds that must be synthesized and tested and thus speeds up the process of drug discovery.

Future developments will continue to improve the efficiency of all aspects of drug discovery. Knowledge about the molecular basis of diseases is rapidly expanding on all fronts and will continue unabated. Molecular biologists will soon be able to provide quantities of receptor molecules and enzymes that have not yet been available to drug researchers. Improvements in x-ray and NMR techniques will yield needed structural information in shorter times and will give more details of the drug-target complex. With these new data will come improvements in computational techniques and their ability to predict the conformational state of a small compound and its macro-molecular receptor. In addition, these techniques will be able to depict more clearly the biological molecules under physiological conditions. Finally, as more and more drug researchers understand and become familiar with the concepts and methods of mechanistic, computer-aided drug design, new applications of the integration of these techniques will emerge and will have a major impact both on basic science and on discovering new drugs for the future.

REFERENCES

1. Propst, C., Modern technologies for the discovery of new pharmaceuticals. In *The World Biotech Report—USA*, Vol. 2. Online Publications, New York, pp. 283–289 (1985).
2. Perun, T., The use of molecular modeling and computer graphic techniques in the design of new cardiovascular drugs. In *The World Biotech Report—USA*, Vol. 2. Online Publications, New York, pp. 313–320 (1985).
3. Newall, C. Injectable cephalosporin antibiotics: Cephalothin to ceftazidime. In *Medicinal Chemistry—The Role of Organic Chemistry in Drug Research*, S. Roberts and B. Price, eds. Academic Press, London, pp. 209–226 (1985).
4. Hopfinger, A., Computer-assisted drug design. *J. Med. Chem. 28*:1133–1139 (1985).
5. Hol, W., Protein crystallography and computer graphics—toward rational drug design. *Angew. Chem. Int. Ed. Engl. 25*:767–778 (1986).
6. Weiss, R., Scientists study the art of protein folding. *Sci. News 28*:344–346 (1987).
7. Ganellin, C., Discovery of cimetidine. In *Medicinal Chemistry—The Role of Organic Chemistry in Drug Research*, S. Roberts and B. Price, eds. Academic Press, London, pp. 93–118 (1985).
8. Young, R., R. Ozols, and C. Myers, The anthracycline antineoplastic drugs. *N. Engl. J. Med. 305*:139–153 (1981).

9. Fischer, E., Einfluss der Configuration auf die Wirkung der Enzyme. *Ber. Deutsch. Chem. Ges. 27*:2984–2993 (1894).

10. Koshland, D., Application of a theory of enzyme specificity to protein synthesis. *Proc. Natl. Acad. Sci. USA 44*:98–104 (1958).

11. Fujino, M., T. Fukuda, S. Shinagawa, S. Kobayashi, I. Yamazaki, R. Nakayama, J. Seely, W. White, and R. Rippel, Synthetic analogs of luteinizing hormone releasing hormone (LH-RH) substituted in positions 6 and 10. *Biochem. Biophys. Res. Commun. 60*:406–412 (1974).

12. Burton, J., R. Cody, J. Herd, and E. Haber, Specific inhibition of renin by an angiotensinogen analog: Studies in sodium depletion and renin-dependent hypertension. *Proc. Natl. Acad. Sci. USA 77*:5476–5479 (1980).

13. Chivvis, A. Jr., D. Mackie, and N. Selby, Playing to win the new game in pharmaceuticals. *Pharm. Exec. 10*:12–16 (1987).

14. Oldham, R., Drug development: Who foots the bill. *Biotechnology 5*:648 (1987).

15. Mannon, J., Developing a new drug: How fast? How safe? *Indust. Chem. 8*:26–29 (1987).

16. Croog, S., S. Levine, M. Testa, B. Brown, C. Bulpitt, C. Jenkins, G. Kierman, and G. Williams, The effects of antihypertensive therapy on the quality of life. *N. Engl. J. Med. 314*:1657–1664 (1986).

Plate I (Chapter 2)

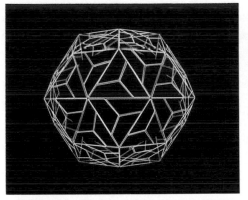

Figure 6 Schematic representation of the TBSV virus particle. The colored quadrilaterals represent different protein subunits on the surface of this icosahedrally symmetric virus.

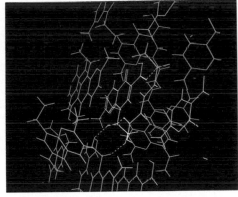

Figure 8 Crystal packing of nalidixic acid. One central molecule is highlighted in red. The neighboring molecules which lie within 5 Å of this central molecule are colored blue. Dashed lines show intermolecular contacts.

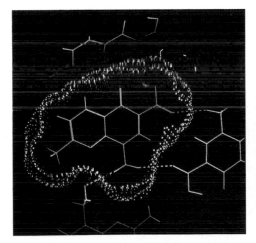

Figure 9 Crystal packing of nalidixic acid showing the surface of the central molecule in red. The composite surface formed by the neighboring molecules is blue. Note the close packing of the two surfaces in this cutaway view.

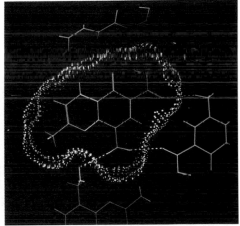

Figure 10 The same crystal packing of nalidixic acid showing the complementarity of the surfaces of the central molecule with that of the neighboring molecules. The surfaces in this figure are color-coded by electrostatic potential showing blue as positive, red as negative, and green as neutral areas on the surfaces. Note complementarity in colors (hence charges) between the two surfaces in this figure.

Plate II (Chapter 2)

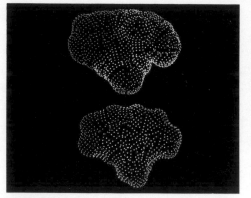

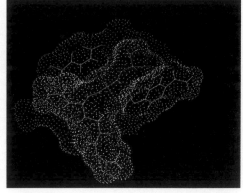

Figure 11   Front view of the electrostatically color-coded surface of the central molecule in the crystal packing of nalidixic acid (bottom) and of the neighboring molecules (top). The surfaces are to be viewed independently and do not attempt to show any intermolecular interactions. Note, however, the complementarity of the two surfaces. These are the same two surfaces shown in Figure 10, but here they are removed from the crystal packing in order to be more easily examined for complementarity of charge.

Figure 12   Interaction of the antibiotic ristocetin (blue) and a tripeptide model of bacterial cell wall (red). The surfaces show the close contact and surface complementarity of this drug-receptor complex.

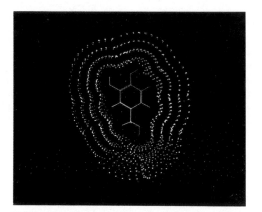

Figure 13   Cutaway view of the surface of nor-epinephrine color-coded by electrostatic potential. The innermost surface is at the van der Waals radius of the molecule. Each successive surface is 1 Å removed from the preceding surface.

Plate III (Chapter 8)

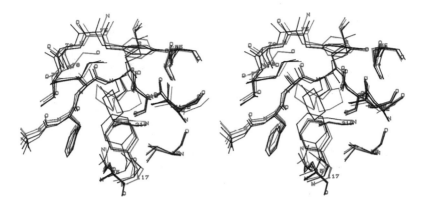

Figure 9   Minimized structures of renin complexed with inhibitors of series C2 highlighting residues of the active site around the P_1 site position. Blue—P_1 = isobutyl. Orange—P_1 = cyclohexyl. Red—P_1 = (cyclohexyl)methyl. Green—P_1 = (cyclohexyl)ethyl.

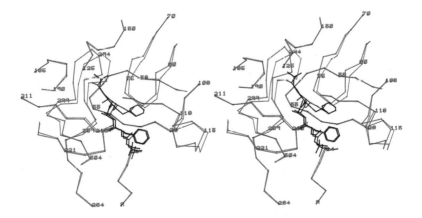

Figure 10   Alpha carbon trace of the active site of renin with two compounds of series C2. P_1 = isobutyl (blue and orange). P_1 = (cyclohexyl)ethyl (red and green).

Plate IV (Chapter 8)

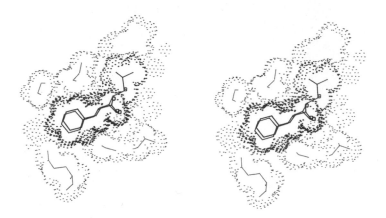

Figure 11   Details of the van der Waals contacts of the C terminus of two inhibitors having P_1 = (cyclohexyl)methyl.   Series C1 (red); series C2 (blue).   The renin molecule is shown in orange.

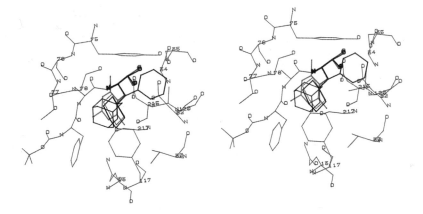

Figure 12   Four large side chains of residue P_1 modeled into the active site of renin orange. Orange—P_1 = (cyclohexyl)methyl.   Green—P_1 = (2,4,6-trimethyl)benzyl.   Red—P_1 = (dicyclohexyl)methyl.   Magenta—P_1 = (adamantyl)methyl.

Methods

2
Uses of Computer Graphics in Computer-Assisted Drug Design

T. J. O'Donnell*
Abbott Laboratories, Abbott Park, Illinois

---

*Present affiliation: O'Donnell Associates, Chicago, Illinois.

I. INTRODUCTION

Science is primarily an experimental endeavor, making constant reference to measurable facts to verify the correctness of its hypotheses. Yet, the greatest contribution of science to the world is not the body of experimental data it produces, but rather the concepts, the ideas, the models of the world that it extracts from those data. Often these models are verbal, more often mathematical, and sometimes graphical. Perhaps more than other fields of science, chemistry uses graphical models to express its concepts. The molecular stick figure has become the language of chemistry, through which chemists communicate and even conceive ideas.

Molecular stick figures carry information about the number and types of atoms that make up a molecule. They most clearly show the ways in which the atoms are bonded to one another, and even show something about the spatial relationships of nonbonded atoms—that is, the conformation of the molecule. Yet they cannot fully express the three-dimensional structure of a molecule or the volume that a molecule occupies. They also cannot show much of the electronic structure of a molecule.

The purpose of this chapter is to explain how molecular models have been constructed that can show three-dimensional and electronic properties of molecules. Although these models are of general use (1–4), the focus of the discussion will be on how these models are used in drug design (5–12). The usefulness of these models in crystallography, NMR, receptor mapping, quantum mechanics, molecular mechanics, and molecular dynamics will be shown.

II. COMPUTER GRAPHIC DISPLAYS

There are a variety of ways of constructing molecular models. Perhaps the simplest types of models are CPK and Dreiding models. CPK models are physical models in which the atoms are represented by color-coded, snap-together, spherically shaped, plastic pieces. These give a good representation of the shape of a molecule. They can be manipulated to produce various conformations of the molecule. They cannot be used to present electronic properties of molecules, and they cannot be superimposed upon one another to compare molecular conformation and shape. The bond lengths and angles cannot be adjusted in these models.

Dreiding models are physical models that use thin metal or plastic rods to represent bonds. Bond lengths and angles are fixed, although rotations around bonds can be easily done. They give a poor representation of molecular volume and cannot be used to show electronic properties. Depending on the complexity of the model, they could possibly be superimposed upon one another for comparison of molecular conformation.

A much better way to represent molecules is with computer models. Computer graphics can be used to draw a virtually limitless variety of molecular representations from stick figures (like Dreiding models) to molecular surfaces (like CPK models). Computer graphics models can also very readily be used to represent electronic properties of molecules. These models can be easily superimposed for comparison. In addition, they can be accurately constructed using any bond lengths, angles, and torsion angles. The greatest benefit of computer models is that they allow one to use other computational methods to construct, evaluate, and modify the models. Computer graphics models can be thought of as a window into the computer through which the chemist expresses ideas for computational evaluation and receives results in a readily understandable form.

A disadvantage of computer models is that they are not physical, three-dimensional models. One of the goals of computer molecular modeling is to portray the computer generated images in a way that seems three-dimensional. The ability to draw good three-dimensional molecular models is heavily dependent on computer technology. Typically, the models are drawn on a cathode-ray tube (CRT), using special-purpose computer hardware. Since the CRT is flat, the image is spatially limited to two dimensions. The third dimension is realized by rapidly displaying slightly different two-dimensional images, as is done in films. In this very effective way, time is used as a parameter to represent the third Cartesian dimension. This technique is referred to as real-time graphics.

Unfortunately for the purposes of this chapter, the print medium is less effective in its ability to display three dimensional models. Stereographic images can also be used in which slightly different images are drawn side by side to be viewed independently by each of the two eyes. The two images are then mentally merged to yield a convincing three-dimensional model. Another technique for viewing three-dimensional models is holography. This may offer new possibilities to molecular modeling in the future, but it is beyond the scope of the present discussion.

Another technique is often used in computer graphics to help give a three-dimensional look. Parts of the image that are "in front" are drawn more brightly than those parts "in back." This optical illusion, called intensity depth cuing, is quite effective. This technique can be used on a CRT but not on a computer plot. To reproduce the depth cuing, the figures in the chapter are photographs from the CRT of an Evans and Sutherland PS350 computer graphics system.

Computer graphics systems such as the PS350 and the Silicon Graphics IRIS work station allow one to combine the techniques of real-time graphics, stereographics, and intensity depth cuing to produce a three-dimensional image that cannot be represented in this book. In addition, they offer the possibility of using color to represent more than just the three-dimensional properties of molecules. Figure 13, which is discussed in later sections of this chapter, shows how color can be used to represent electrostatic potential energy in the volume surrounding a molecule.

A.   Vector Versus Raster Systems

Computer graphics displays are either vector or raster. On vector displays, the lines making up the image are traced on the face of the CRT. The lines are continuous strokes and appear very straight and smooth. However, only lines and dots can be drawn on vector systems. Filled areas, such as molecular surfaces, must be represented by many closely spaced lines or dots, which adds greatly to the complexity of the image.

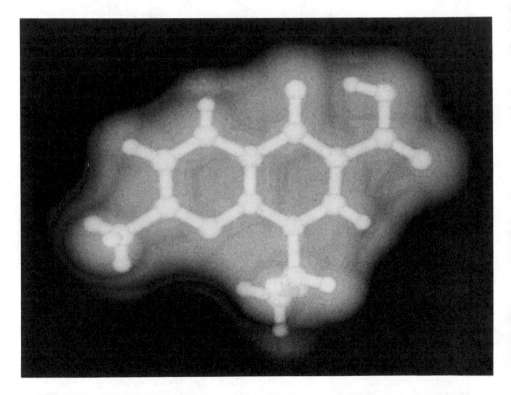

Figure 1   Transparent molecular surface of nalidixic acid showing a ball-and-stick model inside. This was drawn on a raster system and required several minutes of computations on a VAX.

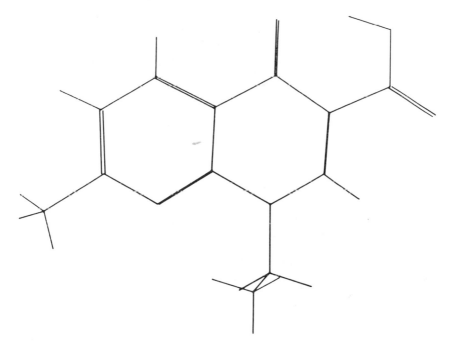

Figure 2 Stick figure of nalidixic acid showing atom connectivity and double bonds. This was drawn on a vector system in real time.

On raster displays, the CRT is repeatedly horizontally scanned, as on a television screen. The image is made up of discrete pixels. Lines (especially diagonal lines) can appear jagged, depending on the resolution of the CRT being used. Because of the pixel method used in raster systems, filled areas are more readily drawn on these systems than on vector systems.

The ability of a computer to show real-time graphics depends on the speed of the hardware and the complexity of the image. Until quite recently, only the special-purpose hardware available in vector graphics systems was able to provide the drawing speed necessary for drawing useful molecular models. A typical protein will contain many thousands of bonds. Since these bonds are handily represented as vectors, vector systems seemed ideal for molecular graphics. Recently, however, raster systems have increased in speed and in the quality of line-drawing capability. The Evans and Sutherland PS390 is a raster system with line-drawing capabilities as good as on vector systems. Within a few years, vector systems will probably be extinct. Figure 1 shows a transparent molecular surface drawn on a raster system using Connolly's analytical molecular surfaces described later in this chapter. Compare this figure to Figures 2 and 3, which were drawn on a vector system.

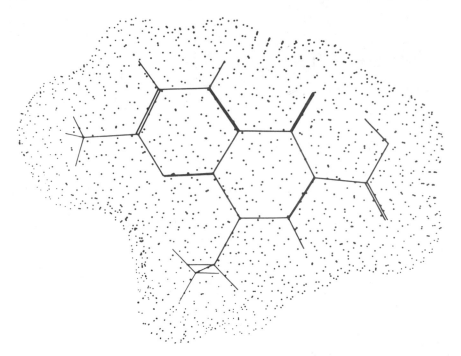

Figure 3 Dot surface of nalidixic acid representing the solvent-accessible surface of the molecule. This was drawn on a vector system in real time.

B. Workstations

Vector systems have been preferred by molecular modelers because of their speed and high quality of line drawing. Since these vector systems use special-purpose hardware, they have been more expensive than raster systems and have been used as display devices separate from the host computer being used to store and modify molecular coordinates. Computer graphics workstations have recently been introduced. Workstations are raster systems in which a computer with a full operating system and mass storage facility is integrated with the graphical display. Examples of these workstations are Silicon Graphics IRIS, Sun Graphics workstations, and Apollo workstations. The Evans and Sutherland PS300 series is not a workstation, since a host computer is required for access to a true operating systems and mass storage.

III. COMPUTED MOLECULAR MODELS

The purpose of molecular modeling is to be able to represent some aspect of molecular structure using a computer graphical model. There are two important aspects of molecular structure that have been found to be useful in drug design. The first is the atomic connectivity and atom types, as are shown in a stick figure. The other is the volume and/or shape of the molecule, as shown in a dot surface representation (13). Other aspects whose usefulness is being investigated include more schematic representations of molecules, such as alpha carbon plots and ribbon diagrams to represent protein structure (14). Electronic aspects of molecular structure can also be represented by models such as dot surfaces that are color-coded according to electrostatic potential energy (15) or contoured surfaces of electron density.

A. Molecular Stick Figures

The most familiar computer molecular model is the molecular stick figure. Figure 2 shows a stick figure of nalidixic acid. The atom types are not shown here. The connectivity is shown by lines representing bonds. The coordinates for the atoms are from a crystal study (16). Using a three-dimensional graphics system, one can view this molecule from any angle. By being able to freely rotate it, one gets a clear impression of the three-dimensional structure.

This structure is not as rigid as it may seem in this model. Several of the bonds in nalidixic acid may be rotated to yield different conformations. Some of these conformations may be undesirable, but this cannot be known without investigating them. It is possible to do a systematic search (17) of most possible conformations, but this technique requires a large amount of computer time which increases exponentially as the number of rotatable bonds increases. Using interactive real-time graphics, one can assign dials to rotate molecular sections around one or more bonds. Turning any combination of these dials, one can instantly see the resulting conformations. These are then evaluated visually by the modeler.

In some conformations, it is clear that nonbonded atoms are too close. Many molecular modeling systems provide the ability to compute distances between selected atoms or to monitor distances for close contacts. Some systems also provide an interactive energy estimation to aid in evaluating the conformational differences. At the very least, a molecular modeling system must provide the ability to record the conformations being viewed, by storing either the rotational angles or the new Cartesian coordinates. These coordinates could then be used in another program to compute the energy.

The advantage of interactive graphics is not in generating lots of configurations or in ruling out conformations. Systematic searches are probably better for that. Generally, one has a hypothesis about the conformation of a molecule. Using interactive graphics, one can mold the conformation of the molecule to cause certain intramolecular interactions, such as hydrogen bonding or hydrophobic interactions to be formed. These selected conformations can then be evaluated, either with an interactive energy estimation or a separate molecular mechanics or quantum mechanics calculation.

For drug design, one must always keep in mind that the molecule acting as a drug does not act alone. It requires a receptor for its pharmacological effect to be expressed. In most cases the drug receptor is unknown. It is very rarely known to the extent that would allow one to construct a molecular model for the receptor. For examples of cases where both the drug and the receptor structures are both known, see Kuyper's Chapter 9 and Bolis and Greer's Chapter 8 in this book. In cases where the receptor is known, one can use interactive graphics to model the intermolecular drug-receptor interactions. Molecular stick figures can be used for this, but judging distances and overlap between two molecules is difficult without having some idea of the volume that a molecule's atoms occupy. Three-dimensional molecular surfaces can also be drawn on a molecular modeling system to help in investigating intermolecular interactions.

B. Molecular Surfaces

The general concept of molecular surfaces was proposed in a paper by Lee and Richards (18). There was a distinction made between molecular surface and solvent-accessible surface. If one imagines the molecule to be made up of spheres of appropriate sizes, the superposition of all these spheres would give rise to the molecular surface (and volume) much like a CPK model of a molecule. The solvent-accessible surface is that part of the molecular surface that is accessible to solvent. In small molecules there is practically no difference in these two surfaces, but in proteins, there are large regions of the molecule that are "inside" and do not contribute to the solvent-accessible surface. There are also other small differences between the molecular surface and the solvent-accessible surface at places where two or three atoms come together. The small crevices between atoms are not accessible to solvent and are represented by dots spanning the point of contact of the probe sphere with the atom spheres.

Connolly published an algorithm (13) and program (19) for computing either molecular or solvent-accessible surfaces. The solvent-accessible surface is generated by using a probe sphere to represent the solvent molecule (say, water with 1.4-Å radius). Starting from outside the molecule, the probe sphere is rolled over the group of atomic spheres making up the molecule.

When the probe sphere just touches an atom sphere, points are generated to record the solvent accessibility of that atom. The outside atoms block the entry of the solvent probe sphere into the inner part of the molecule. In this way only points accessible to the solvent probe are recorded.

These surfaces are represented as a collection of dots on a vector display. Connolly has more recently published a method for the analytical computation and representation of these surfaces (20). These are mathematically more compact and useful representations. They are also used to create filled images of molecular surfaces on a raster display (21). The surfaces used in this chapter are not analytical surfaces, but rather Connolly dot surfaces. Figure 3 shows a Connolly dot surface for nalidixic acid along with molecular stick figure. Figure 1 shows an analytical Connolly surface for nalidixic acid along with a ball-and-stick model. The surface is rendered transparent to allow the ball-and-stick model to show through.

Once a dot surface is generated, it can be displayed interactively using a graphical molecular modeling system. These surfaces give a good representation of the shape and volume occupied by a molecule. They can also be used to evaluate various conformations of a molecule in a way analogous to rotating around bonds in a molecular stick figure. Rather than evaluating energy or distance as bond rotations are made, surfaces are used to give an idea of disallowed overlap between nonbonded atoms—in other words, to indicate atom collisions. The surface can be easily partitioned into those dots that remain fixed and those dots that belong to atoms that move owing to bond rotation. Then the movable part of the surface as well as the molecular stick figure can be rotated in real time on a graphics system. In this way intramolecular contacts can be visualized and evaluated qualitatively.

Surfaces are also very useful for looking at intermolecular interactions, or docking. If one thinks of the probe sphere used in computing the solvent-accessible surface as another (small) molecule, then the surface can be seen as a representation of the limits of potential intermolecular contacts. As described above, it is not favorable to penetrate those limits, but it is also important to realize that maximum surface contact is favorable. This is often expressed in terms of hydrophobic interactions between molecules. It could also be thought of as a geometric expression of the attractive dispersion, or London forces in an empirical force field. For a more detailed description of the forces and parameters used in molecular mechanics force fields, see Burt, Mackay, and Hagler's Chapter 3 in this book. In other words, one can visually and interactively dock two molecules using the criteria that their respective surfaces not interpenetrate and that their surfaces just touch in as many places as possible. This is only a rule of thumb, and more will be said in a later section of this chapter describing the uses of graphics in molecular mechanics calculations.

C.   Color-Coded Surfaces to Represent Molecular Properties

One can also encode information on the molecular surface. For example, one could color the dots to show which type of atom they are closest to (or "belong to"). For example, the dots belonging to carbon atoms would be green, those for hydrogen white, nitrogen blue, oxygen red, and so forth. One might also compute a hydrophobicity index for atoms or groups and color hydrophilic portions of the surface blue and hydrophobic portions red. These schemes could help in visually comparing a set of molecules to detect where and how they are similar or different.

Another useful property that is often used to color-code surfaces is electrostatic potential energy. If one has a set of point charges assigned to each atom in the molecule and one assumes that the probe sphere contains a unit positive charge, then one can easily compute the Coulomb electrostatic potential energy due to the interaction of the probe charge with the collection of point charges in the molecule. If the energy is negative (attractive to the probe charge), then the surface dot is colored red. This means that that portion of the surface is relatively negatively charged. If the energy is zero (neutral), then the dot is colored green. If the energy is positive, then the dot is colored blue. This denotes that that portion of the surface is relatively positively charged and repulsive to the positive probe charge. Intermediate colors may also be used for slightly positive or negative energy values. With this scheme a picture of "reactive" portions of the molecule is obtained. Figure 11, which is explained in more detail in later sections of this chapter, shows an example of this type of coloring scheme.

The general model of drug-receptor interactions is equivalent to the lock-and-key model of enzyme-substrate interactions. With this model in mind, the ideal receptor for a drug would be a molecule whose surface is exactly complementary to the drug's surface, in terms of both shape complementarity and charge or electrostatic potential energy. Examples of this surface complementarity will be given in the sections on the use of graphics in crystallography and molecular mechanics.

D.   Other Molecular Properties

Aside from properties at surfaces, other molecular properties can be represented using computer graphics. One result from a quantum mechanical calculation on a molecule is the electron density. This quantity has a particular value at each point in space surrounding the molecule. If one collects together points of equal value, a contour of equal electron density results. These points could be displayed as dots to represent a surface of equal electron density. A filled surface could also be displayed using a raster system. Figure 4 shows a picture of the electron density around a molecule of uracil. The electrostatic potential energy color-coded surfaces described above are surfaces of fixed geometry with color used to give a feeling of the electronic nature of the area near the surface. In a similar but converse way, the electron density is a surface of fixed electronic nature (constant electron density) with the shape variable according to the size of "electron cloud" near that point in space around the molecule. In both cases the pictures are meant

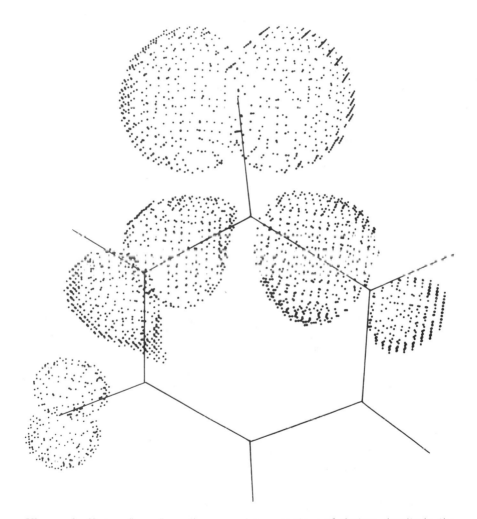

Figure 4 Dot surface of uracil representing a contour of electron density in the highest occupied molecular orbital of the molecule.

to represent the ability of a molecule to use its electrons to interact with another molecule. In the electrostatic potential energy color-coded surface, the color shows the size of the potential interaction at a fixed place. The electron density contour shows how far a given value of electron density can reach out toward another molecule to interact with it.

E. Other Molecular Representations

Although stick figures are the most familiar molecular representation and surfaces are quickly becoming as useful and familiar, there are other ways in which molecules might be represented. For large molecules like proteins, drawing a complete stick figure showing every bond results in a picture that is too cluttered and not very informative. One method of representing proteins that helps avoid clutter is an alpha carbon plot. Because of the regularity of polypeptides, each amino acid can be represented by its alpha carbon. The positions of these atoms are connected by pseudo bonds. The overall shape of

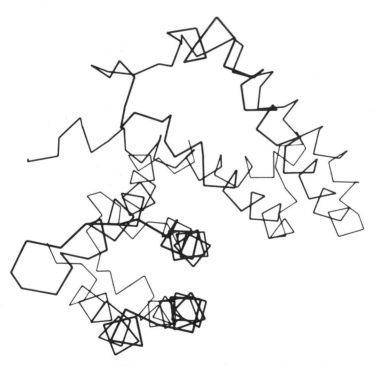

Figure 5   Alpha carbon plot of hemoglobin. The helices in the structure are clearly shown.

the protein can be readily seen, and the point at which the side chain emerges from the main chain is neatly depicted as well, since the alpha carbon is that point. Figure 5 shows an alpha carbon plot of a heme protein cytochrome C. The alpha helical portions of the molecule are readily seen.

As molecules become even larger, even more schematic representations are necessary. A virus is a collection of macromolecules, typically with a protein outer coat. Several viruses have been crystallized, and many details of their structure have been revealed. The tomato bushy virus (TBSV) has an outer coat consisting of 180 nearly identical proteins arranged on an icosohedrally symmetric shell (22). If one were to draw the viral coat in full detail for each protein, or even the alpha carbon plot for each protein, the resulting picture would not reveal the symmetrical relationship among the 180 proteins as clearly as does Figure 6 (see Plate I, facing p. 16). In this figure, a quadrilateral is used to represent an entire protein. The fact that there are three types of proteins (represented by three different colors) and that they stand in a particular symmetric relationship to one another is clearly evident in this schematic picture.

IV. MOLECULAR MODELING SYSTEMS FOR DRUG DESIGN

There are many molecular modeling systems available. Some include a wide variety of features such as statistical packages for QSAR, programs for molecular mechanics and dynamics calculations, and quantum mechanical programs. One thing they all have in common is some sort of graphical display with the ability to produce molecular stick figures and surfaces. Some have additional graphical abilities as well. Some are only commercially available; others are available from academic institutions, probably for a lesser cost. Appendix I lists some molecular modeling systems that are available. A detailed comparison of these molecular modeling systems is beyond the scope of this chapter. Such a comparison might be the subject of future discussions. For the purposes of the present discussion, one should consider any of these molecular modeling systems to have the basic features necessary to accomplish the modeling tasks described in later sections of this chapter. Appendix I is simply intended as a starting point for readers interested in obtaining a molecular modeling system.

A. The CAMD System

The molecular modeling tasks described in this chapter were accomplished using the Computer Assisted Molecular Design (CAMD) system. This proprietary system was designed and written at Abbott Laboratories for the use of molecular modeling researchers. It is described here to provide a good working model system for the discussions in this chapter. Readers who are not familiar with molecular modeling systems can use the descriptions of the CAMD system as a general indicator of what these systems are capable of doing. Readers with more experience with molecular modeling systems can use the description to compare analogous features and productivity among systems. Finally, many sophisticated molecular modelers find there are advantages to building their own molecular modeling system. This description shows how one such system was organized.

CAMD is made up of several pieces which are connected in different ways. It uses GRAMPS (23) to do its graphics, in order to provide as much graphical flexibility as possible in doing molecular modeling. Figure 7 shows an overview of the main pieces of the CAMD system. These are GRAMPS, a general-purpose graphics program for display of arbitrary graphical objects; PDS, a protein modeling system; CMD, a small molecule modeling system; and Interact, a program to coordinate information transfer among GRAMPS/CMD/PDS and provide a convenient user interface. GRAMPS exists as a separate program and runs independently of the other three. CMD, PDS, and Interact are linked together and communicate to GRAMPS using the VAX/VMS mailbox facility for interprocess communication.

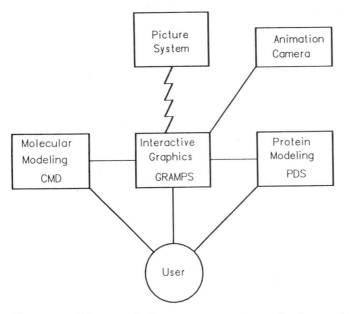

Figure 7 Diagram of the components of a molecular modeling system using GRAMPS as the chemical graphics display driver.

GRAMPS has been converted to run on an Evans and Sutherland PS350 as well as the E&S MPS for which it was originally written. Without changing any code in the other three programs, the CAMD system now runs on both graphics devices. In addition, GRAMPS has been converted to use the TEMPLATE device-independent subroutine library of graphics routines. Although this does not allow full three-dimensional, real-time interactive graphics capabilities, it does allow the use of the CAMD system on an office graphics terminal such as Ramtek, Tektronix, Envision and many other possible devices. It also allows use of a wide variety of hard-copy output devices.

There are many other programs that are used in the CAMD system. These include molecular mechanics (24–26), molecular dynamics, quantum mechanics (27,28), distance geometry (29), Connolly surface generation, and other programs. Rather than bundle all these programs together, they have been left as separate programs, as they arrive from their respective sources. There is a CONVRT program that allows one to read in a file in one format and convert it into a file with the same information in another format. For example, one might retrieve a file from the Cambridge Crystal File (30) data base using only software supplied by them. The resulting file is then CONVRT'ed into an MSF file (molecular structure file—the CMD standard molecule file). This is then read into the CAMD system to be displayed, modified, and evaluated. This modified molecule can be stored in another MSF file. This file might then be CONVRT'ed into an input file for the MM2 program (24), which could optimize the geometry of that molecule.

Clearly, this process involves more steps than would be involved if any "outside" programs were tightly linked into the CAMD system. However, it also provides more flexibility in the following ways. Suppose the molecule to be optimized had an atom type for which a torsional parameter was missing for MM2. If the CAMD system automatically submitted the molecule to MM2, the MM2 optimization would fail because of the missing parameter. Of course the automatic submission could be modified to detect the missing parameter and prompt the user for it, but this requires some degree of programming effort. Using this loosely coupled method, the user would simply edit the MM2 input file which CONVRT had prepared from the MSF file and include the parameter. Of course this requires some time from the user and some thought about what he is actually requesting a program to do, but it also does not restrict the user to using only those features of an outside program that the interface to that program allows. Once the user has determined the correct sequence of programs to use to accomplish the modeling task at hand, the required steps can be knit together using VAX/VMS COM files. This tailor-made file can then be used to automatically process any number of related molecules. In our experience, however, most molecules need to be handled individually, because they are unique in some way. The loosely coupled CAMD system allows this to be done in a straightforward and unrestricting way.

Appendix II shows a list of commands available in the CAMD system and gives a brief description of the function. This table, although it applies specifically to the CAMD system, is representative of the types of commands available in most of the molecular modeling systems described in Appendix I.

V.   USES OF COMPUTER-ASSISTED DRUG DESIGN

Computer graphics has many uses in drug design and related endeavors. This section will give examples of how computer graphics has been used in crystallography, NMR, receptor mapping, quantum mechanics, molecular mechanics and dynamics, and interactively docking molecules.

A.   Crystallography

The primary goal of chemical crystallography is to produce a set of coordinates defining the locations of atoms in a molecule. From this list, a picture can easily be generated as a stick figure using almost any molecular modeling system. There are other, less obvious uses of computer graphics that can be very helpful in the process of interpreting crystal structures.

For example, the environment of a molecule in the crystal can be a clue to what kind of interactions a molecule may prefer in interactions with other types of molecules (31), perhaps with a drug receptor. Based on input from the Cambridge Crystal File, which contains crystal coordinates for over 50,000 compounds, we have written a program to allow one to visualize the environment of a molecule in the crystal. The purpose of this program was to investigate the kinds of intermolecular interactions that a molecule "chooses" when forming a crystal. This may help answer such questions as, "What sort of hydrogen bond donors does a carbonyl oxygen prefer and at what angle does the hydrogen bond prefer to form?" and "What interactions might be responsible for the dimers observed in solution for some particular molecule?" or even "Why is this molecule so insoluble?"

The program uses as input the fractional coordinates of the molecule in the unit cell along with the unit cell dimensions and angles which are easily available from the Cambridge Crystal File. The program generates all symmetrically related molecules within the unit cell as well as outside, up to a distance of, say 5 Å. The resulting picture shows all the intermolecular interactions for a reference molecule in the environment of other molecules in the crystal. These may include solvent as well as other molecules identical to the reference molecule.

As an example of the use of this program, consider Figure 8 (see Plate I, facing p. 16), which shows a picture of nalidixic acid (16) along with every molecule in its crystal that has an atom within 5 Å of the central (red) molecule. This crystal was examined to help figure out why nalidixic acid is so insoluble and what might be done to increase its solubility. The dashed lines show intermolecular interactions. The closest interatomic distances in the crystal occur between the oxygens of the carboxylic acid group and hydrogens bonded to aliphatic or aromatic carbons. One might have expected hydrogen bonding of carboxylic acid groups to one another or to the nitrogen atoms in nalidixic acid. One can also see from this figure the hydrophobic interactions between ethyl groups and methyl groups, at the bottom of the red molecule, forming a little hydrocarbon region in the crystal. The stacking of pairs of aromatic rings is also obvious. Solubility affects directly the concentrations attainable for any drug molecule. Based only on this picture, one could postulate that modifying the ethyl group would disrupt two important interactions in the crystal and make it more soluble.

The study of this crystal described above was extended to investigate an interesting question regarding the interaction of molecules with one another. The model for drug-receptor interactions is an extension of the lock-and-key model for enzyme-substrate interactions. Of course, in some cases the drug receptor *is* an enzyme, with the drug taking the place of the natural substrate in an antagonistic way. When both the drug and its receptor are known, molecular modeling of the bimolecular complex should be carried out. But when the receptor is not known, what can be done? One approach, called receptor mapping, is discussed in a later section of this chapter and in other chapters of this book. Another approach uses the crystal environment as a model for the receptor environment of a molecule.

In this approach, one constructs the local environment of a single molecule in a crystal, as shown in Figure 8. The single reference molecule is then temporarily removed from the crystal. The remaining molecules define the immediate environment of that reference molecule. If one assumes that the molecules surrounding this reference molecule have arrayed themselves in the most favorable way (energetically or otherwise), then the environment of the reference molecule is an optimized environment for that molecule. Without regard to the other special environments (such as the receptor environment) in which this molecule might find itself, we can ask, "What does this ideal environment look like, and do our notions of how intermolecular interactions are modeled hold in this experimentally accurately determined environment?"

To answer this question, a solvent-accessible surface was computed of the cavity (the environment) left in the crystal after removal of the reference molecule. The solvent-accessible surface of the isolated reference molecule was then independently computed. Next, the reference molecule with its surface was returned to the crystal along with the cavity surface. If the surface models we use are exactly correct, then the two surfaces should superimpose exactly. Of course, they do not exactly superimpose, but the similarity in shape is remarkable. There are, however, some free spaces. The volume of the cavity is computed to be 330 $Å^3$. The volume of the reference molecule is 221 $Å^3$. This leaves about one-third of the cavity volume empty! Figure 9 (see Plate I, facing p. 16) shows a cutaway view of the two surfaces and shows that the fit is not as bad as that figure of one-third sounds. If these volumes were spheres, then for the same ratio of volumes, the ratio of radii would be 0.87. Alternately, 330 $Å^3$ corresponds to a spherical radius of 4.9 Å and 221 $Å^3$ to a radius of 4.3 Å, a difference of only 0.6 Å.

Using only this example, one cannot make conclusions concerning how closely two molecules ought to interact and whether empty volume between molecules is allowable or desirable. The numbers reported above used a set of atomic radii from Bondi (32). The volume is very dependent on the choice of atomic radii used, and this choice must be investigated further. Also, in x-ray diffraction crystal studies, the hydrogen atoms are often reported to be too close to the heavy-atom locations. Neutron diffraction studies, or perhaps modified crystal coordinates in which the covalent hydrogen bonds are systematically lengthened, could be used in further studies. Finally, one must look at the intermolecular interactions in crystals of a variety of different molecules.

Aside from the steric fit of molecules, the drug design model requires a complementary electronic fit between molecules. Expanding on the surface-fit model described above, charges were computed by an *ab initio*, quantum mechanical SCF calculation of nalidixic acid. The covalent hydrogen bond distances were lengthened to 1.1 Å for C–H bonds and 1.0 Å for N–H and O–H bonds. The calculation was done for a single, isolated (gas phase) molecule of nalidixic acid. The charges for this reference molecule were used for all molecules in the group of molecules comprising the crystal environment, as described above. The surface of the reference molecules was color-coded according to electrostatic potential energy based on the charges of the reference molecule alone. Then the surface of the cavity was color-coded according to the electrostatic potential energy generated by the point charges assigned to atoms of the molecules comprising the environment of the reference molecule. When the reference molecule and its color-coded surface were restored to the crystal environment, the complementarity of the electronic nature of the surface with that of the cavity surface was remarkably good. Figure 10 (see Plate I, facing p. 16) shows a cutaway view of these two surfaces. Figure 11 (see Plate II, after p. 16) shows the front side of both surfaces. The cavity surface is the top figure, and the reference molecule surface is the bottom figure. The color (electronic) complementarity is seen to be quite good.

Although further work needs to be done with a variety of crystal structures, the above results suggest that the solvent-accessible surface color coded according to electrostatic potential energy using point charges from a reasonable source can truly give a good qualitative picture of how molecules interact.

B. Receptor Mapping

As mentioned above, the drug-receptor model of drug activity is one in which the complementarity of drug and receptor is emphasized (7). If the receptor is perfectly complementary to the drug, then its shape can be inferred from the drug. Because there are many molecules that have the same or similar drug activity, there is no ideal drug fit or ideal receptor. Once one has a group of drugs that are all relatively active, one can hypothesize that the overlap of all those molecules defines a volume that the receptor must be able to accommodate (5). Of course the receptor is not a fixed molecular structure, but is flexible in its geometry to be able to accommodate a range of molecules. This model takes that flexibility into account, although indirectly. The surface that is inferred from the overlap of the active molecules is referred to as a receptor map.

One practical way of constructing such a receptor map is by using the molecular or solvent-accessible surfaces described above. First, one must construct the set of active molecules to be used to compute the volume. Since there are many ways of superimposing any two molecules, much less a large set of them, one must make certain assumptions about which parts of the molecules are to match while making the superposition. This is often not obvious, but in most cases the series of molecules will have certain moieties in common. In fact, a series of drug compounds is suggested based on the idea that an active drug must contain certain pharmacophoric groups to have activity. The surface of the group of superimposed molecules can then be computed in a straightforward manner.

To test whether this surface is a good map of the receptor, one next considers molecules that were tested and found to be inactive yet that retain some or all of the pharmacophoric moieties of the series in question. These molecules should present new volumes, outside the allowed volume for the receptor map formed by the active molecules. These extra volumes then "explain" why a drug is inactive, because of collisions with the intended receptor (33). An advantage of this type of modeling is that it can be continually refined as more and more active drugs are discovered. A disadvantage is that it begs the questions, "What is the conformation of a drug molecule?" and "How do we superimpose two molecules?" However, once such a receptor map is constructed, it should be possible in principle to evaluate an arbitrary molecule that is not necessarily part of the series used to construct the model.

C. Molecular Mechanics and Dynamics

Graphics can be used to great effect in molecular mechanics and dynamics studies. Of course, graphics is used routinely to prepare input structures for these programs and to look at the resulting structures. The use of graphics for looking at results of dynamics programs is particularly important. Molecular dynamics produces a great many molecular conformations. There are statistical ways of analyzing these results to give free energies, entropies, etc. One can also produce plots to show the variation, or transitions in conformations as a function of time. In many cases, however, expecially in large molecules, one cannot know which conformational variables (which bond dihedral angles) are interesting to look at as a function of time. The many conformations produced by molecular dynamics can be displayed on a computer graphics screen in rapid succession if one has a real-time computer graphics system. Just watching these results repeatedly can give one insight into which conformational changes are occurring (either repeatedly or as a single transition). Even though it may be difficult to express these conformational results in a way that would be easy to graph (as a dihedral angle plotted against time), the chemist looking at conformations on a computer graphics screen can categorize them and detect important, or at least interesting, conformational transitions.

The conformations produced by molecular dynamics could be used in many ways. For example, assume one has a hypothetical receptor map into which a molecule under study ought to be able to fit when it is in one of its possible conformations. If the results of a molecular dynamics run show that this conformation is possible, but also shows many other conformations that would not fit the receptor model, then the pictures could lead one to hypothesize new molecules—say, with a methyl "blocking" group or a ring constraint to prevent too much conformational freedom. The analysis of NMR data sometimes leads one to the hypothesis that one or more conformations exist in solution. The graphical and geometric analysis of molecular dynamics results can help in putting this hypothesis on firmer ground. An example of how this was done will be given in a later section of this chapter. As a final example, one can watch the results of a dynamics run and select chosen conformations to be analyzed further—say, with molecular mechanics. One could arbitrarily choose conformations from a molecular dynamics calculation at regular time intervals and minimize those, but that could miss important conformations and duplicate many conformations. Even when one compares the RMS difference between conformations generated in a molecular dynamics calculation, the value of the RMS difference is not a reliable measure of the similarity or difference between conformations, since it is an overall average measure. Yet the chemist's eye can readily distinguish and categorize families of conformations.

Conformations directly obtained from molecular dynamics calculations do not look correct. The bond lengths and angles are "distorted" from what one is used to when looking at results from molecular mechanics minimizations. Perhaps these structures are just as valid as minimized structures, but minimization calculations provide an objective energy value. This energy can be used to compare relative "worth" of several molecular conformations. One of the problems of molecular mechanics is that it minimizes the energy of a starting structure without regard to the overall conformational flexibility of the molecule. In other words, it only finds local minima, not the global minimum. Using results from molecular dynamics calculations as starting points for minimizations is one way to overcome this. Systematic search, in which every rotatable bond is systematically varied, is another. The numbers of possible conformations generated using this technique rise sharply with the size of the molecule. Another way is to use graphics to interact with the molecular model and propose one's own hypotheses about which conformations might be important.

Using this interactive approach to conformational searching will not allow one to examine all possible conformations. It does allow one to quickly propose new conformations, by interactively rotating around bonds. These conformations can be evaluated subjectively and saved for future objective evaluations by a minimization program. The point here is that interacting with the molecule often "suggests" new intramolecular or potential intermolecular interactions which one wishes to pursue further, either with computational evaluation or by synthesizing new molecules that might fix in that interesting conformation. Until a foolproof method is available to locate absolutely the lowest minima (the global minimum is probably not the active conformation in most drug systems), this method of interacting with the molecular structure interspersed with minimizing the structure will continue to be a powerful tool for molecular design.

D. NMR and Computer Graphics

The analysis of NMR/NOE spectra on biological molecules in solution can provide many structural details. For a more detailed description of these techniques, see Fesik's Chapter 5 of this book. One important piece of information available from these experiments is distance between specific hydrogen atoms in a molecule. Using a molecular modeling system, one can easily examine a molecular model and see whether the distances in that model agree with those from the NOE experiment. The CAMD system has a feature that will compute the distance between all pairs of hydrogen atoms and display a dashed line between those pairs whose separation falls within specified limits. This is an easy way to compare model distances with NOE distances, but also to see distances in the model that ought to appear in the NMR spectrum, if the model is correct.

Using such a scheme, an investigation was carried out of the ristocetin pseudo-aglycone molecule bound to Ac_2–Lys–D–Ala–D–Ala (34). The tripeptide is a model for bacterial cell wall. Ristocetin exerts its antibiotic effect by interfering with the cell wall biosynthesis, presumably by binding to the few terminal amino acids in the cell wall and/or its precursors. Before NMR work had begun, we had modeled the binding of ristocetin to the tripeptide based on crystal studies of the tripeptide and on crystal studies of a related antibiotic, vancomycin (35). The docking of the two molecules was carried out interactively based on a qualitative description of the bimolecular complex arrived at from NMR experiments (36). This was then optimized using AMBER molecular mechanics (28). Once the NOE experiment was performed and the data were analyzed to produce about a dozen proton-proton distances, these were compared to distances from the model. Most distances agreed, but there were four that were clearly in disagreement with the NOE work.

One approach taken was to impose the distance constraints on the computer model by introducing pseudo bonds between all the hydrogens whose distances were measured in the spectrum. Minimization including these constraints resulted in a structure that agreed with all the NOE distances. However, once these constraints were relaxed, the model sprang back to nearly its original mimimized conformation. Aside from solvent effects that were ignored in the modeling described here, we postulated that perhaps still another conformation would also produce those distances without being unstable with respect to unconstrained minimization. To investigate other conformations, we performed 10 ps of molecular dynamics on this bimolecular complex.

The results of the molecular dynamics run were examined graphically. One could clearly see a conformational change which occurred repeatedly in the course of the molecular dynamics run. Two representative conformations were selected from the 10,000 that had been generated, and these were then minimized. The four distances in question were substantially different in the two conformations. In fact, the experimental distances fell roughly between these distances measured for the two conformations. From this result, we concluded that the NOE experiment was sampling these two conformations and that the NOE data could not be explained by using only one conformation (34).

E. Molecular Docking, Surfaces, and Hydrogen Bonds

Interactive computer graphics is a great aid in intermolecular docking. There are very many fewer constraints on the way in which two molecules can interact than there are for intramolecular interactions, where bonds serve to limit the possible interactions. For that reason it is not feasible to put two molecules together and let a minimizer find an optimal interaction. The long-range forces responsible for guiding two molecules together into the docked conformation are perhaps not modeled well in existing force fields, or possibly the minimization method is not suited for this task. The chemist's eye is well suited for this task and is the most fruitful way to begin tackling the problem of intermolecular docking.

As was done in the ristocetin problem described above, qualitative NMR results were incorporated into a quantitative model by using interactive computer graphics for docking two molecules. Initially, the graphics system only had dials available for rotations and translations of one molecule relative to another. The process of interactive docking was hindered by the need to use separate devices to control separate graphical operations. Since that time, a three-dimensional tracking device was incorporated into the CAMD system (37). This device can be used in a very natural way to control an object on a computer graphics screen. The ristocetin-tripeptide model was used as a test system to demonstrate the effectiveness of the tracker. With this device, the user has the impression that his hand is wrapped around the molecule and that every movement and twist of the hand is reflected by motions of the object being controlled on the screen. This gives one superb control of the rotational and translational degrees of freedom which must be adjusted when docking two molecules together.

Once one has a good device to do interactive molecular docking, one can use other tools of a molecular modeling system to help arrive at a good hypothesis for how the two molecules dock. If one draws color-coded electrostatic potential energy surfaces for each molecule, then the optimal docked orientation will be that in which the two surfaces are optimally complementary in shape and charge distribution. Figure 12 (see Plate II, after p. 16) shows a cutaway view of the docking of ristocetin with the tripeptide after it had been minimized using molecular mechanics. Notice that the surfaces are very neatly tucked together but that there is some overlap on the bottom right. It is not surprising that the two molecules come closer together than they "ought to" based on the surface description of the molecules. In fact, at other spots where intermolecular hydrogen bonds are formed, the two surfaces interpenetrate.

F. Quantum Mechanics

In some ways, quantum mechanics can be looked on as just another, albeit expensive, way to produce an energy-minimized conformation of a molecule. This is certainly a valid and useful thing. More importantly, quantum mechanics offers a much better description of electronic structure than molecular mechanics can ever do. In fact, parameters used for force fields in molecular mechanics and dynamics are often computed using quantum mechanical methods. Computer graphics can even be of use in this way, by analyzing and assigning normal modes of vibration from quantum mechanical results (38). The correct assignment of these vibrational modes is essential to the analysis of the computational results. Graphical analysis greatly speeds this analysis. The visual representation, as opposed to a table of numbers that are displacements of atoms, clearly and unambiguously verifies that the assignment is being done correctly.

Computer graphics can be used to show some of the results of electronic structure from quantum mechanical calculations (39). Although point charges are routinely used to represent charge distributions in a molecule, this is a poor representation for such things as lone pair electrons. In some studies of structure-activity relationships for drug molecules, it has been shown that the energy of the highest occupied molecular orbital for a molecule correlates with the drug activity (40). If this is true, then the distribution of charge might well be expected to have an important role in the mechanism of the drug molecule's action. One way of representing molecular orbitals is with a contour diagram. This is most often done with flat molecules with the electron density contoured in only some particular plane above the molecular plane. A true three-dimensional (3-D) contour is possible using interactive computer graphics.

Figure 4 shows a representation of the highest occupied molecular orbital in uracil. The electron density from a CNDO wave function was evaluated at a grid of points in the volume surrounding the molecule. If the density fell between some arbitrarily small range of values, then the coordinate of that grid point was saved. When all the saved grid points are displayed, the result is a contour showing the surface in 3-D space. This image can be displayed and rotated in real time to give an even better feel for its 3-D features. This picture is analogous to the 90% orbitals typically seen in chemistry text books for the atomic orbitals of the hydrogen atom. Similar pictures using space-filling raster images of electron density appear in Hout et al. (41). These images are smoother, but they could not be displayed and manipulated in real time with currently available graphics systems.

Another result from quantum mechanical calculations is the electrostatic potential energy evaluated directly using the wave function as opposed to using the point charges extracted from the wave function. If one computes this energy at the points generated from a molecular surface calculation, the resulting color-coded surface can be displayed and used as explained in previous sections describing color-coded surfaces generated from point charges. The two surfaces can be visually compared and evaluated. It is also possible to use the quantum mechanical electrostatic potential energy surface to arrive at a set of point charges that will generate a surface most like the quantum mechanical surface (42).

Regardless of how the electrostatic potential energy surface is computed, the results shown so far are limited to the precomputed molecular surface. Although this surface is valuable as a guide to how two molecules interact, it ignores interactions at larger distances between molecules. If one computes additional surfaces that are successively larger by adding points at 1-Å intervals away from the original surface along the surface normal, one can compute color-coded electrostatic potential energies in areas farther away from the molecule. Figure 13 (see Plate II, after p. 16) shows these shells of electrostatic potential energy for the norepinephrine molecule calculated using the GAMESS *ab initio* program with a 4-31G basis set. As expected, the electronic effect becomes less as one gets farther from the molecule. One can also see that the electronic effect can change from positive to negative or vice versa depending on how far away from the molecule you go. This means that areas of the molecule that are positive when two molecules are docked together may actually act at a distance as a negative charge for orienting the incoming molecule. This is not a mysterious effect, but results simply from the potential shielding effect of, for example, the many protons surrounding a "buried" electronegative atom.

VI. EXTENDING MOLECULAR MODELING

As in all fields of science, molecular modeling is always changing. The tools described above to create and use molecular models must be constantly updated to accommodate new ideas and new models of intra- and inter-molecular interactions. Rather than viewing a molecular modeling system as a black box and accepting its limitations, many molecular modelers are anxious to extend the capabilities of their system. Some of the systems in Table 1 will allow this more easily than others, and some users will be more ingenious in their understanding of the features of those systems that allow interesting and useful extensions. The most important feature of a molecular modeling system can be its flexibility to allow the user to test out new ideas quickly and easily. This section provides two examples of the ways one might like to extend a molecular modeling system to accommodate new types of molecular models.

The CAMD system described above uses GRAMPS (23) as a common graphics tool. This allows graphics output to a wide variety of different graphics devices. More importantly, it allows graphics input from a wide variety of sources as well. As the system is currently assembled, both the small-molecule program (CMD) and the protein display program (PDS) contribute pictures to GRAMPS. These pictures can be viewed and graphically manipulated together. In addition, any other program could be used to create additional pictures to be read in by GRAMPS without concern for the inner workings of CMD, PDS, or even of the graphics computer being used. GRAMPS provides a common, user-oriented, interactive interface between the user or his program and the graphics computer. GRANNY is another example of a protein modeling system that uses GRAMPS as a graphical base (43).

Consider as an example two features of the CAMD system described in previous sections. Receptors have been modeled as the overlap of active compounds' volumes. This feature was not originally in the design of the CAMD system. Without having to pay attention to any details of the CMD or PDS system, a program was written to read many molecular structure files, compute molecular surfaces, and produce either the intersection or union of specified molecular surfaces (44). The program-produced GRAMPS picture files that are written using straightforward, well-documented methods. These files were then used in addition to picture files produced by the CMD program to verify that the molecular surfaces were being computed in a way that was compatible with the molecules drawn by CMD. GRAMPS was a convenient tool for program development and the testing of the idea of molecular overlap as a way of representing receptor maps. Ultimately the program was turned over to a CMD programmer who incorporated it into the CMD system as an automatic feature.

The color-coded electrostatic potential energy shells computed from *ab initio* wave functions were done in the same way (45). A programmer familiar with GAUSSIAN80 code modified it to produce GRAMPS picture files containing dots colored according to electrostatic potential energy. The results were verified, and when it was seen to be a useful tool for many other scientists in the group, it was incorporated by another programmer into the CMD system.

Finally, molecular dynamics results are handled in a similar way. The molecular dynamics analysis program already had a feature to output a GRAMPS picture file containing frames of data representing the coordinates at selected time steps in the dynamics run. We are simply able to read those files into GRAMPS, which may also be displaying other molecules at the same time.

The point of these examples is to show how graphics is necessary as a tool for programmers as well as users. Having a common graphics tool of communication allows people who concentrate in different specialties to communicate in a very effective way. For example, a quantum chemist can communicate his results to a molecular modeling chemist as a picture, or better yet a program to produce a picture. This is then able to be incorporated into the modeling system. In a similar way, the modeling chemist is able to express his ideas in pictures that can be quickly and accurately conveyed to a synthetic medicinal chemist. Graphics provides a common language for a wide variety of scientific researchers and encourages productive collaborations among them.

Computer graphics will continue to be an essential part of molecular modeling. The current tools of molecular modeling are sometime seen as too approximate by many, but this does not limit the effectiveness of molecular modeling per se. As more accurate methods become available, they can be incorporated into modeling systems. Graphics serves as a valuable focal point to express the results of those new methods. In summary, graphics is a window into the computer. Regardless of which computational methods are being employed, graphics allows the researcher to see what the computer method is producing and to guide those computer methods by being able to input molecular models in a clear, consistent way.

As supercomputers become cheaper and more readily available, graphics will become even more important. The huge amount of information that can be produced quickly by supercomputers cannot be interpreted by examining columns of numeric data. The goal of computer graphics in chemistry should be to use real-time manipulations of appropriately color-coded stick figures or space-filled images to succinctly represent the multidimensional results produced by computer methods. This goal is recognized by designers of the current computer hardware. Only a few years ago, graphics was seen as an add-on to a computer. Today the graphics workstation integrates a powerful graphics system with a powerful computational system. As the computational and graphical components become more completely integrated, graphics will be more widely used as a way to involve the researcher with the progress of the computation. As this happens, the results of molecular modeling studies will grow increasingly more valuable.

Appendix I Some of the Molecular Modeling Systems Available, Brief Description of Their Capabilities, and Person or Organization to Contact for More Information

---

AMBER—Molecular Mechanics and Dynamics
Professor Peter Kollman
Department of Pharmaceutical Chemistry
University of California
San Francisco, CA 94143

CAMSEQ—Molecular Mechanics and Molecular Display
Weintraub Software Design Associates, Inc.
P.O. Box 42577
Cincinnati, OH 45242

CHEMLAB—Molecular Mechanics, Quantum Mechanics, Molecular Display
Molecular Design Limited
2132 Farallon Drive
San Leandro, CA 94577

CHEM-X—Molecular Mechanics, Dynamics and Display
Chemical Design Ltd.
200 Route 17 South
Suite 120
Mahwah, NJ 07430

DISCOVER—Molecular Mechanics and Dynamics
INSIGHT—Molecular Display
BIOSYM Technologies
9605 Scranton Road
Suite 101
San Diego, CA 92121

FRODO—Molecular Display (especially macromolecular crystallography)
Dr. Flo Quiocho
Department of Chemistry
Rice University
Houston, TX

GRAMPS—General Graphical Display System
Abbott Laboratories
D-47E AP9
Abbott Park, IL 60064

HYDRA—Molecular Mechanics, Molecular Dynamics, Molecular Display
Polygen Corporation
200 Fifth Avenue
Waltham, MA 02154

MACROMODEL—Molecular Mechanics and Molecular Display
Dr. Clark Still
Columbia University
New York, NY

Appendix I

MIDAS—Molecular Display
Professor Robert Langridge
Computer Graphics Lab
Department of Pharmaceutical Chemistry
University of California
San Francisco, CA 94143

MMS—Molecular Display
Steve Dempsey
Department of Chemistry Computer Facility
Department of Chemistry B-014
University of California at San Diego
La Jolla, CA 92093

SYBYL—Molecular Mechanics and Molecular Display
MENDYL—Macromolecular Mechanics and Molecular Display
Tripos Associates, Inc.
6548 Clayton Road
St. Louis, MO 63177

Appendix II Commands Available in the CAMD System and Brief Descriptions of Their Functions

CMD commands

ADDH	Add hydrogen atoms to a particular atom
BANGLE	Compute bond angle
BREAK	Break a bond
CHARGE	Display atom charges
CLOSE	Compute all close contacts
COLOR	Color a molecule, solid or by atom type
CONNECT	Make a bond
COORD	List a particular atom coordinate
DISTANCE	Compute an atom-atom distance
DREIDING	Make a Dreiding-type picture (ball and stick)
DSTORE	Store two molecules in one output file
ENANTIOMER	Make the molecule into its enantiomer
ENERGY	Compute electrostatic and Lennard-Jones energy
FETCH	Read in a molecule from MSF file on disk
FILL	Display a CPK (filled) picture
FIX	Fix molecular conformation (remove bond rotations)
FUSE	Fuse two molecules into a new one
GPLUCK	Remove a group of atoms
INPLANE	Position the molecule into the XY plane
JOIN	Join two molecules into a new one

Appendix II

KILL	Remove a molecule from the work space
MOLRENAME	Rename a molecule
MOVIE	Display a movie (dynamics) file
NAME	Show the atom names
NMR	Compute NMR coupling constants
NOMENU	Turn off the display of molecule names in the menu
NUMBER	Rename atoms according to sequence in input file
PLUCK	Remove an atom from a molecule
REDRAW	Redraw a molecule (without hydrogens)
RENAME	Rename an atom
REPLACE	Replace an atom with a template (methyl, phenyl, etc.)
RINGFLIP	Flip a ring (chair to boat)
RMS	Superimpose molecules to minimize RMS distances
ROTATE	Allow torsion angle change (interactively or by value)
SELECT	Select default molecule name for subsequent commands
SET	Set system parameter (e.g., STEREO, COLLECT commands)
STORE	Output new MSF file to disk
SURFACE	Display a surface (Connolly, color-coded, etc.)
SYMBOL	Display atomic symbols for atoms
TANGLE	Compute a torsion angle
UNSELECT	Don't have a default molecule name
USE	Read commands from a disk file
VOLCOMP	Compute molecular volume and overlap between molecules
WINDOW	Center viewing window on some atom

PDS commands

ADDMAP	Add a chain conformation to a map file
ADDRES	Add a residue to an existing chain
ADDSYMB	Add a symbolic name to represent a group of atoms
ADVICE	A brief help command
ALIAS	Specify an alias for an atom or residue
APPEND	Append one chain onto another
ATTACH	Attach GRAMPS dials to manipulate a molecule
BUILD	Build a molecule from the residue library
CLOSE	Compute distances between sets of atoms
CLRFLAG	Clear an atom's flag
CMPLIB	Compare data in library with input molecule data
COPCHN	Create a new chain as a copy of an existing one
COPMOL	Create a new molecule as a copy of an existing one
COUNT	Display the count of matched molecules, atoms, etc.
CROSS	Make a cross-link between residues
DELALIAS	Delete a previously specified alias name

Appendix II

DELATM	Delete an atom
DELCHN	Delete a molecule
DELCRS	Delete a cross-link
DELJIG	Delete a jiggle (bond rotation)
DELLIB	Delete a library residue
DELMAP	Delete a chain conformation from a map file
DELMOL	Delete a molecule
DELRES	Delete a residue from a molecule
DELSYMB	Remove a symbolic name for a group of atoms
DETACH	Detach GRAMPS dials assigned using ATTACH
DIFFERENCE	Compare two sets of residues
DRAWSURFACE	Display a section of a precomputed dot surface
FINDCRS	Find unconnected cross-links and form cross-links
FIXJIG	Fix molecule's jiggled (rotated) bond angles
FLAG	Allow logical operations on atoms using flags
FORCES	Display forces between specified atom pairs
GETCOORD	Read molecule coordinates from a file
GETLIB	Add residues from a library file to working library
GETRES	Create new molecules from residue in working library
GETSURF	Read a precomputed dot surface file
GETXYZ	Replace coordinates with those from a disk file
HBOND	Find possible hydrogen bonding partners
HELP	On-line help using VAX/VMS help libraries
HMOMENT	Draw hydrophic moment vectors for specified residues
INITLIB	Return working library to initial state
JIGGLE	Modify conformation of molecule by bond rotations
JIGSURF	Modify conformation of dot surfaces by bond rotations
MAKESURF	Create a van der Waals dot surface
MAPCONF	Compare conformations against map file conformations
MODATM	Modify atom coordinates
MODCHN	Modify chain names
MODH	Add or remove hydrogens from residues
MODMOL	Modify information about a specified molecule
MODRES	Change a residue to its enantiomer
MUTATE	Change one residue into another type of residue
NBROF	Display distances between two sets of atoms
NEWVFF	Create a new VFF library from existing library
NOROCK	Stop automatic rocking (rotation) of GRAMPS objects
NOTRWORLD	Deassign GRAMPS rotation and translation commands
PCENTER	Center the GRAMPS display window on specified atom
PDRAW	Draw a GRAMPS picture file of atoms and bonds
PDRAWGUIDE	Draw a GRAMPS picture file of alpha carbon atoms
PPOINT	Pick a point using GRAMPS tablet
PRMS	Calculate RMS difference between sets of atoms

Appendix II

PSCALE	Set GRAMPS scale factor to accommodate specified atoms
READMSF	Read residue coordinates from disk file in MSF format
REDRAW	Reexecute a previous PDRAW command
RENUMBER	Renumber residues within a specified range
REPAIR	Try to restore "correct" bond lengths and angles
REPRANGE	Replace a set of residues with another set
ROCK	Continuously rock images on GRAMPS screen
SCAN	Restricted systematic search of conformational space
SCCENT	Modify GRAMPS window to center all displayed atoms
SELMAP	Select previously stored configurations from map file
SETANG	Set the standard angles of selected residues
SETCHA	Set atom charges according to charges in library
SETCONF	Set residues to standard conformation
SETDASH	Set style of dashing desired
SETDRAW	Set default drawing parameters
SETFLAG	Set specified atom flags
SHOALIAS	Show the list of alias names
SHOANG	Show the standard angles for residues
SHOATM	Show information on selected atoms
SHOCHN	Show information on selected chains
SHOCOMP	Show composition based on frequency of residue type
SHOCONF	Partition chains into regions of secondary structure
SHOCRS	Show current cross-links
SHODASH	Show currently selected dashing style
SHODRAW	Show currently selected drawing parameters
SHOFLAG	Show previous command lines that modified atom flags
SHOJIG	Show current jiggles (bond rotations)
SHOWLIB	Show residue and atom information in working library
SHOMAP	Print conformations in map file
SHOMOL	Show information on specified molecule(s)
SHONUM	Show numbers of molecules, residues, atoms, etc.
SHOPDRAW	Show objects created by PDRAW command
SHORES	Show information on selected residues
SHOSEQ	Show amino acid sequence of specified chain
SHOSURF	Show objects created by DRAWSURF command
SHOSYMB	Show symbolic names for a group of atoms
SPLIT	Split one chain into two
SUMCHARGE	Report sum of charges assigned to specified atoms
SURFAREA	Display surface area by atom or residue
SURFFLAG	Set atom flag based in surface area of atom
TRANSFORM	Matrix-multiply specified atoms' coordinates
TRWORLD	Translate and rotate GRAMPS objects

Appendix II

UNATTACH	Like DETACH, but return objects to original state
VALJIG	Display current rotation values of jiggled bonds
WEIGHT	Report sum of atoms' molecular weights
WRITECOORD	Write a disk file of coordinates for a set of atoms
WRITELIB	Write a disk file of residues from working library
WRITEMOL	Write a disk file of coordinates file for a molecule

Interact commands

AMACRO	Append to a macro definition
CSCALE	Set scale factor for GRAMPS pictures
DCL	Spawn a subprocess to use VAX/VMS/DCL
DEFDIR	Define a default directory for subsequent files
DKEY	Define a function key on user terminal
DMACRO	Define a macro
EMACRO	End a macro definition
ERASE	Clear user terminal screen
ESCAPE	Define file name for store definition of function keys
EXIT	Leave the program
IHELP	Get help with Interact commands
KEYS/NOKEYS	Use/don't use function keys on terminal
LAST	List last 20 commands (can be recalled and executed)
LIST	List the names of commands available
LMACRO	List the contents of a macro definition
MACTAB	Define a table of macro command names
MAIL	Access VAX/VMS mail utility
PASSALL	Pass commands directly to CMD/PDS/GRAMPS
PROFILE	Define file name for profile file (start up file)
QUIT	Like exit, but don't save any function keys, etc.
RDEXT	Set default input file extension (type)
RECORD	Start a file to record output from the program
REVDAT	List date of last program revision
SKEY	Show function key definitions
SMACRO	Show macro definitions
STEP	Single step through macros when they are used
STEXT	Set default output file extension (type)
SUGGEST	Send a suggestion or bug to programmers
TMACRO	Type contents of a macro
UMACRO	Use (execute) a macro definition
WARNING	Allow warning messages to be output

REFERENCES

1. Brickmann, J., Raster computer graphics in molecular physics. *Int. J. Quantum Chem. Quantum Chem. Symp. 18*:647–659 (1984).
2. Gavezzotti, A., Molecular free surface: A novel method of calculation and its uses in conformational studies and in organic crystal chemistry. *J. Am. Chem. Soc. 107*:962–967 (1985).
3. Namasivayam, S., and P. M. Dean, Statistical method for surface pattern-matching between dissimilar molecules: Electrostatic potentials and accessible surfaces. *J. Mol. Graphics 4*:46–50 (1986).
4. Crippen, G. M., Conformational analysis by scaled energy embedding. *J. Comput. Chem. 5*:548–554 (1984).
5. Marshall, G. R., Computer graphics and receptor modeling. In *Quantitative Approaches to Drug Design*, J. C. Dearden, ed. Elsevier, Amsterdam, pp. 129–136 (1983).
6. Ghose, A., and G. M. Crippen, Use of physicochemical parameters in distance geometry and related three-dimensional quantitative structure-activity relationships: A demonstration using *Escherichia coli* dihydrofolate reductase inhibitors. *J. Med. Chem. 28*:333–346 (1985).
7. Kuntz, I. D., J. M. Blaney, S. J. Oatley, R. Langridge, and T. E. Ferrin, A geometric approach to macromolecular-ligand interactions. *J. Mol. Biol. 161*:269–288 (1982).
8. Cody, V., Computer graphic modelling in drug design: Conformational analysis of dihydrofolate reductase inhibitors. *J. Mol. Graphics 4*:69–73 (1986).
9. Liebman, M. N., Approach to modelling specificity determinants in receptor-ligand complexes: Congeners of serotonin. *J. Mol. Graphics 4*:61–68 (1986).
10. Hansch, C., B. Hathaway, et al., Crystallography, quantitative structure-activity relationships and molecular graphics in a comparative study of dihydrofolate reductase from chicken liver and *Lactobacillus casei* by 4,6-diamino-1,2-dihydro-2,2-dimethyl-1-(substituted-phenyl)-s-triazenes. *J. Med. Chem. 27*:129–143 (1984).
11. Gund, P., J. D. Andose, J. B. Rhodes, and G. M. Smith, Three-dimensional molecular modelling and drug design. *Science 208*:1425–1431 (1980).
12. Langridge, R., T. Ferrin, I. D. Kuntz, and M. Connolly, Real-time color graphics in studies of molecular interactions. *Science 211*:661–666 (1981).
13. Connolly, M. L., Solvent-accessible surfaces of proteins and nucleic acids. *Science 221*:709–713 (1983).
14. Carson, M., Ribbon models of macromolecules. *J. Mol. Graphics 5*:103–106 (1987).
15. Weiner, P. K., R. Langridge, J. M. Blaney, R. Schaefer, and P. A. Kollman, *Proc. Natl. Acad. Sci. USA 79*:3754 (1982).
16. Huber, C. P., D. S. S. Gowda, and K. R. Acharya, Nalidixic acid. *Acta Crystallogr.* Sect. B 36:497 (1980).
17. Mayer, D., C. B. Naylor, I. Motoc, and G. R. Marshall, A unique geometry of the active site of angiotensin-converting enzyme consistent with structure-activity studies. *J. Comput.-Aided Mol. Design 1*:3–16 (1987) and references therein.

18. Lee, B., and F. M. Richards, The interpretation of protein structures: Estimation of static accessibility. *J. Mol. Biol. 55*:379–400 (1971).

19. Connolly, M. L., *QCPE Bull. 1*:75 (1981). Quantum Chemistry Program Exchange, Department of Chemistry, Indiana University, Bloomington, IN 47405.

20. Connolly, M. L., Analytical molecular surface calculation. *J. Appl. Crystallogr. 16*:548–558 (1983).

21. Connolly, M. L., Depth buffer algorithms for molecular modeling. *J. Mol. Graphics 3*:19–24 (1985).

22. Harrison, S. C., A. J. Olson, C. E. Schutt, F. K. Winkler, and G. Bricogne, Tomato bushy stunt virus at 2.9 angstroms resolution. *Nature 276*:368–373 (1978).

23. O'Donnell, T. J., and A. J. Olson, GRAMPS—A graphics language for real-time, interactive, three-dimensional picture editing and animation. *Comput. Graphics 15*:133–141 (1981).

24. Burkert, U., and N. L. Allinger, *Molecular Mechanics,* American Chemical Society, Washington, D.C., 1982.

25. Weiner, S., P. A. Kollman, D. A. Case, U. C. Singh, C. Ghio, G. Alagona, S. Profeta, and P. Weiner, A new force field for molecular mechanical simulation of nucleic acids and proteins. *J. Am. Chem. Soc. 106*:765–784 (1984).

26. Hagler, A. T., E. Huler, and S. Lifson, *J. Am. Chem. Soc. 96*:5319 (1974).

27. Dupuis, M., J. Rys, and H. King, HONDO, programs available for a variety of computers from Quantum Chemistry Program Exchange, Department of Chemistry, Indiana University, Bloomington, IN 47405. *J. Chem. Phys. 65*:111 (1976).

28. Binkley, J. S., R. A. Whiteside, R. Krishnan, R. Seeger, D. J. DeFrees, H. B. Schlegel, and J. A. Pople, GAUSSIAN 80 programs available for a variety of computers from Quantum Chemistry Program Exchange, Department of Chemistry, Indiana University, Bloomington, IN 47405. GAUSSIAN 82 programs available from Carnegie-Mellon University.

29. Crippen, G., *Distance Geometry and Conformational Calculations.* Chemometrics Research Studies Series, D. Bawden, ed. Wiley, New York (1981).

30. Allen, F. H., O. Kennard, D. S. Motherwell, W. G. Town, and D. G. Watson, The Cambridge Crystallographic Structural Data File. *J. Chem. Doc. 13*:119 (1973).

31. Taylor, R., and O. Kennard, Hydrogen-bond geometry in organic crystals. *Accounts Chem. Res. 17*:320–326 (1984).

32. Bondi, A., Van der Waals volumes and radii. *J. Phys. Chem. 68*:441 (1964).

33. Martin, Y. C., and E. A. Danaher, Molecular modeling of receptor-ligand interactions. In *Receptor Pharmacology and Function*, R. A. Glennon, ed. Marcel Dekker, New York (1987) (in press).

34. Fesik, S. W., T. J. O'Donnell, R. T. Gampe, and E. T. Olejniczak, Determining the structure of a glycopeptide–diacetyl–Lys–D–Ala–D–Ala complex using NMR parameters and molecular modelling. *J. Am. Chem. Soc. 108*:3165–3170 (1986).

35. Sheldrick, G. M., P. G. Jones, O. Kennard, D. H. Williams, and G. A. Smith,

Structure of vancomycin and its complex with acetly–D–alanyl–D–alanine. *Nature 271*:223–225 (1978).

36. Kalman, J. R., and D. H. Williams, An NMR study of the interaction between the antibiotic ristocetin A and a cell-wall peptide analogue. Negative nuclear Overhauser effect in the investigation of drug binding sites. *J. Am. Chem. Soc. 102*:906–912 (1980).

37. O'Donnell, T. J., and K. Mitchell, 3D Docking device for molecular modelling. *J. Mol. Graphics 5*:75–78 (1987).

38. Oie, T., G. H. Loew, S. K. Burt, J. S. Binkley, and R. D. MacElroy, *Ab initio* study of catalyzed and uncatalyzed amide bond formation as a model for bond formation: Ammonia–formic acid and ammonia-glycine reactions. *Int. J. Quantum Chem. Quantum Biol. Sym. 9*:223–245 (1982).

39. Kahn, S. D., C. F. Pau, A. R. Chamberlin, and W. J. Hehre, Modelling chemical reactivity 4. Regiochemistry and stereochemistry of electrophilic additions to allylic double bonds. *J. Am. Chem. Soc. 109*:650–663 (1987).

40. Martin, Y. C., *Quantitative Drug Design.* Marcel Dekker, New York, pp. 103–107 (1978).

41. Hout, R. F. Jr., W. J. Pietro, and W. J. Hehre, *A Pictorial Approach to Molecular Structure and Reactivity.* Wiley, New York (1984).

42. Singh, U. C., and P. A. Kollman, An approach to computing electrostatic charges for molecules. *J. Comput. Chem. 5*:129–145 (1984).

43. Connolly, M. L., and A. J. Olson, GRANNY, a companion to GRAMPS for the real-time manipulation of macromolecular models. *Comput. Chem. 9*:1–6 (1985).

44. Sanathanan, L., personal communication.

45. O'Donnell, T. J., and C. F. Chabalowski, Computer graphics applied to molecular modelling. In *New Methods in Drug Research*, Vol. 2, A. Makriyannis, ed. J. R. Prous, Barcelona, Spain (1986) (in press).

3

Theoretical Aspects of Drug Design: Molecular Mechanics and Molecular Dynamics

Stanley K. Burt
Sandoz Research Institute, East Hanover, New Jersey

Donald Mackay and Arnold T. Hagler
The Agouron Institute, La Jolla, California, and Biosym Technologies, Inc., San Diego, California

I. INTRODUCTION

It has long been recognized that peptides and proteins play a crucial role in biological function and regulation. Newer techniques in isolation, purification, and separation, as well as in molecular biology and genetic engineering, have spurred research efforts in this field. These new techniques have also accelerated interest in development of new therapeutic agents such as peptideomimetics, artificial enzymes, and diagnostic agents.

The fundamental problem when dealing with any molecule that elicits a biological response is to understand the relationship between molecular structure and the physiochemical properties of the molecule that are ultimately responsible for its mechanism of action. In the case of peptides, the number of degrees of freedom makes the determination of the spatial arrangement of the functional groups especially difficult. This spatial arrangement then determines the bioactive conformer. To determine the bioactive conformer, information about both structure and function is necessary.

Peptide chemists have recently made great strides in designing analogs that probe both structure and function. Structural features can be probed by geometrical constraints—for example, macrocycles, lactam bridges between adjacent residues, introduction of proline residues, and substitution with rigid individual amino acids. Function, on the other hand, can be probed by replacement of L amino acids by D, substitution of polar amino acids for nonpolar, and replacement of amide bonds. All of these modifications can be useful in helping to determine those features necessary for bioactivity, but they are expensive in labor and time. Theoretical techniques, in conjuction with these experimental techniques, can greatly speed the process of determining the bioactive conformation.

The rapid increase in computer power, combined with molecular graphics and improved potential energy functions, has made the use of computer-assisted drug design a potentially powerful tool in designing new drugs. These techniques are fast and reliable and therefore can be incorporated into efficient searching strategies and can aid in keeping costs within reasonable limits. There have been many applications of empirical energy calculations for the determination of peptide conformations, but new theoretical techniques, combined with new experimental techniques, offer even more hope that these methods can be useful in drug design. In this chapter we discuss the foundations of empirical energy methods and the newer techniques in the field and discuss how they can be used in searching for bioactive conformers.

The function of conformational calculations on biomolecules and the information available from these calculations depends on how well the potential functions used actually represent the energy of the biomolecule as a function of its atomic displacements. The precision required of the potential function is related to the question asked of the calculations. For example, if one wants to know what values of (θ, ϕ) for a given peptide are excluded owing to "steric hindrance," a hard-sphere representation (1,2) of the energy as a function of distance is probably sufficient. A hard-sphere approach would also be able to give a good idea as to whether a given substrate would fit into an enzyme active site or not. If, however, one were to ask whether the active site could expand somewhat to accommodate a substrate or what is the most favorable position of the substrate in the active site, then a potential function that included more terms would be required. At this level of inquiry the potential function would have to reflect the fact that electrostatic effects are probably important and that large, highly polarizable groups, such as aromatic rings and aliphatic side chains, exhibit a strong Van der Waals attraction. To account for the relaxation of both the substrate and the enzyme, the potential function would have to include terms allowing for relaxation of bond lengths and bond angles. In general, as the questions that one asks become more specific and more mechanistic, the potential functions must reflect the underlying physics.

The potential energy of the system, since we are dealing with interacting particles, should, in principle, be suitable for study by quantum mechanical methods. However, this is not true for most calculations involving biomolecules. Quantum calculations are not yet feasible for these calculations for several reasons. First, in quantum mechanics, since we are dealing with both nuclei and electrons, the number of particles to be considered increases rapidly. Second, the computational expense is prohibitive even for molecules as small as tetrapeptides. Third, semiempirical calculations, which would have to be the method of choice for large molecules, are not necessarily sufficiently accurate for these problems and may be worse than properly parameterized empirical potential functions.

For the above-cited reasons, most calculations on biomolecules are carried out using empirical potential functions. These functions have several advantages. One of the main advantages is that they are conceptually simpler and the energy expression can be considered in a framework with which most persons are familiar. These simpler expressions lead to analytical expressions for the derivatives that make energy calculations rapid. Also, if properly parameterized, these methods can yield results that are more accurate than quantum mechanical calculations.

There have recently been numerous reviews on the application of empirical potential functions (3–6). These reviews have dealt with conformational analysis, enzyme-substrate interactions, molecular dynamics of proteins, Monte Carlo calculations, and linear free-energy calculations. In this chapter we restrict ourselves to a description of the empirical potential functions, and applications of these functions and complementary techniques to the calculation of peptide and protein structures that are drug related.

II. POTENTIAL ENERGY FUNCTION

Empirical potential energy functions, or molecular mechanics, are analytical expressions that express the potential energy in terms of valence interactions. The most common forms of these potentials employed today are known as valence force fields. The valence force fields are composed of energy terms which can be divided into three main groups: nonbonded energy, electrostatic energy, and intramolecular energy. A general expression for the potential energy is given by the following expression:

$$
\begin{aligned}
V = {} & 1/2 \sum K_b (b - b_0)^2 + 1/2 \sum K_\theta (\theta - \theta_0)^2 + 1/2 \sum K_\phi (1 + s \cos n\phi) \\
& + 1/2 \sum K_\chi \chi^2 + \sum \sum F_{bb'} (b - b_0)(b' - b_0') \\
& + \sum \sum F_{\theta\theta'} (\theta - \theta_0)(\theta' - \theta_0') + \sum \sum F_{b\theta} (b - b_0)(\theta - \theta_0) \\
& + \sum F_{\phi\theta\theta'} \cos \phi (\theta - \theta_0)(\theta' - \theta_0') + \sum \sum F_{\chi\chi'} \chi\chi' \\
& + \sum \left(\frac{B_{ij}}{r_{ij}^{12}} - \frac{A_{ij}}{r_{ij}^{6}} + \frac{e_i e_j}{r_{ij}^{2}} \right)
\end{aligned}
\tag{1}
$$

This equation reflects the energy necessary to stretch bonds (b), to distort bond angles (θ) from their reference values, and to generate strain in the torsion angles by twisting about bonds. Here K_b, K_θ, K_ϕ, K_χ, $F_{bb'}$, $F_{\theta\theta'}$, $F_{b\theta'}$, and $F_{\phi\theta\theta'}$ are force constants for the corresponding deformations, such as bond stretching, angle bending, torsional barriers, out-of-plane deformations, and the coupling between various movements such as bond stretch and angle bending. The last summation in Eq. (1) contains terms for the nonbonded energy and the electrostatic energy. There are many variations on the above expression, but, with the exception of the cross terms ($F_{bb'}$; $F_{\theta\theta'}$;...), most potential functions employed today such as Amber (7), Charmm (8), and Discover (9) are variations on this type of empirical equation.

As seen in Eq. (1), there are numerous parameters that must be found for the potential function. Reference values for the geometrical variables and force constants must be determined by experiments or quantum mechanical calculations and then fitted by least-squares methods. One way to reduce the number of parameters is to allow the bond lengths and/or bond angles to remain fixed. In the case of bond lengths, this procedure may be justifiable, since bond stretching requires a large energy penalty, but for bond angles this is more questionable (10).

Even if the cross terms are ignored and bond angles and bond lengths are fixed, the problem of parameter determination is not substantially easier.

Cross terms, which are also numerous, are necessary for fitting spectroscopic data and can be important for precise calculation of geometries and energy (11). As applications of molecular mechanics in all areas of science increase, the determination of the proper form of the potential energy function and the proper values of the parameters for them become a critical problem.

III. NONBONDED ENERGY TERMS

The energy of interaction between two nonbonded atoms is probably the most extensively studied term in Eq. (1). There have been numerous reviews devoted to this subject (12—14). In principle, these molecular forces are well understood and are essentially electrostatic in nature. Quantum mechanical calculations have become a major source of information about molecular interactions, but accurate results are limited to systems with only a few electrons. Usually it is impossible to obtain exact solutions, and for larger systems approximate methods must be used. Information about nonbonded interactions can also come from crystal packing data (15).

The important contribution of quantum mechanics has been to indicate the form of the intermolecular potential rather than to calculate the potential for all systems of interest. Despite the level of approximation used, or whether a power law or exponential is used ro represent the repulsive part of the potential, all interatomic nonbonded potentials exhibit the qualitative dependence on interatomic distance shown in Figure 1. At long distance the atoms attract each other owing to dispersion forces, whereas at short distances there is a strong repulsion due to overlap of the atoms' electronic clouds. Between the two regions there is a minimum.

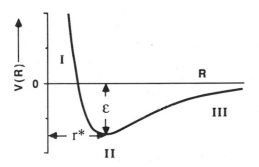

Figure 1 A typical Lennard-Jones potential energy curve. r^* is the interatomic distance at which the energy is a minimum, and ε is the energy at the minimum. The short-range region is labeled I, the intermediate region II, and the long-range region III.

It is convenient to define r^* as the interatomic distance at which the energy is a minimum and ε as the energy at the minimum. In the long-range region $r \gg r^*$, there is a negligible overlap of the electronic charge clouds (schematically, III in Fig. 1). In the short-range region (I in Fig. 1), the charge clouds overlap and strongly perturb each other. In the intermediate region (III in Fig. 1), the charge clouds overlap only slightly.

In the long-range region, even electroneutral molecules exert attractive forces on each other. These forces are functions of the intermolecular distances as well as of the electronic structures. The theory of attractive interactions is due to London (16,17), and the forces acting on the system of particles are called dispersion forces. Although the mathematical derivation of the theory of these forces is complex, the qualitative origin of the force is straightforward. At any given moment, instantaneous dipoles are created because of nuclear and electronic fluctuations. These fluctuating dipoles induce dipoles in other atoms, and the interaction of these two dipoles creates a net attraction.

From London's theory the dispersion term can be represented by an r^{-6} dependence, where r is the distance between two atoms, i and j. The dispersion energy can be related to polarizabilities and various other macroscopic properties such as ionization potentials. Slater and Kirkwood (18) derived a relationship for the dispersion energy

$$V_{\text{disp}} = \frac{-1}{r^6} \frac{3e\hbar}{2M_e^{1/2}} \frac{\alpha_a \alpha_b}{(\alpha_a/N_a)^{1/2} + (\alpha_b/N_b)^{1/2}} \tag{2}$$

where α_a is the polarizability of atom a, N_a is the number of electrons in the outer shell of atom a, and similarly for atom b. This expression is frequently used by various groups in determining the dispersion terms (19,20).

The short-range forces are repulsive forces. The qualitative explanation for these forces is that when atoms are close, there is considerable overlap of their electronic clouds and these clouds are distorted owing to the Pauli exclusion principle. The net effect is a repulsion between the two atoms. For the short-range force there is much less guidance for the analytical form. From quantum mechanical calculations the repulsive energy is expressed in the form

$$V_{\text{rep}} = P(r)e^{-br} \tag{3}$$

where $P(r)$ is some slowly varying function of r such as a polynomial and b is a constant that determines the steepness of its repulsion.

The above expression is not suitable for conformational calculations and is often expressed as

$$V_{\text{rep}} = Ae^{-br} \tag{4}$$

The exponential function in Eq. (4) reproduces for the most part the repulsive potential for the region of interest in conformational calculations. This functional form, however, is not computationally efficient for large molecular systems. For this reason most potential functions employ either a r^9 or r^{12} dependence for the functional form (21,22) of the short-range term.

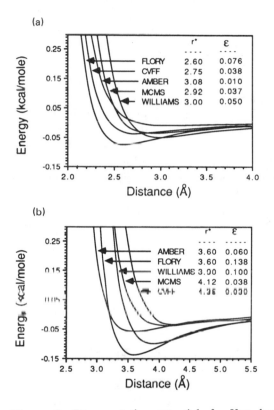

Figure 2 Representative potentials for Van der Waals interactions of aliphatic carbons (panel a) and hydrogens (b). The parameters are taken from the following references: AMBER—Weiner et al., *J. Comp. Chem.* 7:230–252 (1986); CVFF—Hagler et al., *J. Am. Chem. Soc.* 96:5319–5327 (1974); FLORY—Brant et al., *J. Mol. Biol.* 23:47 (1967); MCMS—Momany et al., *J. Phys. Chem.* 79:2361–2381 (1975); WILLIAMS—Williams and Starr, *Comput. Chem.* 1:173–177 (1977). r^* is the location of the energy minimum, and ε is the value of the energy at r^*. (a) Plot of nonbonded potential for C...C interactions from representative potential functions. r^* is the location of the potential minimum; ε is the energy of the well at the minimum. (b) Plot of nonbonded potential for H...H interactions from representative potential functions. r^* is the location of the potential minimum; ε is the energy of the well at the minimum.

The expressions for the coefficients of the r^{-6} term for like atoms, A_{aa}, A_{bb}, and for unlike atoms, i.e., A_{ab}, are interrelated. It is therefore useful to express A_{ab} in terms of A_{aa} and A_{bb} in order to reduce the number of independent energy parameters that must be determined in constructing a force field. The simplest method is to use a geometric mean combination rule

$$A_{ab} = (A_{aa}A_{bb})^{1/2} \tag{5}$$

Another combination rule (23) is

$$A_{ab} = 2A_{aa}A_{bb}/[(A_{aa}\alpha_b/\alpha_a) + (A_{bb}\alpha_a/\alpha_b)] \tag{6}$$

where α_a and α_b are the polarizabilities of atoms a and b.

It is inconsistent to mix parameters from one potential function with those of another without the assurance that the potential functions are entirely homogeneous. Figure 2 shows the C...C nonbonded potentials and the H...H potentials from various potential functions. Notice in Figure 2 that whereas the H...H potentials are fairly similar, the location of the minimum is different by about 0.4 Å. For the C...C potentials, the situation is much worse, and the minimum differ by as much as 0.75 Å between the Amber force field and the VFF force field. This points out the need for extensive further work in deriving and testing of force fields against a large array of experimental data.

IV. ELECTROSTATIC ENERGY (V_{es})—THEORETICAL CONSIDERATIONS

In the previous section on nonbonded forces, we discussed the intermolecular forces between neutral, nonpolar atoms or molecules. However, proteins and other biological macromolecules contain highly polar substituents, and often even charged groups. The electrostatic interactions are important and must be taken into account in conformational calculations.

A. Coulomb's Law

The form of the electrostatic potential is given by Coulomb's law

$$V_{es} = q_a q_b / Dr \tag{7}$$

where q_a and q_b are the charges on the particles a and b, r is the distance between the particles, and D is the dielectric constant.

The electrostatic potential for the interaction of polar molecules is sometimes expanded in a series of multipole interactions. For example, the next two higher-order terms are

$$V_{q\mu} = -q\vec{\mu} \cdot (\vec{r}/r)/Dr^2 \tag{8}$$

$$V_{\mu_a\mu_b} = (1/Dr^3) \cdot [\vec{\mu}_a \cdot \vec{\mu}_b - 3(\vec{\mu}_a \cdot \vec{r})(\vec{\mu}_b \cdot \vec{r})/r^2] \tag{9}$$

where $\vec{\mu}$ is the dipole moment and r is the vector of length r connecting the two dipoles (or the charge and dipole). Higher-order terms contain contributions from the quadrupole moments, octupole moments, etc. (24).

In the case of the electrostatic potential, as with dispersion forces, the analytical form of the potential is known and presents no problem. For a system of charges interacting in a macroscopic medium the constant q_i and D are also readily available. For example, for the interaction of two ions in a solution, the charges are known, and the dielectric constant of a substance is available from standard measurements (25).

Unfortunately, for the case of intramolecular interactions, such as those that occur in proteins, neither the charges of the interacting groups nor the local dielectric of the "medium" between these groups is known unambiguously. Thus, as in the case of nonbonded forces, approximations to the constants (namely the charges and dielectric constant) must be made. The common approximations made in conformational analysis in order to obtain values for these constants will be discussed below.

B. Second-Order Effects—Induction Forces

When a charged particle, a, interacts with a neutral, nonpolar atom or molecule, b, the charged particle induces a dipole moment in the nonpolar atom. This induced dipole moment is due to the relative displacement of the nuclei and electrons by the field of the charged particle. The moment induced is directly proportional to the field, E_a due to the charge q_a acting on atom b, where the constant of proportionality is the polarizability of atom b, α_b, i.e.

$$\mu_b = \alpha_b E_a \tag{10}$$

The interaction of this charge with the induced dipole then leads to a net attractive force. The energy of charged-induced dipole interaction $V_{q-\mu\alpha}$ is given by (24)

$$V_{q-\mu\alpha} = -q_a^2 \alpha_b/2Dr^4 \tag{11}$$

namely, it goes as the inverse fourth power of the distance.

A permanent dipole also induces a dipole moment in nonpolar atoms and likewise with higher moments. The potential energy $V_{\mu-\mu\alpha}$, of the interaction between a permanent dipole and the dipole it induces is (24)

$$V_{\mu-\mu\alpha} = (\mu_a^2 \alpha_b/2De^6)(3\cos^2\theta + 1) \tag{12}$$

where μ_a is the permanent dipole moment of molecule a and θ is the angle between μ_a and the line connecting it to the induced dipole. Thus this interaction goes as the inverse sixth power of the intermolecular distance. Interactions involving dipole-induced quadrupole go as the inverse eighth power and so on for still higher-order interactions.

C. Total Electrostatic Energy

The total electrostatic energy for the interaction of two polarizable atoms, a and b, separated by a distance r bearing partial charges q_a and q_b of opposite signs is then given by

$$V_{es} = -q_a q_b/r - q_a \mu_b/r^2 - q_b \mu_a/r^2 + \mu_a^2/2\alpha_a$$
$$+ \mu_b^2/2\alpha_b - 2\mu_a \mu_b/r^3 + \cdots \tag{13}$$

where the terms in Eq. (13) correspond in order to: the Coulomb interaction; the attraction between the charge on a and the dipole it induces in b; similarly for charge on b and induced dipole in a; the energy of inducing the dipole in a; similarly for b; and finally the interaction between the two induced dipoles on a and b*. Solving for the induced dipoles by requiring that the energy be a minimum (26) one obtains

$$V_{es} = -q_a q_b/r - (1/2r)[(q_b^2 \alpha_a + q_a^2 \alpha b)/r^3 + 4q_a q_b \alpha_a \alpha b/r^6]$$
$$\times (1 - 4\alpha_a \alpha b/r^6)^{-1} \tag{14}$$

where again the first term is the Coulomb term, the second is the charge-induced dipole interaction, and the last is the induced dipole-induced dipole interactions. Higher-order terms have been omitted, and we have assumed unlike charges. For like charges the first and third terms have opposite signs.

To give an idea of the relative order of magnitude of the terms in Eq. (14), we can consider an interaction between two "typical" atoms in a protein (i.e., H, C, N, O, etc.). To get an upper estimate for the importance of the induction terms, which go as r^{-4} and r^{-7}, respectively, a relatively small, although not unreasonable value of 3 Å is chosen for the interatomic interaction distance. The polarizabilities of the atoms are of the order of 1 Å^3, while the partial charges are taken as ~ 0.33 electrons for the purpose of this rough estimate. It should be noted that the value of the partial charges does not affect the relative values of the terms. For this case the three terms have the values $q_A q_b/r \sim 10$ kcal/mole, $\alpha_b q_a^2/r_4 \sim 0.5$ kcal, and $4q_a q_b \alpha_a \alpha_b/r^7 \sim 0.05$ kcal/mole.

---

*For a clear discussion of the induction energy, see Ref. (26).

From this rough estimate it is seen that typically the last term is not significant ($<1\%$), while the value of the charge-induced dipole interaction is on the order of 5% of the Coulomb energy.

The relation given in Eq. (14) represents the interaction between an isolated pair of polarizable charges. The situation is much more complicated in a protein or in other biological macromolecules, where the dipole induced in a given atom is due to a field of the charges on all the other atoms in the molecule as well as the induced moments in these atoms. Thus in general the induced dipole in an atom due to the field of all the other atoms would have to be calculated by minimizing the total energy given by an expression analogous to Eq. (14) except that the energy is now a sum over all possible interactions in the protein. Arridge and Cannon (27) have considered this polarization (induction) energy in a treatment of the lattice energy of amides, polyamides, and peptides. They were only able to solve for the exact polarization energy in the one-dimensional case of a collinear array of polarizable dipoles. For the general three-dimensional lattice, the problem became intractable, and numerical methods are required.

D. Relative Magnitude of Electrostatic and Nonbonded Interactions

London (17) and Hirschfelder et al. (24) have considered the relative magnitude of the various contributions to the intermolecular potential, for representative polar molecules, ranging from carbon monoxide with a dipole moment of 0.12 D to water with a dipole moment of 1.84 D. In the majority of cases, the dispersion forces are most important. However, in highly polar molecules the Coulomb, or dipole-dipole forces are more important. In water these forces account for approximately 80% of the total interaction energy, but even here the dispersion forces are not negligible, accounting for another 16%.

The induction effect is never very important for polar molecules, accounting for at most approximately 5% of the energy (in the case of NH_3). However, the case of interactions between ions and nonpolar (although polarizable) molecules is different. For these systems, the induction forces become a dominant contribution to the energy (24), although here again the dispersion forces are not negligible, being also related to polarizability. There are often highly polarizable moieties in proteins such as tryptophan, histidine, and tyrosine and ionizable $-NH_2$ and COOH groups as well as other ions in the media. In cases where these groups interact, the effects of induction energy could be significant.

E.   Dielectric Constant and Partial Atomic Charges

The macroscopic dielectric constant, which attenuates charge interactions, arises from permanent or inducible multipole moments between interacting charges and is related to the dielectric permittivity of the medium. In conformational calculations the dielectric is used to account for the effect of solvent in attenuating the electrostatic interactions of charged groups in an aqueous environment. Rather than attribute any physical significance to the dielectric constant, in molecular mechanics it is often considered an empirical parameter.

In the past the dielectric constant was taken as unity for those systems where the partial atomic charges were taken from crystal packing studies (28), and as a value of 2 or 4 in systems where the partial charges were obtained from quantum mechanical calculations (29,30). The value of 2 was choosen by Scheraga and co-workers (30) to yield reasonable results for hydrogen-bonded dimers, and since the CNDO charges used underestimate dipole moments, this value was considered approximately equal to an effective dielectric of 4–8. Other studies on proteins have seen values of $D = 20$ applied in interactions of charged side chains in order to account for counterion shielding (33).

More recently a distance-dependent dielectric has been employed in empirical potential functions (7,8). The relationships have ranged from a linear dependence on r to an inverse second-power dependence. The rationale is that by using a distance dependence the polarization effects for closer interactions are weighed more heavily and longer-range interactions are dampened more than shorter-range interactions. Macroscopic dielectric functions have recently been replaced by modeling the electric field numerically through a finite element approach (31,32). This model accounts for different parts of a macromolecule having completely different dielectric properties. Of course, if explicit solvent molecules are included in the simulation, an empirical dielectric may be unnecessary. For example, in a full-scale simulation including many explicit waters, the dielectric shielding is accounted for by the physics of the interacting waters as they reorient their dipoles to counteract the local electrostatic field.

The most widely used method for obtaining partial atomic charges is by performing a quantum mechanical calculation and doing a Mulliken population analysis (34). Mulliken population analysis is usually done in both semiempirical or ab initio calculations. While Mulliken population analysis is a standard technique, there are theoretical objections to its use, because problems arise as to how to partition the overlap charges between atoms of different electronegativity (in a Mulliken analysis the two atoms are weighed equally). Usually partial atomic charges are derived from STO3G calculations CNDO (35) or MNDO (36) calculations or derived along with Van der Waals parameters from fitting to crystal geometries and parameters. Alternate schemes for obtaining partial atomic charges, especially for larger molecules, include the Del Re (37) method and the Gasteiger (38) method. The Del Re method is an older molecular orbital calculation that obtains charges in sigma bonds, whereas the Gasteiger method is based on charge neutrality. Both of these methods have the advantage that they are very fast and give reasonable estimates of physical properties associated with charge. However, the Del Re method is insensitive to molecular structure and conformation, and the Gasteiger method is equivocal for charge distributions of resonance structures.

Point charge models, in general, are not good representations of the true charge distribution, and higher-order terms such as dipole and quadrupole terms are needed to provide reliable representations. In addition, atomic charge is not physically observable, so partial atomic charges must be inferred by experimentation or other means. Researchers are now attempting to derive partial atomic charges by fitting to quantum mechanically calculated electrostatic potentials. First suggested by Tomasi (39,40), some of the recent work in this area is due to Cox and Williams (41) and Kollman's group (42). Momany (43) found that partial atomic charges fitted to the electrostatic potential are a better representation of the SCF unperturbed electrostatic potential than those obtained from a Mulliken population analysis. The major drawback to these approaches is that they require more effort to obtain partial charges, and if electrostatic potentials of fragments of molecules are fitted, then these must be smeared together to form a molecule. Also, if additional centers of charge must be placed on the fragments to reproduce the electrostatic potential, then computational time is increased, and transferability between fragments is more difficult.

V. HYDROGEN BONDS

The description of hydrogen bonding in empirical potential energy function is problematic. The original theories of the hydrogen bond were mainly electrostatic (24,44,45), while some have argued that the effect is primarily due to charge transfer (46). Most efforts to include hydrogen bonding in empirical energy functions are to use properly choosen partial atomic charges and Lennard-Jones parameters to reflect the strength of hydrogen bonding. Poland and Scheraga (47) developed an empirical hydrogen bond function which is of the form shown below.

$$V_{hb} = \frac{d}{r^{12}} - \frac{c}{r^6} \tag{15}$$

for the interaction of the O...H atoms participating in the hydrogen bond. The values of d and c were obtained by requiring that the total interaction energy for a pair of hydrogen-bonded molecules at a specified minimum distance be equal to an estimated experimental dimerization energy. McGuire et al. (48) proposed a hydrogen bond potential which describes the O...H interaction by

$$V_{HB} = \frac{A}{r_{OH}^{12}} - \frac{b}{r_{OH}^{10}} \tag{16}$$

This potential was obtained by subtracting from the CNDO/2 energy of two hydrogen-bonding molecules, calculated as a function of r, the empirical nonbonding and electrostatic interaction for all atoms except the O...H atoms. The differences between the two energy curves for many molecules were fit by a least-squares procedure with a potential of the form

$$V_{HB} = \frac{A}{r_{OH}^{12}} - \frac{b}{r_{OH}^{m}} \tag{17}$$

A best fit was found for $m = 10$, although different A's and B's were needed for each molecule. This procedure was carried out only in the attractive region of the curve, since the CNDO/2 procedure underestimates the repulsive interactions and leads to very short O...H distances. The resultant value for the parameters A and B were then adjusted further to fit the gas phase heat of dimerization and the equilibrium geometry of the formic acid dimer.

A study of the amide hydrogen bond by calculation of the crystal structure and sublimation energies of amide crystals led Hagler et al. (49,50) to the conclusion that the hydrogen bond could be represented well with only electrostatic and nonbonded interactions. In an effort to determine the transferability of potential parameters between similar molecules, Hagler and Lapiccirella (51) used population analysis and the shape of the spatial electron density as a guide for transferability and similarity of similar functional groups. As shown in Figure 3a, contours of constant electron density in the plane of the amide group in N-methylacetamide show that the amide proton is essentially embedded in the spherical electron density of the nitrogen. In Figure 3b, the density obtained from superposition of spherical atoms is shown. The similarity between the two density plots shows that there is little change in electron distribution upon molecular formation and suggests that the use of spherical atoms to represent the Van der Waals interaction is justified. This conclusion is in agreement with the proposed dominance of the electrostatic interaction suggested by ab initio calculations (52–54). In another study on hydrogen-bonded crystals of adipamide (55), it was also demonstrated that the potential function, without Van der Waals

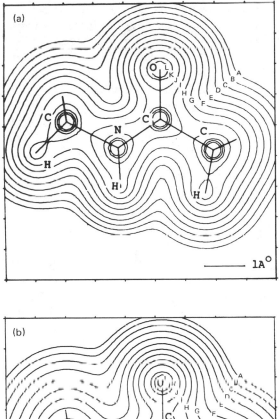

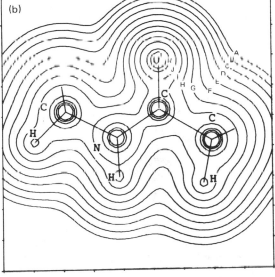

Figure 3 (a) Contour map of the electron density of N-methylacetamide calculated by 6-31 G basis set. Note the amide proton is located in the sphere of the electron density of the nitrogen. (b) Electron density of N-methylacetamide obtained by superposition of spherical atoms.

parameters for the amide hydrogen, were able to correctly predict the hydrogen bond geometry. One of the central features that emerged from the crystal calculations is the necessity of a small "Van der Waals radius" of the amide hydrogen (corresponding to a particularly short range of repulsion) to account for the properties of the hydrogen bond. This allows the oxygen to approach the hydrogen more closely, thus contributing to the large electrostatic energy.

In general, most current empirical force fields include an "explicit" hydrogen-bonded potential and assume that the proper choice of Lennard-Jones parameters and partial charges will not adequately represent the hydrogen bond interaction. Some programs allow the scaling of hydrogen-bonded terms to enhance their ability to form, whereas others reduce the repulsion on hydrogens involved in hydrogen bonding.

VI. ENERGY MINIMIZATION

Once we have a set of molecular coordinates, the energy of the system can be calculated by using the molecular mechanics force field. Most often one is interested in determining minimum energy structures. This can be done by finding the coordinates at which the first derivative of the potential function is equal to zero. If one calculates the second derivatives of the energies, then the eigenvalues of the second derivative matrix will provide the vibrational frequencies, and the corresponding eigenvectors will yield the normal modes. From the vibrational frequencies, using statistical thermodynamics, the vibrational entropy can be calculated.

There are numerous algorithms available for geometry optimization. The simplest and most straightforward of these is the method of steepest descent. In steepest descent we move down the gradient in a direction parallel to the net force. Steepest descent will lead directly to the nearest local minimum by following a path that is determined by moving from the previous value to a new value by some constant k times the direction in which the energy is decreasing. Another move is made, and the step size k is adjusted according to the result. If the new move decreases the energy, the new structure is accepted, and the process is repeated. If, on the other hand, the energy increases, the previous structure is restored, and the step size is decreased. Steepest descent is a very fast procedure for correcting "bad" initial geometries, but this method has poor convergence properties, since the derivatives become increasingly small near the minimum.

The conjugate gradient method (56,57), unlike steepest descent, utilizes information from the previous gradients along with the current gradient to locate the minimum. Conjugate gradient methods take the second search direction to be a linear combination of the current gradients and the previous ones. Conjugate gradient methods are more efficient than steepest descent and require fewer energy evaluations and gradient calculations. Conjugate gradient methods can also induce large changes in the coordinates while searching for a minimum, but the convergence characteristics are better than with steepest descent.

The Newton-Raphson procedure (22) is a powerful, convergent minimization procedure. In the Newton-Raphson algorithm, one needs to have the second derivative matrix available. Then the new coordinates in each

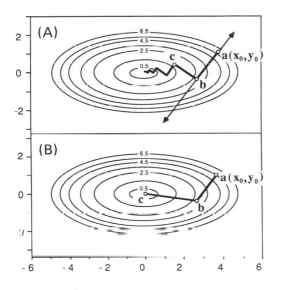

Figure 4 (A) Example of a minimum-energy search using steepest descents. Starting at the initial point (a) with coordinates (x_0, y_0), the gradient direction (represented by the arrowed line) is calculated and followed "downhill" until the energy begins to increase (point b). Note that the gradient direction does not point directly to the minimum and that it is tangent to the energy contours at (b). At (b), a new gradient direction is calculated and followed until point (c). The process is repeated until the minimum is reached. Note that each gradient direction is orthogonal to the previous gradient. (B) Example of a minimum-energy search using conjugate gradients. Starting at the initial point (a) with coordinates (x_0, y_0), the minimum (c) is found in only two steps. The step from (a) to (b) is identical to that in steepest descents of Figure 4A. However, instead of following the gradient direction away from point (b), a direction conjugate to the previous direction is derived (thus the term "conjugate gradient"), which, unlike steepest descents, is not necessarily orthogonal to the previous direction. By constructing and following mutually conjugate directions, this algorithm will find the minimum of an N-dimensional harmonic system in N steps.

iteration can be found by the following equation

$$\Delta X = F_s^{-1} \frac{\partial V}{\partial x_i}$$
(18)

where F is the matrix of the second derivative with respect to the coordinates and $(\partial V)/(\partial x_i)$ are the first derivatives. The Newton-Raphson method is based on the assumption that the energy is quadratically dependent, i.e., behaves like a classical spring. If the energy function were quadratic, the increments x would lead directly to the minimum in one step. This is, of course, almost never the case for the potential surface of complex biomolecules. Newton-Raphson methods do not need to do linear interpolations like conjugate gradient, so energy evaluations can be speeded up by a factor of about 2–3. The major drawback of the Newton-Raphson method is that one must spend the time to calculate the second derivatives, which is computationally expensive, and, to save time, one would have to be able to express the second derivatives in an analytical form, which is not necessarily easy for complex potential functions.

The difference between steepest descent and conjugate gradient methods can best be illustrated by Figure 4. In Figure 4A, steepest descent is shown for a simple two-dimensional case. The new gradients are all shown to be orthogonal to the previous gradient. Thus, the process of minimization occurs in a stepwise manner and will proceed to the minimum. In Figure 4B, the method of conjugate gradient is shown for the two-dimensional case. Note that for the case shown here, that of a quadratic function, the method converges in two steps. Conjugate gradient methods will, in general, converge in N iteration (where N is the dimensionality of the system) for harmonic systems.

The best compromise is to use the method of Fletcher and Powell (58). This algorithm combines the advantages of steepest descent with Newton-Raphson and requires only the first derivatives, but builds up the second derivatives by successive approximations. This method is both quadratically convergent and efficient.

VII. APPLICATIONS OF THEORETICAL TECHNIQUES TO DRUG DESIGN

The basic equations for calculating the conformational energy of biomolecules have been known, as seen in the previous sections, for some time, although derivation and testing of force constants have lagged. The increase in computer power and speed at a reasonable cost has spurred the use of theoretical techniques for biological applications. Since the late 1970s new theoretical tools have emerged from treating the complex problems involved in studying peptide conformational and dynamic properties. These techniques include vibrational normal mode analysis, Monte Carlo methods, total geometry optimization, and molecular dynamics. These techniques, combined with computer graphics, give promise to a greatly expanded role of computer-assisted molecular design.

A. Monte Carlo

The Monte Carlo technique is a stochastic method in which chains of configurations are generated and the average structural features and thermodynamic properties are obtained by weighted averages. For the statistics to yield accurate results, this usually requires the generation of several million configurations (61,62). Using these configurations, the average of some desired property can be calculated by the following relationship:

$$\langle x \rangle = \frac{\sum_i x_i \exp(-E_i/kT)}{\sum_i \exp(-E_i/kT)} \tag{19}$$

where x is the property of interest, x_i is the value of the property in the configuration i, E_i is the energy of the configuration, k is the Boltzmann constant, and T is the temperature. The factor $\exp(-E_i/kT)$ is the Boltzmann factor and thus weighs the property x. Unlike energy minimizations, Monte Carlo does not find an energy minimum but rather samples an ensemble of states, just as the actual molecular system does, with higher energy states being sampled as temperature increases. Even though some high energy states will be sampled, their contributions to the value of the property X is small. This is because as the energy of the system increases, the term $\exp(-E_i/kT)$ becomes small. The problem of efficiently sampling configuration space was addressed by an algorithm due to Metropolis et al. (59). Efficient sampling of conformational space is achieved in this algorithm by generating each configuration at random but with the random step taken from a previous configuration (61,62).

There are various ways to optimized the sampling algorithm in Monte Carlo calculations. As opposed to molecular dynamics techniques, where the equations of motion are integrated numerically and thus small time steps are necessary, in Monte Carlo one can take larger steps to optimize the efficacy of the method. Furthermore, we can take different steps for rotation, translation, and internal coordinates, each optimized independently. In addition, one can bias the sampling to concentrate on regions of interest, such as the solvent in proximity to a peptide molecule. These types of biasing are known as importance sampling or umbrella sampling (60).

Monte Carlo calculations have been performed on a wide variety of biological problems, especially the study of solvent around peptides and proteins (61,62). Monte Carlo has also been applied to the study of conformational statistics of oligopeptide chains (63). In later calculations a Metropolis algorithm was not used, but rather sampling was performed from a limited set of preselected single-residue conformations. This type of calculation has also been used to calculate conformational entropy for met-enkephalin by Paine and Scheraga (64). Other applications of the Monte Carlo method have been carried out by Premilat and Maigret (65) on met-enkephalin and adrenocorticotrophic hormone (66). Demonte et al. (67) also performed Monte Carlo calculations on substituted met-enkephalin analogs.

B. Molecular Dynamics

Molecular dynamics is a deterministic process as opposed to the Monte Carlo stochastic process. If one expresses the energy of the system by an analytical potential as described above, then by calculating the first derivative of the energy with respect to the cartesian coordinates and solving for the case where these derivatives are zero, one can obtain a minimum energy conformation. We note that the negative of the first derivative of the potential with respect to the coordinate gives the force on each atom. Thus, from Newton's law, we can write that

$$F = ma = -\frac{dV}{dr} \tag{20}$$

or

$$-\frac{dV}{dr} = m\frac{d^2r}{dt^2} \tag{21}$$

where m is the mass of the atoms and a is the acceleration, t is the time, and r represents the cartesian coordinates of atom i. One can then integrate the equations of motion and compute a trajectory for each atom as a function of time. There are two algorithms used to integrate the equations of motion. These are the second-order predictor method of Verlet (68) and a fifth-order method due to Gear (69). The Gear algorithm is the more accurate and more stable algorithm for small time steps ($< 10^{-15}$ seconds), but smaller time steps require more simulation time and thus are more computationally expensive to achieve a trajectory of equivalent time. Time steps chosen in molecular dynamics simulations are usually on the order of 10^{-15} sec, and as a general rule should be significantly smaller than the period of the fastest local motion in the system in order for the numerical integration to remain stable.

In the computer environment of today, simulations of 20–30 psec (20,000–30,000 steps) are routine for protein systems (70). Constraints on bond lengths and bond angles have been used to increase the time step (as these remove the fastest motions in the system). However, these constraints carry the implied assumption that they are only weakly coupled to the remaining motions. The SHAKE algorithm (71) is capable of constraining these motions. It has been reported that constraint of bond lengths and angles speeds computations by a factor of 2 when all atoms are treated explicitly and by a factor of 3 when a united atom approach is taken (72). Bond angle constraints, however, have not been found to be acceptable, because these motions are intimately coupled to other motions in the molecules (72).

Simulations can be carried out in vacuo or in solution. If the simulations are performed in solution, atoms near the surface will be distorted by vacuum boundary conditions unless edge effects are taken into account. Edge effects are minimized by using periodic boundary conditions. In periodic boundary conditions the molecule of interest is placed in the center of a box, and then the box is replicated in all directions. All interactions with atoms in the central box or images in surrounding boxes are taken into account, provided they lie within the cutoff distance. To eliminate the possibility of an atom interacting with another atom or its image, the box size should be larger than twice the cutoff radius.

Usually in molecular dynamics simulations, the system is first partially minimized to relieve strain in the system such that excessive forces and accelerations are not present. Then by taking small time steps and integrating the equations of motion, new forces and accelerations are calculated. This procedure is then repeated iteratively to produce a trajectory. Conformational changes can be monitored either by computer graphics or by graphical analysis of variables of interest. If the trajectories are carried out for a sufficiently long time, one can obtain statistical thermodynamical properties by calculating time-averaged quantities. Correlation functions can also be obtained (73).

C. Use of Theoretical Simulations in Drug Design

Computer simulation techniques can aid medicinal chemists in designing new analogs in several ways. The first is in obtaining structures of minimum energy, dynamic trajectories of analogs, or a series of Monte Carlo configurations and displaying these on a stereographic display. The knowledge of the accessible structures and insight into accessible spatial relationships observable from movies or still pictures may allow the chemist to postulate the importance of a given conformation in interacting with the receptor. Analogs may then be synthesized to lock in a certain conformation to enhance stability.

A second complementary and more quantitative approach is to use the computational techniques to analyze the results of the simulation and characterize similarities and differences between the conformational and energetic properties of various analogs. If we minimize various geometries of a peptide, we can compare the energy differences among these conformations. From the mass-weighted second derivatives matrix of the energy with respect to the cartesian coordinates, we can calculate the eigenvalues and eigenvectors, which yield the vibrational frequencies and normal modes, respectively. Using statistical thermodynamics we can use these frequencies to calculate the entropy, vibrational energy, and free energy of a given conformational state. Therefore, by being able to calculate the energy of a molecule we can determine the structure, dynamics, vibrational spectra, energetics, and other properties (74).

One of the most powerful uses of molecular dynamics in drug research is to aid in the determination of the bioactive conformation. This goal is different from those addressed in most molecular dynamics simulations, where one is interested in time-averaged phenomena and the reproduction of an ensemble average. Because molecular dynamics runs of 20–30 psec and longer are now easily performed on an array of modern, widely available computers like a Vax 8600, molecular dynamics trajectories provide a method by which accessible conformational space can be explored and characterized (75,76). The purpose of these trajectories is to arrive at an initial hypothesis in a relatively short time and to generate ideas for the chemists to test by synthesis of new analogs.

The first application that took this approach was a study on gonadotrophin-releasing hormone (GnRH). GnRH, pGlu–His–Trp–Ser–Tyr–Gly–Leu–Arg–Pro–Gly–NH, is a member of the class of peptide hormones secreted by the hypothalamus to regulate pituitary hormone levels. It controls the release of luteinizing hormone and follicle-stimulating hormone which, in turn, are involved in regulating ovulation and spermatogenesis. Although thousands of analogs have been synthesized and both experimental and theoretical research has been carried out, there is little consensus on the conformation of the peptide. To answer the question of how closely the relative spatial orientations of corresponding functional groups in two flexible molecules can be, one can use the technique of "template forcing." This solves for the conformation that optimizes the overlap of these functional groups while maintaining the lowest potential energy cost to the molecule (77). With this tool we can then examine the similarities and differences between analogs quantitatively as well as graphically by displaying molecules on interactive graphics systems that have been optimally superposed to observe differences systematically. From the template forcing we can look for the common conformation of two analogs directly and also begin to ask why a desired conformation is inaccessible to a given analog. We can then prepare modifications that introduce favorable interactions to stabilized the target conformation.

In template forcing we minimize the energy of the molecule to be superposed onto an analog (the template), along with a penalty function that is proportional to the RMS distance between the common atoms to be superposed (77). For a review of the use of such constraints in strategies for simulations, see Mackay et al. (6). That is, we minimize the energy of the molecule, subject to an external force which forces the common atoms together.

$$F = V + K \left[\sum_i^N (x_i - x_i^0)^2 / N \right]^{1/2} \qquad (22)$$

In this equation F is a function which is the sum of the energy V from the normal valence force field plus the penalty function, a constant K, times the root-mean square deviation between the coordinates of the corresponding atoms of the template (x_i^0) and the forced molecule (x_i) (N is the total number of atoms forced). As the distance between the atoms goes to zero, the contribution of this penalty function vanishes. The balance between the degree to which the superposed molecule is forced onto the template and strain energy caused by the forcing is governed by the value of the constant K, which can be chosen arbitrarily to give any desired degree of fit.

To study the conformations of GnRH, a cyclic analog that was bridged between residues 1 and 10 was examined by molecular dynamics techniques (77). By comparing the structures of the cyclic molecule and the linear analog that adopted the same structure, information could be gained about the conformation, which may be the bioactive form. Molecular dynamics were run for 24 psec, and every picosecond the instantaneous configuration was extracted and minimized. From the minimizations 18 unique structures were found. The cyclic antagonist was much more highly constrained than the linear analog of GnRH. It was noticed, however, that several of the folded structures of GnRH appeared to have conformations that were similar to those adopted by the cyclic antagonist.

Using the technique of template forcing, GnRH was forced into a conformation which best superimposed residues 4–8 and 4–9 onto the corresponding residues of the cyclic structure. The superposition of residues 4–8 within 0.29–0.38 Å of the cyclic structure is shown in Figure 5. The forcing of residues 4–8 or 4–9 onto the cyclic structure can be achieved at a relatively low cost in energy (see Table 1). The energy required to force residues 4–8 with an RMS value of 0.29 Å was 5.2 kcal/mol, whereas forcing residues 4–9 cost only 4.9 kcal/mol. Generally, the more exact the structures are required to overlap, the higher the energy required will be. The energy

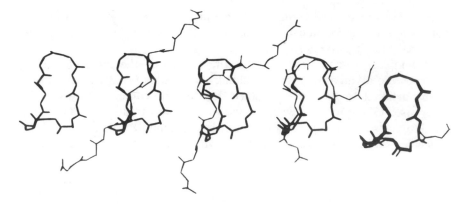

Figure 5 Template forcing of GnRH onto a constrained analog. The forcing is shown from left to right. At first only a few residues of the linear structure are aligned, but as the simulation proceeds, the linear structure is almost completely superimposed onto the cyclic analog. The final structure of the linear analog is low in energy, implying that the conformation of the cyclic structure could be adopted at the receptor.

Table 1　Template Forcing of GnRH onto the Cyclic Antagonist

Residues forced	RMS	Energy of GnRH in forced conformation[a]
4–8	0.29	61.5 (5.2)[b] kcal/mol
4–9	0.38	61.2 (4.9) kcal/mol

[a]A stiffness constant of $K = 10$ was used for this forcing.
[b]Number in parentheses is the difference in energy between the forced conformation and the lowest-energy GnRH conformation.

values obtained here are not of an unreasonable magnitude to be expected to be induced in a ligand by the receptor, and in addition, the latter can still adjust to accommodate the ligand. This conformation, then, remains a viable candidate in the search for the binding conformation. Thus, using template forcing, one can find common conformations of two molecules and compare their relative stabilities.

With template forcing we are not limited solely to the comparison or consideration of minimum energy structures. Indeed, the dynamic fluctuations of a molecule are fluctuations about minimum energy conformations, and the actual minimum energy structure itself may seldom be adopted. More important, binding to the receptor may well induce limited strain into the ligand and possibly into the receptor as well. Therefore, we see that when comparing two molecules it may be important not only to compare the geometric distance between minima, but to compare the difference between conformations close to but not necessarily located at local minima. Template forcing gives us a method by which we can directly find the common conformations of two molecules and compare their relative stabilities. In fact, by minimizing the energy of both molecules together with the superposition function, one can find common conformations neither of which corresponds to rigorous minima.

D. Use of NOE Data from NMR

Recent advances in NMR techniques have made it possible to determine the structure of numerous polypeptides, proteins, and oligonucleotides (78–80). With these techniques it is possible to obtain a large number of approximate interproton distances, which can be used as structural constraints. Unfortunately, the number and range of the experimentally determined distances is limited (those less than 5 Å) and are usually insufficient to obtain an unequivocal structure. To generate structures that satisfy the distance constraints, distance geometry methods (81) are commonly used. In this method, covalent bonding information such as bond lengths and angles are used as input along with the distance information to generate structures. Chirality constraints can also be included to eliminate structures with the incorrect stereochemistry. Distance geometry methods, employed alone, have several disadvantages. First, the method requires large amounts of memory and storage for large molecules, and second, the structures generated by distance geometry may well be energetically unfavorable. By using complementary energy minimizations and molecular dynamics coupled with the interproton distances, one has the advantage that the structural refinement is carried out with energetic criteria as well.

When using energy minimization and molecular dynamics along with NOE data for structural refinement, another term is added to the potential energy function (6) such that the total energy is expressed as

$$E_{\text{total}} = E_{\text{empirical}} + C_{\text{NOE}} \tag{23}$$

where C_{NOE} is a harmonic term that constrains the interproton distances r_{ij} to the experimentally determined distances r_{ij}^0. Thus the contrary function C_{NOE} is given by

$$C_{\text{NOE}} = K (r_{ij} - r_{ij}^0)^2 \tag{24}$$

and the force constant K is expressed as

$$K = \frac{kTS}{2(\delta_{ij})^2} \tag{25}$$

where k is the Boltzmann constant, T is the temperature in degrees kelvin, S is a scale factor, and δ_{ij} is the estimated error in the interproton distance. S is usually adjusted so that K has a value of 40–50 kcal mol^{-1}Å^{-2}.

Although the harmonic form of the potential, given above, is commonly used, there are other functional forms that have been employed. One technique is to use a square-well effective potential, and another is to use the combination of a linear and harmonic potential (82). This latter is used such that beyond a certain distance the forces between atoms will become constant. Also the curvature of the potential can be adjusted to suit the range in the interproton distances that are consistent with experiment, and the scale factors for the force constants can be adjusted for uncertainty in the NOE data. Finally, the nonobserved NOEs can be included in the simulation as a constraint on the lower bound of the distances allowed (82). One has to be careful in the choice of force constants, because high values of the force constant may inhibit the flexibility of the molecule and distort the structure. A low value of the force constant, on the other hand, may lead to slow convergence.

Several examples of the applications of these techniques have recently been reported. These include applications to crambin (83), human growth hormone releasing factor (84), aridicin (85), phoraroxin (86), and renin inhibitors (80). The results of these studies show that constrained energy minimization and constrained dynamics may help to determine the 3-D structure and, in some cases, be the mode of choice. Constrained energy minimizations will not provide as many different structures as dynamics, and the convergence depends on the starting structure (80). Constrained molecular dynamics, on the other hand, will cross more energy barriers because of the kinetic energy available in the calculation. Constrained dynamics are less sensitive than constrained minimization to the starting structure for small molecular systems, but for large systems, suitable starting structures might be necessary (80). In general, if the dynamics are run at higher temperature with lower forcing constants, then the averaged structures yield results that satisfy the NOE constraints and provide energetically reasonable structures (80).

E. Use of Simulated Annealing

One of the major problems with all searching techniques including either Monte Carlo methods or molecular dynamics methods is that of adequately searching conformational space. Monte Carlo samples the space well, but at the expense of extremely long simulations. Molecular dynamics is typically carried out at 300°K, and under these conditions, it takes a very long time to overcome even modest energy barriers, so conformational space is sampled slowly. Higher temperatures, however, can distort the geometries such that subsequent energy minimizations result in local minima with relatively high energies, and the system can become unstable (bonds may break and asymmetric centers can invert) (76).

By accounting for these negative aspects of high-temperature dynamics, however, increased thermal energy can significantly increase the efficiency with which conformational space is sampled. This application has recently been applied to the determination of structural families of the biologically active peptide atrial natriuretic factor (ANF). The protocol is to run the dynamics at a high temperature so that there is sufficient thermal energy to cross energy barriers and then to cool down the system and equilibrate it at a lower temperature to allow the system to escape from high-energy minima. The concept is reminiscent of annealing wherein a substance is first heated to a higher temperature and allowed to cool slowly to find more stable (harder, more crystalline) configurations.

A closer examination of the ANF example will illustrate the advantages and caveats of simulated annealing. The active component of ANF is a 28-amino acid fragment having the sequence:

```
SER–LEU–ARG–ARG–SER–SER–CYS–PHE–GLY–GLY–ARG–MET
                              |                 ASP
                              S                 ARG
                              S                 ILE
                              |                 GLY
TYR–ARG–PHE–SER–ASN–CYS–GLY–LEU–GLY–SER–GLN–ALA
```

A disulfide bridge between residues 7 and 23 divides the molecule into three fragments, two tail regions and a closed ring from residues 7–23. Starting with an extended backbone structure and standard side-chain conformations, an initial structure was created by constructing a beta turn at GLY 16 (thereby bringing the cysteine disulfide to within bonding distance). Subsequently this structure was minimized at 300 and 600°K for 20 psec each. Then the dynamics were continued at 900°K for 100 psec with periodic randomization of the atomic velocities (every 5–10 psec). To evaluate the effectiveness of high-temperature dynamics to induce conformational transitions, minimizations were performed every picosecond, and the resulting structures were compared both energetically and structurally.

A useful structural comparison is to optimally superimpose the backbone atoms of the ring domain of each minimized structure onto each of the other 99 minimized structures. The root mean square deviation between these atoms following superposition is a quantitative measure of the three-dimensional similarity of two conformations. Figure 6 displays the RMS superposition values in a 100×100 matrix. Each element of the matrix represents the RMS value converted to a gray scale for the two structures

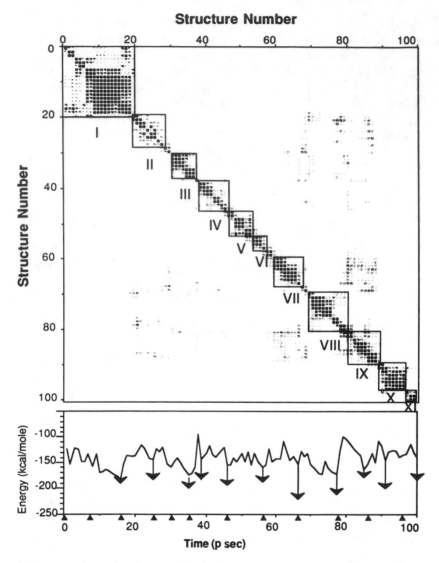

Figure 6 A matrix of RMS deviations between backbone atoms in the ring region of ANF (residues 7–23) for 100 minimized conformations with each other. Every structure is compared with every other structure, giving a matrix of 100 × 100 points. Structures exhibiting small RMS deviations and closeness in time are delineated by boxes, indicating 11 structural families. The bottom graph shows the minimized energy of each picosecond sampled structure for the 100 structures (open circles). The solid structures represent the lowest energy found by annealing.

making up the column and row. The structures are ordered temporally; that is, the first structure is the conformation minimized from the first picosecond, and the last structure from the 100th picosecond. The RMS values are converted to a gray scale such that a low value is darker than a high value. Thus, similar conformations are characterized by dark squares, and dissimilar values by lighter squares.

Several conclusions can be drawn for Figure 6. Elements close to the diagonal are darker than elements off the diagonal. This simply means that structures close in time are also similar in conformation. A striking observation is that these dark regions tend to occur in blocks. This suggests that a conformational state will persist for some time before undergoing a rapid transition to a new conformational state. By studying in detail those structures making up the blocks of the "persistent" conformations, one sees that they can often be classified as a single conformational family with only minor differences compared to the differences between conformational families. By this criterion, 11 distinct conformational families were classified.

One of the risks of performing high-temperature dynamics is that the structures can get stuck in high-energy local minima. The minimized energies of all the structures compared in Figure 6 are plotted below the RMS superposition matrix. The range of these minimized energies suggests that at least some of these energies are unrealistically high. Therefore, to complete the annealing process, representative structures from each family were subjected to additional 300°K dynamics for 20 psec.

Figure 7 shows the RMS superposition matrix and energy profile of minimized conformational states during this annealing phase for three of the 11 families. Convergence is characterized by a leveling out of the energy and by cessation of change in the RMS values (recognized as a dark block in the lower right-hand corner of the matrix). The equilibration procedure resulted in as much as a 60 kcal/mol drop in the energy of the initial structures. In Figure 7, the energy achieved during equilibration for each of the families is depicted by an arrow beneath the energy of the structure used as the initial point. As one can see, the relative ordering of the structures by energy has changed during equilibration. Clearly, one must not draw conclusions from the relative energies of structures sampled from high-temperature dynamics until low-temperature equilibration has been performed. In addition, the following points should be kept in mind when performing high temperature dynamics.

1. Unrealistic conformational perturbations. Peptide bonds at 900°K often undergo trans to cis conversions. To avoid this artifact, a biasing potential can be added to the peptide bond potential. A harmonic force of 5 kcal/radian^2 is adequate to maintain trans peptide bonds. For ANF, this was the only detrimental conformational consequence observed.

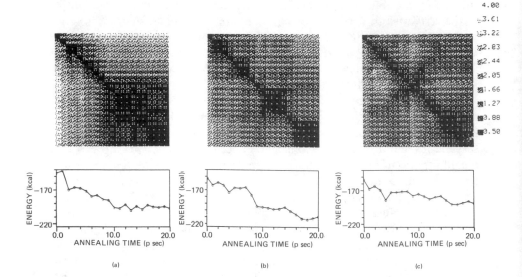

(a)   (b)   (c)

Figure 7 Examples of RMS and energy changes that occur during the annealing process. (a) Annealing of family 10. A rapid drop in energy occurs from −146 kcal/mol to −200 kcal/mol in approximately 10 psec. This is the behavioral pattern in five of the 11 families—a rapid fall in energy followed by a stabilization of energy. (b) Annealing of family 7. This structure falls into four different local minima indicated by the four boxed areas in the RMS plot. (c) Annealing of family 5. The "X" pattern indicates that the molecule has reflected from a barrier and is retracing some of its trajectory. Notice that the 15-psec structure is more similar to the 2-psec structure than to the 8-psec structure, but the energy continues to fall. A longer simulation would probably lead to a different deep minimum.

2. Rerandomization of the atomic velocities every 5–10 psec helps move the system into new areas of conformational space whicg would not normally be explored by dynamics. For ANF, new conformational families were identified within 2–3 psec after each randomization.

3. Minimization of structures during dynamics is only necessary to study the conformational states sampled during the trajectory. When one is only interested in the best-quality minima, expensive minimizations can be avoided until the end of the annealing/equilibration procedure.

In addition to the ANF example, we have also simulated the annealing process for cyclic opiates. Similar results were obtained: annealing found better-quality (lower-energy) structures whether the initial conformations were generated by molecular dynamics or distance geometry. After simulating the annealing process, other strategies can be integrated to use the structures found in the drug design process. The most likely candidate for the bioactive conformations can be sorted from the others by the use of SAR data. Repeating the dynamics for active molecules and introducing backbone constraints will greatly aid the search. Using several of these active analogs, an RMS fitting between appropriate groups on the set of molecules should help identify an appropriate candidate. The next step is to try to reduce the flexibility of the molecule further such that the preferred conformation is that of the receptor-bound conformation. This can be simulated before the chemists actually make the proposed analog. This process will aid in a more advantageous selection of candidates, since prescreening will be done on the computer.

A second approach is to try and enhance the binding of the analog by increasing the enthalpy of binding. In this process the candidate conformer can be substituted by different functional groups, based on the existing SAR data, such that the binding to the receptor is tighter and a greater enthalpy is achieved.

VIII. FUTURE DIRECTIONS

The success of theoretical efforts in application to biological problems depends on many interrelated fields. The accuracy of the potential expressions and the parameters derived from them are central. The general methodology is decades old but has been spurred on by the advent of modern high-speed computers. Older empirical force fields were developed when computer capabilities were more limited, and therefore the energy expressions remained simpler. With today's myriad of supercomputer technologies, it is necessary to take advantage of these new technologies and increase the accuracy of the empirical force fields as well as extend the range of their applications.

Implicit in improving the accuracy of the force field is more rigorous and comprehensive comparison with experimental reality. Lack of adequate experimental checks has been a valid criticism of most all molecular mechanics and dynamics calculations. To be sure, such comparisons are difficult. The differences in scale, both in size (single-protein molecules in a simulation vs. fractions of a mole in a crystal) and time (picosecond simulations of millisecond events), are often insurmountable challenges for even the fastest computers and the most sensitive apparatus. Progress is being made, however. With the recent advent of free-energy calculations (87), direct comparisons with thermodynamic data are now becoming possible (88,89). Not surprisingly, these comparisons are turning up inconsistencies in force fields and parameters (89). Progress in experimental areas has been equally impressive. Site-directed mutagenesis now probes the intricate balances of protein structure and function at a level of resolution rivaling theoretical modeling and is proving to be an uncompromising judge.

Related to the accuracy of the force field is the completeness of the model. Just as limited computer power restricted the sophistication of the force field, calculations of comprehensive macromolecular systems including solvent, counterions, and crystal symmetry have been unthinkable until recently, simply because of the massive computational requirements. Most macromolecular calculations have ignored solvent, not because the effects are assumed to be insignificant, but because no one can afford the computer time to even evaluate their contribution.

Faster computers will not solve all the problems. There are problems such as protein folding which will not succumb to a brute force approach. Better algorithms must be invented for searching the conformational space of large flexible molecules. Some modeling problems cannot be approached with classical physics alone. Quantum effects are essential in any making or breaking of bonds. How to model such quantum effects in tandem with classical calculations is an exciting and potentially fruitful area for the future. The analysis of the voluminous data generated by simulation programs must also be improved. Pattern recognition techniques will become important in recognizing and classifying the literally thousands of structures sampled in a Monte Carlo or molecular dynamics ensemble.

The ultimate though often unstated objective of molecular modeling is to understand the microscopic basis for macroscopic function. Armed with a detailed and accurate model for the molecular interactions that lead to substrate recognition, enzymatic catalysis, and competitive inhibition, the drug designer of tomorrow will be able to test his ideas at the computer terminal and perhaps even accept advice from his analysis programs as to potential likely drug candidates. To achieve this goal, however, will require theoretical, computational, and experimental advances on many fronts.

REFERENCES

1. Scheraga, H. A., Calculations of conformations of polypeptides. *Adv. Phys. Org. Chem. 6*:103 (1968).
2. Ramachandran, G. N., and V. Sasisekharan, Conformation of polypeptides and proteins. *Adv. Protein Chem. 23*:283 (1968).
3. Hermans, J., *Molecular Dynamics and Protein Structures.* University of North Carolina Press, Chapel Hill (1985).
4. Karplus, M., and J. A. McCammon, Dynamics of proteins: Elements and function. *Annu. Rev. Biochem. 52*:263 (1983).
5. McCammon, J. A., and S. C. Harvey, *Dynamics of Proteins and Nucleic Acids.* Cambridge University Press, Cambridge (1987).

6. Mackay, D. H. J., A. J. Cross, and A. T. Hagler, The role of energy minimization in simulation strategies of biomolecular systems. In *Prediction of Protein Structure and the Principles of Protein Conformation*, J. Fasman, ed. (in press).

7. Weiner, S. J., P. A. Kollman, D. A. Case, U. C. Singh, C. Ghio, G. Alagona, S. Profeta, Jr., and P. Weiner, A new force field for molecular mechanical simulation of nucleic acids and proteins. *J. Am. Chem. Soc. 106*:765 (1984).

8. Brooks, B. R., R. E. Bruccoleri, B. D. Olafson, D. J. Stales, S. Swaminathan, and M. Karplus, CHARMM: A program for macromolecular energy, minimization, and dynamics calculations. *J. Comput. Chem. 4*:187 (1983).

9. Biosym Technologies, Inc., Barnes Canyon Road, San Diego, CA 92121.

10. van Gunsteren, W. F., and M. Karplus, Effect of constraints on the dynamics of macromolecules. *Macromolecules 15*:1528 (1982).

11. Maple, J. R., U. Dinur, and A. T. Hagler, Derivation of force fields for molecular mechanics and dynamics from ab initio energy surfaces. *Proc. Natl. Acad. Sci. USA* (1988) (in press).

12. Hirschfelder, J. O., Nature of intermolecular forces. *Adv. Chem. Phys. 12* (1968).

13. Buckingham, A. D., and B. D. Utting, Intermolecular forces. *Annu. Rev. Phys. Chem. 21*:287 (1970).

14. Claverie, P., Elaboration of approximate formulas for the interactions between large molecules: Application in organic chemistry. In *Intermolecular Interactions*, B. Pullman, Wiley Interscience, New York, p. 69 (1981).

15. Dauber, P., and A. T. Hagler, Crystal packing, hydrogen bonding, and the effect of crystal forces on molecular conformation. *Accts. Chem. Res. 13*:105 (1980).

16. London, F., Properties and applications of molecular forces. *Z. Physik Chem. B11*:222 (1930).

17. London, F., The general theory of molecular forces. *Trans. Faraday Soc. 33*:8 (1937).

18. Slater, J. C., and J. G. Kirkwood, Van der Waals forces in gases. *Phys. Rev. 37*:682 (1931).

19. Brooks, C. L., III, and M. Karplus, Deformable stochastic boundaries in molecular dynamics. *J. Chem. Phys. 79*:6312 (1983).

20. Wipff, G., A. Dearing, P. Weiner, J. Blaney, and P. Kollman, Molecular mechanics of enzyme-substrate interactions: The interaction of L- and D-N-acetyl tryptophanamide with α-chymotrypsin, *J. Am. Chem. Soc. 105*:997 (1983).

21. Lennard-Jones, J. E., Forces between atoms and ions. *Proc. Roy. Soc. London A106*:463 (1924).

22. Ermer, O., Calculation of molecular properties using force fields. Applications in organic chemistry. *Struct. Bonding (Berlin) 27*:161 (1976).

23. Moelwyn-Hughes, E. A., *Physical Chemistry*. Pergamon Press, New York (1957).

24. Hirschfelder, J. O., C. F. Curtiss, and R. B. Bird, *Molecular Theory of Gases and Liquids*. Wiley, New York, (1954).

25. Smyth, C. P., *Dielectric Behavior and Structure*. McGraw Hill, New York (1955).

26. Moelwyn-Hughes, E. A., *Physical Chemistry*, Revised ed. Pergamon Press, Oxford, pp. 308, 445 (1964).

27. Arridge, R. G. C., and C. G. Cannon, Calculations of the COHN dipole contribution to lattice energies of amides, polyamides, and polypeptides. *Proc. Roy. Soc. 278*:106 (1964).

28. Hagler, A. T., E. Huler, and S. Lifson, Energy functions for peptides and proteins. I. Derivation of a consistent force field including the hydrogen bond from amide crystals, *J. Am. Chem. Soc. 96*:5319 (1974).

29. Bolis, G., E. Clementi, M. Ragazzi, D. Salvedera, and D. R. Ferro, Preliminary attempt to follow the enthalpy of enzymatic reaction by ab initio computations: Catalytic action of papain, *J. Quant. Chem. 14*:815 (1979).

30. Pincus, M., A. W. Burgess, and H. A. Scheraga, Conformational energy calculations of enzyme-substrate complexes of lysozyme. I. Energy minimization of monosaccharide and oligosaccharide inhibitors and substrates of lysozome. *Biopolymers 15*:2485 (1976).

31. Warwicker, J., Continuum dielectric modeling of the protein-solvent system, and calculation of the long-range electrostatic field of the enzyme phosphoglycerate mutase. *J. Theor. Biol. 121*:199 (1986).

32. Gilson, M. K., A. Rashin, R. Fine, and B. Honig, Secondary structure of the alpha-amylase polypeptide inhibitor tendamistat from streptomyces tendae determined in solution by proton nuclear magnetic resonance. *J. Mol. Biol. 183*:503 (1985).

33. Rees, D. C., Experimental determination of the effective dielectric constant of proteins. *J. Mol. Biol. 141*:323 (1980).

34. Mulliken, R. S., Electronic population analysis on LCAO-MO [linear combination of atomic orbital-molecular orbital] molecular wave functions. *J. Chem. Phys. 23*:1833 (1955).

35. Pople, J., and D. Beveridge, *Approximate Molecular Orbital Theory*. McGraw-Hill, New York (1978).

36. Dewar, M. J. S., and W. Thiel, Ground states of molecules. 38. The MNDO method approximations and parameters. *J. Am. Chem. Soc. 99*:4899 (1977).

37. Del Re, G., A simple MO-LCAO method for the calculation of charge distributions in saturated organic molecules. *J. Chem. Soc. 4031* (1958).

38. Gasteiger, J., and M. Marsili, Iterative partial equalization of orbital electronegativity—A rapid access to atomic charges. *Tetrahedron 36*:3219 (1980).

39. Scrocco, E., and J. Tomasi, Electronic molecular structure, reactivity, and intermolecular forces: An heuristic interpretation by means of electrostatic molecular potentials. *J. Adv. Quant. Chem. 11*:115 (1978).

40. Politzer, P., The role of electrostatic potential in chemistry. In *Chemical Applications of Atomic and Molecular Electrostatic Potentials*, P. Politzer and D. G. Truhlar, eds. Plenum Press, New York, p. 1 (1981).

41. Cox, S. R., and D. E. Williams, Representations of the molecular electrostatic potential by a net atomic charge model. *J. Comput. Chem. 2*:304 (1981).

42. Singh, U. C., and P. A. Kollman, Energy component analysis calculations on neutral atom base interactions. *J. Comput. Chem. 5*:129 (1984).

43. Momany, F. A., Determination of partial atomic charges from ab initio molecular electrostatic potentials. Applications to formamide, methanol, and formic acid. *J. Phys. Chem. 82*:592 (1978).

44. Pauling, L., *The Natural of the Chemical Bond*, 3rd ed. Cornell University Press, Ithaca, NY, p. 450 (1960).

45. Pimentel, G. C., and A. D. McCellan, Hydrogen bonding. *Annu. Rev. Phys. Chem. 22*:347 (1971).

46. Bratoz, S., Electronic theories of hydrogen bonding. *Adv. Quant. Chem. 3*:209 (1967).

47. Poland, D., and H. A. Scheraga, Energy parameters in polypeptides. I. Charge distributions and the hydrogen bond. *Biochemistry 6*:3791 (1967).

48. McGuire, R. F., F. A. Momany, and H. A. Scheraga, Energy parameters in polypeptides. V. Empirical hydrogen bond potential function based on molecular orbital calculations. *J. Phys. Chem. 76*:375 (1972).

49. Hagler, A. T., E. Huler, and S. Lifson, Energy functions for peptides and proteins. I. Derivation of a consistent force field including the hydrogen bond from amide crystals. *J. Am. Chem. Soc. 96*:5319 (1974).

50. Hagler, A. T., and S. Lifson, Energy functions for peptides and proteins. II. The amide hydrogen bond and calculations of amide crystal properties. *J. Am. Chem. Soc. 96*:5327 (1974).

51. Hagler, A. T., and A. Lapiccirella, Spatial electron distribution and population analysis of amides, carboxylic acid, and peptides, and their relation to empirical potential functions. *Biopolymers 15*:1167 (1976).

52. Kollman, P., and L. C. Allen, The nature of the hydrogen bond. Dimers involving electronegative atoms of the first row. *J. Am. Chem. Soc. 93*:4991 (1971).

53. Del Bene, J., Molecular orbital theory of the hydrogen bond. Dimers of hydrogen bonded alkanol-formaldehyde. *J. Chem. Phys. 58*:3139 (1973).

54. Port, G. N., and A. Pullman, Quantum mechanical studies of environmental effects on biomolecules. II. Hydration sites in purines and pyrimidines. *FEBS. Lett. 31*:70 (1970).

55. Hagler, A. T., and L. Leiserowitz. On the amide hydrogen bond and the anomalous packing of adizamide. *J. Am. Chem. Soc. 100*:5879 (1978).

56. Fletcher, R., *Practical Methods of Optimization, Unconstrained Optimization*, Vol. 1. Wiley, New York (1980).

57. Fletcher, R., and C. M. Reeves, Function minimization by conjugate gradients. *Comput. J. 7*:149 (1964).

58. Fletcher, R., and M. J. D. Powell, A rapidly convergent descent method for minimization. *Comput. J. 6*:163 (1963).

59. Metropolis, N., A. W. Rosenbluth, M. N. Rosenbluth, A. Teller, and E. Teller, Equation of state calculation by fast computing. *J. Chem. Phys. 21*:1087 (1953).

60. Valleau, J. P., and G. M. Torrie, A guide to Monte Carlo for statistical mechanics. 1. Highways. In *Statistical Mechanics*, Part A, B. Berne, ed. Plenum Press. New York, p. 169 (1977).

61. Hagler, A. T., and J. Moult, Computer simulation of the solvent structure around biological macromolecules. *Nature (London) 272*:222 (1978).

62. Hagler, A. T., J. Moult, and D. Osguthorpe, Monte Carlo simulation of the solvent structure in crystals of a hydrated cyclic peptide. *Biopolymers 19*:395 (1980).

63. Warvari, H. E., W. K. Knaell, and R. Scott, Monte Carlo calculation on polypeptide chains. *J. Phys. Chem. 57*:1161 (1972).

64. Paine, G. H., and H. A. Scheraga, Prediction of the native conformation of a polypeptide by a statistical mechanical procedure. III. Probable and average conformations of enkephalin. *Biopolymers 26*:1125 (1987).

65. Premilat, S., and B. Maigret, Statistical molecular models for angiotensin II and enkephalin related to NMR coupling constants. *J. Phys. Chem. 293*:1980 (1984).

66. LeClerc, M., S. Premilat, and A. Englert, Nonradiative energy transfer in oligopeptide chains generated by a Monte Carlo method including long-range interactions. *Biopolymers 17*:2459 (1978).

67. Demonte, J. P., R. Guillard, and A. Englert, Theoretical conformational analysis of enkephalin analogs related to fluorescence and NMR measurements in aqeuous solution. *Int. J. Pept. Protein Res. 18*:478 (1981).

68. Verlet, L., Computer experiments on classical fluids. I. Thermodynamical properties of Lennard-Jones molecules. *Phys. Rev. 159*:98 (1967).

69. Gear, C. W. *Numerical Initial Value Problems in Ordinary Differential Equations.* Prentice-Hall, Englewood Cliffs, NJ (1980).

70. McCammon, J. A., and M. Karplus, Simulation of protein dynamics. *Annu. Rev. Phys. Chem. 31*:29 (1980).

71. van Gunsteren, W. F., and H. J. C. Berendsen, Algorithms for macromolecular dynamics and constraint dynamics. *Mol. Phys. 34*:1311 (1977).

72. van Gunsteren, W. F., and M. Karplus, A method for constrained energy minimization of macromolecules. *J. Comput. Chem. 1*:266 (1980).

73. McCammon, J. A., P. G. Wolynes, and M. Karplus, Picosecond dynamics of tyrosine side chains in proteins. *Biochemistry 18*:927 (1979).

74. Hagler, A. T., P. S. Stern, R. Sharon, J. M. Becker, and F. Naider, Computer simulation of the conformational properties of oligopeptides. Comparison of theoretical methods and analysis of experimental results. *J. Am. Chem. Soc. 101*:6842 (1979).

75. Hagler, A. T., D. J. Osguthorpe, P. Dauber-Osguthorpe, and J. C. Hempel, Dynamics and conformational energetics of a peptide hormone: Vasopressin. *Science 227*:1309 (1985).

76. Rodgers, J., D. H. J. Mackay, W. Ghoul, and A. T. Hagler, Molecular dynamics of atrial natriuretic factor (ANF) (in preparation).

77. Struthers, R. S., A. T. Hagler, and J. Rivier, Design of peptide analogs: Theoretical simulation of conformation, energetics, and dynamics. In *Conformationally Directed Drug Design: Peptides and Nucleic Acids as Templates or Targets*, J. A. Vida and M. Gordon, eds. American Chemical Society, Washington, DC, p. 239 (1984).

78. Clore, G. M., A. T. Brunner, M. Karplus, and A. M. Gronenborn, Application of molecular dynamics with interproton distance constraints to three-dimensional protein structure determination. *J. Mol. Biol. 191*:523 (1986).

79. Levy, R. M., R. P. Sheridan, I. W. Keepers, G. S. Dubey, S. Swaminathan, and M. Karplus, Molecular dynamics of myoglobin at 298°K. Results from a 300-ps computer simulation. *Biophys. J. 48*:509 (1985).

80. Fesik, S. W., G. Bolis, H. Sham, and E. T. Olejniczak, Structural refinement of a cyclic peptide from two-dimensional NMR data and molecular modeling. *Biochemistry 26*:1851 (1987).

81. Havel, T. F., I. D. Kuntz, and G. Crippen, The theory and practice of distance geometry. *Bull. Math. Biophys. 95*:665 (1983).

82. de Vlieg, J., R. Boelens, R. M. Scheek, R. Kaptein, and W. F. van Gunsteren, Restrained molecular dynamics procedures for protein tertiary structure determination from NMR data: A lac repressor headpiece structure based on information on J-coupling and from presence or abscence of NOE's. *Isr. J. Chem. 27*:181 (1986).

83. Brunger, A. T., G. M. Clore, A. M. Gronenborg, and M. Karplus, Three-dimensional structure of proteins determined by molecular dynamics with interproton distance restraints. Application to Crambin. *Proc. Natl. Acad. Sci. USA 83*:3801 (1986).

84. Brunger, A. T., G. M. Clore, A. M. Gronenborg, and M. Karplus, Solution conformations of human growth hormone-releasing factor: Comparison of the restrained molecular dynamic and distance geometry methods for a system without long-range distance data. *Prot. Eng. 1*:399 (1987).

85. Jeffs, P. W., L. Muller, C. Debrosse, S. L. Heald, and R. Fisher, The structure of Aridicin A. An integrated approach employing 2D NMR, energy minimization and distance constraints. *J. Am. Chem. Soc. 108*:3063 (1986).

86. Clore, G. M., D. K. Sukumaran, M. Nilgos, and A. M. Gronenborg, Three-dimensional structure of phoratoxin in solution: Combined use of nuclear magnetic resonance, distance geometry, and restrained molecular dynamics. *Biochemistry 26*:1732 (1987).

87. Mezei, M., and D. L. Beveridge, Free energy simulations. *Ann. NY Acad. Sci. 482*:1 (1986).

88. Jorgensen, W. L., and C. Ravimohan, Monte Carlo simulation of differences in free energies of hydration. *J. Chem. Phys. 83*:3050 (1985).

89. Mezei, M., The finite difference thermodynamic integration, tested on calculating the hydration free energy difference between acetone and dimethylamine in water. *J. Chem. Phys. 86*:7984 (1987).

4

X-Ray Crystallography and Drug Design

Donald J. Abraham
Medical College of Virginia, Virginia Commonwealth University,
Richmond, Virginia

I. INTRODUCTION

The most foolproof structure elucidation of complex molecules comes from an x-ray crystallographic investigation. It is the only technique at present that will give the complete three-dimensional structure in detail at high resolution including bond distance, angles, stereochemistry, and absolute configuration. The use of such a powerful technique for drug design was recognized over a decade ago (1).

To arrive at an understanding about the role of x-ray crystallography in rational drug design, we review past, current, and new methodologies involved in the determination of complex structures by x-ray methods. Small- and large-molecule crystallography contributions are presented. Examples of research problems that detail the elucidation of the mechanism of action of known drugs at the molecular level and studies aimed at the design of new drugs are illustrated. Finally, hemoglobin is discussed as a model drug receptor.

II. METHODOLOGY

A. Theory

Crystals are made up of repeating units of molecular structure. This order gives rise to a periodicity that can be analyzed at the atomic level with the appropriate wave length of radiation. X-ray radiation is ideal, since the wavelengths obtainable are of the order of 0.75 Å, which is about one-half the distance of an aliphatic carbon-carbon bond.

A crystal placed in an x-ray beam will diffract according to Bragg's law:

$$n\lambda = 2d \sin \theta$$

where n is the order of the diffraction, λ the wavelength of the radiation, d the distance between a given family of planes, and θ the angle of the diffraction. A diffracted beam will only appear when this equation is satisfied so that the angle between the incident beam and the plane normal satisfies a set of discrete values.

A lattice of the diffraction showing a periodicity will emerge if a special precession camera recording device is employed. Such a pattern is shown in Figure 1. Each diffraction intensity arises from a single solution of the Bragg equation and can be numbered in three dimensions to give a unique identification. These identification numbers are known as Miller indices (h, k, l) for each reflection (diffraction) and are easy to label in the two-dimensional lattice which was recorded with $k = 0$ (Fig. 1a). The first spot in the vertical direction from the film's center is labeled 100, and the first spot in

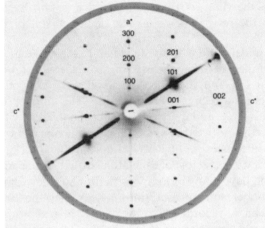

(a)

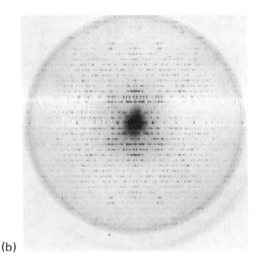

(b)

Figure 1 (a) Diffraction pattern from a crystal of a small-molecule natural product with MW 222. The reflections (diffraction spots) are numbered along both axes to illustrate the method of assigning Miller indices. (b) Diffraction pattern for carbomonoxy hemoglobin with MW 64,500. Notice the symmetry around the axes, unlike that observed in Figure 1a. The symmetry around the axes and certain absent reflections determine the space group (geometrical packing of molecules in the crystal). There are only 230 geometrical ways (space groups) that molecules can pack to form three-dimensional crystals.

the horizontal direction to the right, 001, etc. This lattice is known as a reciprocal lattice, and it is the reciprocal or inverse of the crystal or real lattice.

One important point to understand without delving into the mathematics is that the greater the distance between the spacings on the film (d), the smaller the size of the real cell and therefore the smaller the size of the molecule contained; i.e., there is a reciprocal relationship. The unit cell that contains a protein molecule is large, and therefore the spots on the film will be close together (see Fig. 1b). Also notice that some spots on the film are weak and some are strong. The differences in intensity arise from the addition or subtraction of the diffraction wave (vector) of each atom at that Bragg angle. A protein or virus crystal will have many more spots on the film than a small-molecule crystal exposed under similar conditions. The higher the Bragg angle, the more spots that can be recorded, and the higher the resolution of the structure. At the maximum Bragg angle of 90°, sin θ is 1.0, and $\lambda = 2d$. Therefore, with Cu radiation, $\lambda = 1.54$ Å, the maximum resolution obtained is $1.54/2 = 0.77$ Å. At this resolution, atoms are completely resolved.

It is no simple task to appreciate or understand the ideas presented above if one has not been exposed previously to x-ray diffraction theory. The take-home lesson, however, is that one does not have to master the details of crystallographic analysis to use the information (coordinates of structures of interest) for drug design purposes. The steps that one goes through to solve a crystal structure are enumerated below with the hope of providing non-crystallographers with an overview of the process.

B. Crystallization

Linus Pauling once entitled one of his lectures "The Importance of Being Crystalline" (2). Crystallization is a major bottleneck hindering the advance of structural molecular biology, and structural molecular biology is the foundation for rational drug design based on the nature of the receptor. It is ironic that such quantitative and precise analyses as found in crystallography are entirely dependent on the far less sophisticated art of growing crystals.

Although discovering crystallization conditions for a biological molecule can be a tedious task, relatively unexperienced workers have succeeded once the conditions have been worked out. The details in setting up crystal preparations can be obtained from the literature cited for individual studies in this chapter or from general treatises on crystallization techniques (3,4). Some of the most successful methods to crystallize macromolecules include vapor diffusion in cavities on slides or via hanging drops; precipitation from salt solutions or from mixtures of organic agents that are miscible with buffers; microdialysis; and layering organic liquids not miscible with buffers containing the macromolecule.

The vapor phase diffusion method is detailed here, since it could help medicinal and organic chemists who wish to prepare single crystals for x-ray analysis. This method, in our hands, has achieved by far the greatest success, even with a milligram or less of material. In the vapor phase method, the compound to be crystallized is dissolved in a small amount of solvent in a tube or small flask (Fig. 2a). This tube is placed inside a larger tube containing a second solvent that is miscible with the first solvent but that normally precipitates the compound if added dropwise. The larger, outer tube is sealed, and the vapors are left to mix in a quiet place. Typical solvent systems for organic compounds include ethanol-ether and ethyl acetate-petroleum ether. Crystals should appear within a few days. Protein crystallographers use this same technique but in a modified manner. For example, we have crystallized

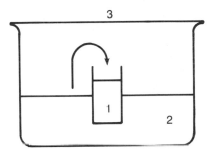

(a)

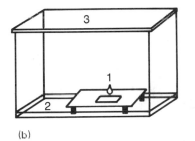

(b)

Figure 2 (a) Vapor phase setup for growing single crystals suitable for x-ray diffraction: (1) vial with MeOH and compound; (2) vial with ether; (3) capped top. This top can be fashioned from aluminum foil which is covered with a plastic material such as parafilm and secured to the outside chamber with a rubber band. (b) Vapor phase setup used for macromolecules: (1) 40-λ drop with 0.5 mg t-RNA; (2) 12% isopropanol solution; (3) Capped top. In this case, the top is Plexiglas which is sealed against a Pyrex dish with grease and putty.

0.4 mg or less of tRNA^{Phe} in 40-μl drops of buffer in small cavities on microscope slides at 4°C. The slides are propped up off the bottom of the sandwich box, and 10% isopropanol as a precipitating agent is added to the bottom of a sandwich box (Fig. 2b). Good crystals, 1 mm long, appeared in a few days to 3 weeks (5).

The hanging drop method (a modification of the vapor phase diffusion method) is suited for screening a variety of conditions when only small amounts of material are available. A microdroplet as small as 5 μl can be inverted on a microscope coverslip over a well containing about 1 ml of the precipitating solution. Siliconized coverslips are necessary to prevent spreading of the drops. Airtight sealing of the coverslip over the well is usually accomplished with silicon grease. Special tissue culture trays with level ground rims are ideal for this methodology.*

C. Data Collection

Once good single crystals of a molecule of biological interest are in hand, they must be mounted in glass capillaries with a small amount of solvent near the crystal, the sealed capillary placed in front of the x-ray source, and the intensities of the diffraction spots measured. The longer a crystal of a biological molecule is immersed in the x-ray beam, the greater the crystal damage and diffraction pattern deterioration. The intensities can be measured with a diffractometer or recorded on film and measured with an optical film scanner. The advent of modern data collection systems, such as the area detector,† has enabled the solution of the complex structures described above in very short time frames. The accuracy of the structure determination depends on the quality of the crystal diffraction and the accuracy of the measurement of the intensities. The higher the angle observed for diffraction intensities, the higher the resolution of the structure determination. Rotating anodes as a source for high-intensity x-ray beams have increased the resolution of the data and decreased the time the crystal needs to be exposed. Even higher-powered sources of energy such as that at the Cornell High Energy Synchrotron Source (CHESS) can produce a full set of virus data in 600 min of exposure time on crystals not suitable for analysis with weaker sources (6). The data collection system used at the University of Pittsburgh is shown in Figure 3.

---

*See ref. 132 for information about a new crystallization plate sponsored by the American Crystallographic Association (ACA) and an automated Protein Crystallization system called Apocalypse that uses the ACA crystalplate.

†An area detector records the intensities of a large number of diffraction spots simultaneously.

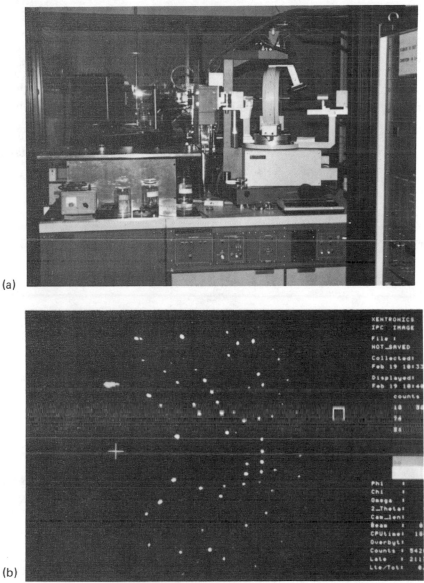

(a)

(b)

Figure 3 (a) The area detector-diffractometer system. The diffractometer (white) is on the right; the area detector (black) is on the left. The rotating anode is in the center under the light. The generator is housed under the table. The computer and other peripherals necessary for the data collection are not shown. (b) A still diffraction pattern of ricin or as recorded by our Nicolet X-100A area detector. The crystal-to-detector distance is 14 cm. The reflection shown in the box has a *d*-spacing of 2.8 Å. The cross marks the position of the direct beam with a detector swing angle of 15° (Courtesy of Dr. B. C. Wang, University of Pittsburgh.)

D.   The Phase Problem

The most crucial operation in accurately imaging a molecule from x-ray diffraction data involves the inclusion of the correct *phase angles* with the diffraction intensities (amplitudes) in a Fourier transform. The phase angle of every diffraction intensity must be known in relation to a common origin so that the resulting transform will produce an accurate electron density map of the molecule (see Fig. 4). In the case of large macromolecules such as proteins, the backbone of the protein is first traced in the map, and then the side chains

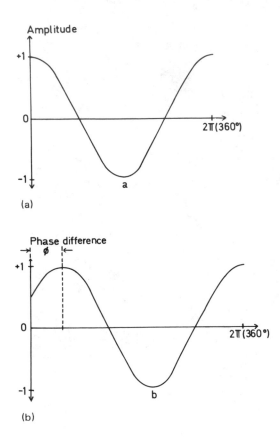

Figure 4   (a) This cosine curve represents a diffraction wave with an intensity (amplitude) of +1 and a phase of zero. (b) This second curve represents a second diffraction wave with the same intensity as in Figure 4a but differs in phase (φ) by a fraction of 2π. The phase angles for all reflections are determined to obtain the correct three-dimensional structure.

are fitted. The stereochemistry of the side chains in the fitting process is a powerful constraint in assuring that the electron density derived from the phases is correct.

The solution of the phase problem for proteins was discovered by Perutz in 1953 (7) using the multiple isomorphous heavy-atom derivative method, which is still the primary technique used to solve large-molecule structures. Other methods for producing accurate phases with one heavy-atom derivative include anomalous scattering (8) and solvent flattening (9). If a protein or virus has a similar shape to one whose structure is already known, a molecular replacement method can be used to solve the structure of the unknown macromolecule (10).

Direct methods for the solution of the phase problem, pioneered by Karle and Hauptmann (11,12), have made crystallography the premier method for structure elucidation of small molecules. Direct methods are usually successful for molecules under MW 1000. The upper end of this scale ($\sim$700–1500 MW and above) can require the use of a heavy atom in combination with direct methods. One of the most notable small-molecule structures, accomplished over a decade ago (MW $\sim$2000) using this latter technique, was the solution of an actinomycin-deoxyguanosine complex by Sobell and co-workers (13). In many cases it can be just as quick (but more expensive), if even tiny single crystals are available, to get an x-ray structure of a small organic molecule as it is to send it for a carbon hydrogen analysis.

On the other end of the size scale, the nucleosome core particles (14) have required heavy-metal clusters to deduce the phases. Five heavy-atom derivatives were used in the solution of the crystal structure of the photosynthetic reaction center (15). In summary, this step had not posed serious problems for structural analysis of the most complex molecules in the majority of cases.

E. Computing

Another major factor for the proliferation of solved crystal structures can be directly linked to advances in computing. The latest developments in rapid computing in crystallography arise from the use of supercomputers for large-scale data processing such as with viruses and the refinement of macromolecular structures. To give a rough idea concerning the importance of computers in the revolution that occurred in the output of x-ray structures, consider the following test of the difference between humans and computers. In 1974, it required about 3 days with a hand calculator (and many mistakes) to calculate one axial Fourier peak (one grid point) of a natural product, MW 222 (16). The top-line computer of that day took 14 sec to calculate the whole axis row of 50 grid points. If one were to attempt to calculate *one* virus electron density map (using a hand calculator, at 3-Å resolution, and at the same speed as the natural product calculation, which is not actually possible), it would require 156 million years.*

F. Resolution and Refinement

The value of crystallography to those interested in drug design lies in the resolution and accuracy of the coordinates obtained from the x-ray structure. The greater the Bragg angle of diffraction, the higher the resolution of the electron density map, and the more detail that can be seen. For small molecules that diffract well, the highest resolution attainable is one-half the wavelength of the x-ray source. For Cu-produced x-ray radiation, the maximum resolution is 0.77 Å. Most molecules under 1000 MW can be imaged at or near this resolution; the electron density around each atom including hydrogens is distinct, so atomic resolution is obtained. Protein and nucleic acid crystals contain large amounts of water and do not usually diffract to better than 1.5 Å. Most of the macromolecule structures are solved at 2- to 3-Å resolution. Hydrogen atom positions are not determined at the resolution obtained for macromolecules. A 5- or 6-Å map of a protein will usually produce the shape of the molecule; a 3-Å map permits the placement of most if not all of the backbone and side chains readily.

To obtain the highest level of assurance of the position of the atoms, one must refine the structure. For small molecules including hydrogen atoms, the observed and calculated values for the intensities and phases (structure

---

*To calculate one electron density of the whole natural product by hand, one would have about 7800 grid points and at 271 hr per nonaxial grid point and 2000 reflections, it would take about 2.11×10^6 hr or 241 years. The vast majority of grid points in a lattice are nonaxial. Axial grid points are calculated in a much shorter time than required for nonaxial grid points. To calculate, by hand, one electron density map of the mengo virus with 19.8 million grid points for a 300-Å sphere with 509,915 unique reflections (3 Å) and 69,000 hr per grid point would require 1.37×10^{12} hr or 156 million years.

	Natural product	Virus
Space group	P2$_1$/c	P2$_1$2$_1$2$_1$
Unit cell	8,16,8 Å	220,427,211 Å
Unique cell	1/2a,b,1/2c	1/2a,1/2b,1/2c
Grid points	$12 \times 50 \times 13 = 7800$	$220 \times 427 \times 211 = 1.98 \times 10^7$
Total data (reflections)	2000	509,915
Time/axial reflection by hand	44 sec	44 sec
Time/nonaxial reflection by hand	8 min	8 min
Summation for fourier	4 hr	1×10^3 hr
Resolution	0.77 Å	3.0 Å

factors) for all the measured data usually agree to 6% or less: this agreement percentage is known as the R factor. To get this good an agreement, a least-squares refinement procedure is used.

For protein structures, the values of R range from 30% for low-resolution structures to 15% or better for very high resolution structures. The refinement of each atom independently in protein structures by nonlinear least squares is too large a problem for even the fastest computers. Alternate methods of refinement have been developed by Hendrickson and Konnert (17,18) utilizing a "constrained" or "restrained" least-squares procedure. For example, penicillopepsin, an aspartyl protease, has been refined by restrained-parameter least squares to an R factor of 13.6% at 1.8 Å resolution (19).

G. Data Bases

There are two x-ray crystallographic data bases that are being used with increasing frequency by scientists in allied fields, especially those interested in drug design. These data bases contain molecular coordinates and other crystallographic information that can be read directly into the most popular graphics software packages.

The Cambridge Structural Database (CSD) was initiated by Olga Kennard, University Chemical Laboratories, Cambridge University, U.K.* The CSD contains the coordinates for some 2 million atoms with 50% of this material published since 1980. The January 1987 version contains 56,642 crystal structures. The importance of this data base in generating new leads for drug design was highlighted during a 1-day workshop at the recent meeting of the Drug Information Association (20). I. D. Kuntz described a search of the CDS to discover all molecules having a shape complementary to a known binding site. Examination of the first 3000 entries produced 150 templates for that site, which could be used as a starting point for drug design.

The Brookhaven Protein Data Bank is the depository for macromolecular crystal structures and contains the coordinates of protein and nucleic acid structures. There are at present 293 structures deposited.† Both data bases provide coordinates, connectivity features, and references.

---

*To get the CSD in the United States, contact Dr. William L. Duax, Medical Foundation of Buffalo, Inc., 73 High St., Buffalo, NY 14203-1196.
†To get information, except in Australia and Japan, contact the Protein Data Bank, Chemistry Department, Brookhaven National Laboratory, Upton, NY 11973 (BITNET address: ABOLA@BNLDAG).

III. EXAMPLES OF CRYSTALLOGRAPHIC STUDIES

The role of X-ray crystallography in medicinal chemistry and drug design is divided into five categories. These include studies that (1) are aimed at the structure elucidation of complex biological molecules that have interesting pharmacological properties; (2) compare the conformational aspects of x-ray structures with solution and protein-bound states; (3) map out the structure of the receptor or binding site; (4) attempt to define the molecular mechanism of action of drugs; and (5) are focused primarily on the design of new agents by discovering general characteristics and rules related to drug binding.

Crystallographic studies of both small and large molecules contribute to the success of the approaches. A number of examples will be cited to illustrate these categories. Many of the examples in categories 4 and 5 overlap, combining mechanism of action and drug design investigations.

A. Use of Small-Molecule Crystallography to Determine the Structure of Biologically Active Molecules

The literature is so extensive in this area that no examples are covered. The *Journal of the American Chemical Society*, the *Journal of Natural Products* (Lloydia), *Acta Crystallographica*, and the *Journal of Medical Chemistry* routinely report x-ray structures of important biologically active small molecules. As mentioned at the beginning of the chapter, x-ray analysis is the premier method for structure elucidation of complex molecules. It has been our experience to initiate three separate x-ray analyses on complex natural products in which possible structures based on NMR, mass spectra, IR, and UV had to be reassigned from the x-ray-produced structure (1). This was before the recent advances in spectroscopy, for example, the advent of two-dimensional NMR, and obviously does not imply that one should abandon spectral techniques in favor of an x-ray analysis. In the majority of cases, the most productive use of x-ray crystallography for complex small molecules is to solve one structure by x-ray analysis and solve the derivatives and/or analogs of this class using mass spectrometry, NMR, etc.

B. Conformational Analysis of Drug Molecules

Equating x-ray crystallographic structures with the minimum energy conformation of small molecules in solution has been under scrutiny since the first x-ray structures of organic or biological molecules of interest were published. Several reasons for a great lack of assurance that solid-state and solution structures are equivalent can be suggested. On the other hand, several studies have found the solid-state and solution state conformational structures to be identical or similar (see below). We can not solve this debate here. We can, however, demonstrate the use of x-ray-determined conformations in aiding drug design efforts and in postulating drug interactions with receptors or macromolecules. We must also keep in mind the advances in NMR that permit the comparison of accurate solution state structures with the solid state.

Is there a difference between the conformation a drug crystallizes in, the conformation of the drug in solution, and the conformation of the drug at the receptor? The molecules could have the same conformation in all three states, differ in each state, or be alike in two and not in the other. This makes correlations of theoretical predictions of interactions with receptors using x-ray analysis a difficult one. Answers to questions concerning the conformation in different states are starting to emerge. For example, the three-dimensional structure of a complex of an antibody with influenza virus neuraminidase (MW 60,000) has been solved by Colman and co-workers (16). The structure of the complex is inconsistent with the old idea of a rigid lock-and-key fit for the antigen-antibody binding. The antibody and possibly the antigen conformations are reshaped upon binding.

On the other hand, Todd Wipke recently reported (20) that the Cambridge Structural Database could be used as the initial starting conformations for energy refinement, and, in fact, if the desired molecule was not available in the data bank, it was preferable to assemble fragments of several structures together. The conformations of the patched molecules in many cases were quite close to those obtained via energy calculations (20,21). Earlier studies by Lotter et al. comparing solution structures by NMR with crystal structures indicated no major differences (22,23). Duax and colleagues have reported that over 800 x-ray crystal structure determinations (24,25) have provided accurate data on steroid conformation, geometry, and flexibility of low-energy forms, the existence of conformational isomers, and the influence of specific substituents on conformation and conformational isomerism (26).

Other studies have indicated that x-ray structure conformations of small molecules can contribute to the understanding of drug binding to macromolecules. For example, the molecular structures of the two antibiotics formycin and 2-methyl formycin (Fig. 5) were known prior to x-ray analysis. Of these two compounds, 2-methyl formycin (2MF) is more active than formycin (F), and this activity difference has been attributed to the fact that adenosine deaminase (AD) requires an anticonformation of the nucleoside base to deaminate the antibiotic. It was proposed that the presence of the 2-methyl group in 2MF causes the molecule to reside exclusively in the *syn* form (because of steric hindrance). 2MF is more active than F and cannot be detoxified as readily as F by deamination. It was proposed that the *syn* form cannot be deaminated by AD as readily as F and accounts for the difference in activity. X-ray analyses confirmed these conclusions, showing F to be between the classical *syn* and anticonformations (high-anti) (27) and 2MF to be in the *syn* form (28).

Final answers on conformational analysis and drug interaction in most instances will not be revealed until the detailed nature of the receptors is known. In at least two cases in our work, we have been able to compare the small-molecule crystal structure conformation of a drug with the conformation of the drug bound to hemoglobin (see Fig. 6). The small-molecule structure of the diuretic agent ethacrynic acid (ECA) is almost identical to the conformation of ECA found bound to Cys 93β on hemoglobin (Hb); the crystal conformation of the antilipidemic drug bezafibrate (BZF) is only altered slightly in making over 40 contacts in the central water cavity of Hb

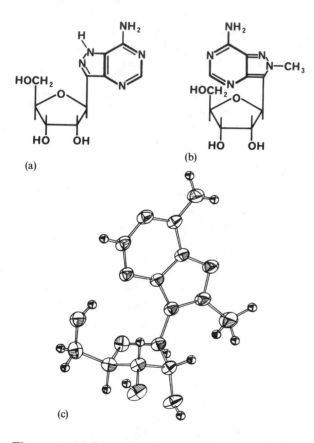

(a)

(b)

(c)

Figure 5 (a) Formycin. (b) 2-Methylformycin. (c) A computer plot of 2-methylformycin showing the thermal vibration ellipsoids, which indicate the movement of various atoms in the structure (28).

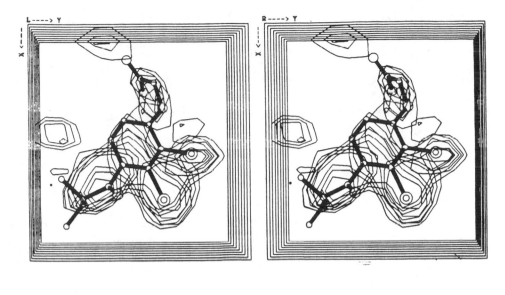

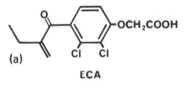

(a)

ECA

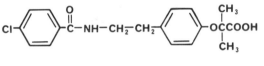

BZF

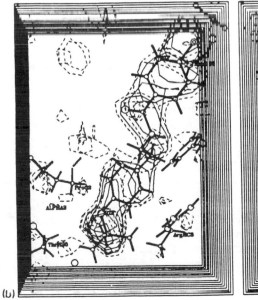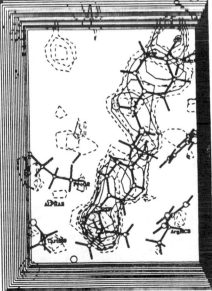

(b)

(29). Hegde et al. have recently found that the conformation of BZF in the small-molecule crystal structure is different than that found for BZF bound to HbA (30).

C. Mapping the Receptor Site from Agonists and Antagonists

The stereochemical nature of most of the pharmacologically interesting receptors has not been characterized at the atomic level. Therefore the use of agonists and antagonist to map the size and shape of a receptor site using small-molecule x-ray structures has proved necessary. Robert Sheridan of Lederle Laboratories has calculated molecular shapes of agonists and antagonists and searched the Cambridge Structural Database to derive new candidates for drug development (20). Duax and colleagues have superimposed compounds that compete for the estrogen receptor. They discovered that significant differences occur in the D ring of steroids and that it would appear that identification by the estrogen receptor occurs with rings A and B. They conclude that the receptor is either flexible in the D ring region or insensitive to it (31,32).

Marshall and colleagues have developed the technique of receptor mapping to determine the volume adjacent to the pharmacophore that must be available for drug binding (33). The addition of the volume for each active drug appropriately maps out the minimum volume necessary for binding. Inactivity of compounds can be rationalized if the inactive compound contains a unique new volume not derived from the active molecules. It is assumed that the new volume of the inactive compound is sterically incompatible with the receptor. The pitfalls and limitations of receptor site by deduction method have been clearly stated in a recent review by Marshall (34).

D. Elucidating the Molecular Mechanism of Action of Drugs

There are several structures being studied that are germane to the topic at hand. The following examples are not meant to be exhaustive but

---

Figure 6 (a) Stereo view of ECA, bound to the sulfhydryl of Cys F9(93)β of human deoxyhemoglobin. Model fitted to the difference electron density that arises from the subtraction of the modified intensities (structure factors) of native hemoglobin from the modified intensities (structure factors) of the drug-hemoglobin complex. (b) Stereo view of BZF fitted to the difference electron density found between the two α chains. Only positive difference electron density is shown: solid contours are drawn at intervals of 3σ or $0.06\,e/\text{Å}^3$, and broken contours are drawn at intervals of 2σ or $0.04\,e/\text{Å}^3$ (29).

representative of the kinds of information that can be obtained from studying drug-DNA or drug-protein interactions. Table 1 summarizes these and other macromolecular systems that may be of interest in the design of new therapeutic agents.

1. DNA-Drug Interactions

Dickerson and colleagues have studied the antitumor antibiotic netropsin (35) and the DNA stain and carcinogen Hoechst 33258 (36) bound to B DNA. Both molecules bind within the minor groove of DNA to displace the spine of hydration and replace it with a covalently bound molecular backbone that is even better at holding the double strands together (Figs. 7b,c). The disruption of the spine of waters is a necessary first step in the B to A helix transition (Fig. 7a). The covalently bound molecules inhibit both replication (to make new DNA) and transcription (to make messenger RNA). The observed A–T base pair preference observed for netropsin does not arise directly from hydrogen bonding but rather from close Van der Waals nonbonded contacts that arise when the drug molecule is oriented in the proper position by hydrogen bonds. Interestingly, the small-molecule crystal structure of netropsin shows it to be in the same overall banana shape as that observed in the DNA-netropsin crystal complex (37).

The general rule that appears to be emerging from various DNA structural studies is that antibiotics and small molecules prefer to bind to the minor grove, whereas proteins such as the restriction enzyme ECOR1 (38) prefer the major grove of B DNA.

Wang, Quigley, Rich, and co workers have shown that the interaction of drugs with DNA is a complex process (39 42). The DNA-drug interactions can result in considerable distortions of both drug and DNA compared to their isolated crystal or solution structures. The stability of the complexes can include numerous Van der Waals interactions, hydrogen bonding, hydrophobic bonding, intercalation, and ion pairing or salt bridges. Both the strength of interaction and sequence specificity can be substantially altered by small changes in drug structure. Several daunomycin- and adriamycin-related crystal structures have been determined (43), as have a number of the corresponding native DNA structures (44). Daunomycin and adriamycin are monointercalators. The drug-DNA complexes reveal a number of interactions including several hydrogen bonds to DNA, both direct and mediated by water. They also demonstrate a complex set of Van der Waals interactions that involve the conjugated intercalator with the stacked bases and the adjacent DNA backbone as well as with the remainder of the drug with the groove. Echinomycin and triostin A (39–42) are related cyclic octadepsipeptide antitumor antibiotics containing two aromatic quinoxaline side chains. These drugs interact as *bis* intercalators and shape themselves and the DNA to provide a complex set of hydrogen bonds and Van der Waals

Table 1   Macromolecular X-Ray Crystal Structures of Interest in Drug Design

Structure	References
Viruses	
Polio	86
Mengo	6
Rhino	87,88
Influenza neuraminidase	16
Nucleic Acids	
DNA-netropsin	35, 36
DNA-triostin A	42
DNA-eco R1	38
β-DNA-H$_2$O	89
DNA-antibiotic	39,41–43
Chromatin	90,91
tRNA	92
Proteins	
Photosynthetic receptor	15,93
Penicillopepsin	19
Penicillin target enzyme	46
β-Lactamase (penicillinase)	45
Purine nucleoside phosphorylase	48,94,95
Calmodulin	96
Renin inhibitor	97,98
Renin	99
Thymidylate synthetase	100
Dihydrofolate reductase	101–105
Elastase	106
α_1-Proteinase inhibitor	107
Trifluoroacetyl dipeptideanilide inhibitor	108
Rhizopus chinensis carboxyl proteinase and	
pepstatin	109,110
Subtilisin Carlsberg and the Inhibitor Eglin	111,112
Thermolysin	113
Thermolysin inhibitor complexes	114–118
Trifluoperazine binding site on troponin C	119
Troponin C–trifluoperazine	120
Mercaptan–thermolysin	117
Inhibitor complex of carboxypeptidase	121
complex with glycly-1-tyrosin	122
Inhibitors of angiotensin I converting enzyme	123
Phospholipase A2	124–128
Carboxy peptidase A	121,122,129
C–H ras p^{21}	131

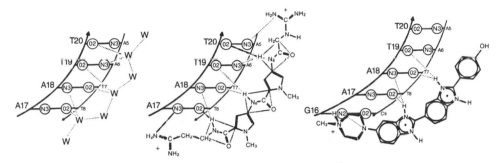

Figure 7 Schematic representations of the minor groove of β-DNA, showing hydrogen bonding. (a) Spine of hydration (130); (b) Netropsin (35); (c) Hoechst 33258 (130).

interactions involving at least four consecutive base pairs. The triostin A-DNA octamer complex has four Watson-Crick base pairs and four Hoogstein base pairs, two of which are G–C pairs that contain protonated cytosines (Fig. 8) (39).

2. Protein-Drug Interactions

Table 1 documents a number of studies that are focused on understanding the nature of protein-drug interactions. The work on the elucidation of the binding site and interactions of potential antiviral drugs with the rhino (common cold) virus has progressed rapidly and is presented in Chapter 10. As we show below in the section on hemoglobin, understanding protein-drug interactions can be directly coupled with the design of new agents. The following example illustrates a systematic study that uses structural knowledge derived from crystallographic analyses to explain both drug activity and drug deactivation.

Knox and colleagues (45–47) are studying two kinds of penicillin-binding enzymes: (1) those target enzymes normally involved with bacterial cell wall biosynthesis and inhibited by β-lactam type antibiotics, and (2) those β-lactamase enzymes that inactivate any β-lactam antibiotic in the cell's vicinity.

The 1.6-Å data on the target enzyme from *Streptomyces* R61 (MW 37.500) and 1.8-Å data on the acyl complex with cephalosporin C (Fig. 9a) were recorded at the University of California at San Diego (UCSD) area detector facility. Ser 62 at the N-terminal end of a helix in the catalytic site (in the 2.25-Å map) is the nucleophile responsible for attacking D-alanyl substrates or β-

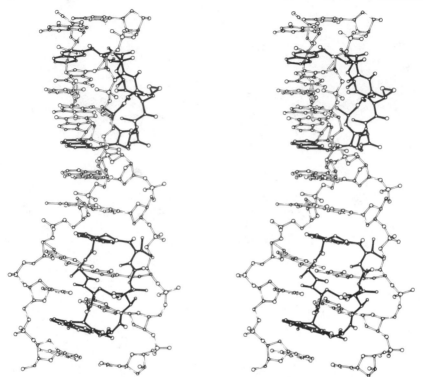

Figure 8   A stereo diagram showing triostin A (solid bonds) complexed to the right-handed DNA octamer (open bonds). The cyclic peptide fills the minor groove at the bottom of the diagram. The extent of intercalation by the quinoxaline rings is seen in the upper part of the diagram. The helix shows no apparent discontinuity when it changes from Watson-Crick to Hoogsteen pairing between the bases (39).

lactam inhibitors. It is speculated that the helix dipole contributes to the labilization of the Ser hydroxyl proton prior to nucleophilic attack on the carboxyl.

Area detector data (2.0 Å) from the University of Virginia facility on the β-lactamase enzyme from *Bacillus licheniformis* (MW 29,300) has been recorded. The 3.5-Å map also depicts the same ser-x-x-lys sequence at the catalytic site (45).

Knox and colleagues found a strong similarity in the tertiary structures of both the penicillin target enzyme and the β-lactamase. The two enzymes have only 19% sequence homology and differ considerably in size and catalytic behavior (45,46,48). These workers believe that what is obtained from the advanced structural analysis of the target enzyme can be applied with some justification, for the purposes of drug design, to the β-lactamase whose complexes are less stable. The rational design of specific β-lactamase

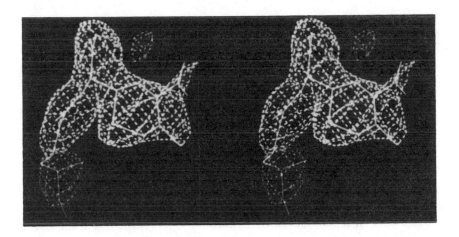

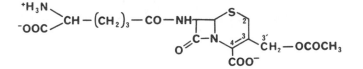

Figure 9 (a) Experimental difference electron density (2.25-Å resolution) of enzyme-bound cephalosporin C. The chemical structure of the ring-opened 3' exo-methylene form of the antibiotic has been fitted to density (46). (b) Cephalosporin C, a representative of the large cephalosporin family of β lactams, was chosen for binding experiments because it has a long half life of binding (7.5 days) to the target enzyme. The envelope of difference density (Fig. 9a) is consistent with the size of cephalosporin C (46).

inhibitors using x-ray structure data is an ideal test case for this methodology and if successful could produce pharmaceutically important agents that lengthen the lifetime of β-lactam antibiotics in patients.

E. Drug Design

The importance of the use of x-ray crystallography in drug design is best illustrated by reference to Table 1, the section below on hemoglobin, and other chapters in this text. Molecular modeling and computational chemistry (Chapter 3) routinely use the x-ray crystal data bases. Two-dimensional NMR studies of the structure of drugs (Chapter 5) and proteins (49) compare their results with the x-ray-determined structures. The design of the blood pressure-reducing drug captopril (Chapter 7) from the x-ray-determined binding site of carboxypeptidase A was a landmark event. The work on the elucidation of the binding site and interactions of potential antiviral drugs with the rhino (common cold) virus has progressed rapidly (Chapter 10).

IV. HEMOGLOBIN AS A MODEL SYSTEM FOR DRUG–PROTEIN INTERACTIONS AND DRUG DESIGN: ANTISICKLING AND ANTIISCHEMIC AGENTS

A. The Structure of Hemoglobin

Hemoglobin is a tetramer made up of two α chains and two β chains with 141 and 146 amino acid residues, respectively. The α chains contain seven, and the β chains eight helical segments designated as A to H (starting from the N terminus). The nonhelical segments are denoted NA (from the N terminus to the A helix), AB (between helix A and B) etc. to HC (after the H helix to the C terminus). Residues within each helix are numbered from the N terminus A14 etc., which denotes the 14th amino acid of the A helix (Fig. 10a). The mutation site Val would be designated Val A3 (6) β which indicates it is at position 3 on the A helix and position 6 on the β chain. A true molecular twofold axis relates the chains; α1 to α2 and β1 to β2. Each subunit binds one heme. In the deoxy state(T), looking down the twofold axis, a large, water-filled cavity can be observed. This is designated as the central water cavity (Fig. 10b). This cavity is substantially closed in the oxy state (R).

B. Stereospecific Design of Antigelling and Antisickling Agents

Sickle cell anemia is a painfully devastating disease with no known treatment for the underlying problem. It is ironic that more is known about the molecular bases of this disease than any other. Pauling and co-workers were the first to define sickle cell anemia as a molecular disease (50). Sequence of the β chain of Hb by Ingram (51) demonstrated that the sixth amino acid (Glu) in normal hemoglobin (HbA) had been replaced by a hydrophobic amino acid (Val). The x-ray crystal structure of mutant HbS is known (52–54) and has been related to the polymeric fiber structure (55–60), so the intermolecular contact sites are known. The mutant Hb polymerizes distorting the erythrocyte shape. The rigid sickled cells eventually become occluded in the capillaries and give rise to painful episodes called "crises." Symptomatic treatment for pain, strokes, and infection coupled with frequent transfusions for the most serious cases provides only temporary relief. Major drawbacks from symptomatic treatment include addiction from frequent use

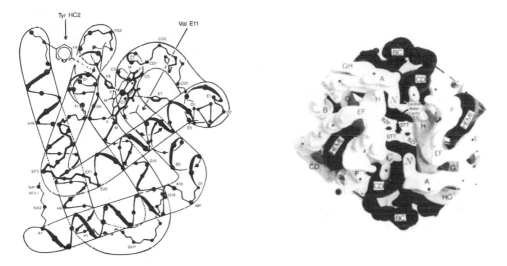

Figure 10 Structure of hemoglobin. (a) Tertiary structure of the α chain, showing the notation of helical and nonhelical segments, the heme pocket with the proximal histidine F8 forming a covalent link to the iron, and the distal histidine E7 and valine E11; also the hydrogen bond between the penultimate tyrosine HC2 and the carbonyl of valine FG5 that stabilizes the tertiary structures of both oxy- and deoxyhemoglobin (29). (b) A model of the quaternary structure of hemoglobin. This view is taken parallel to the dyad axis that runs through the central water cavity of the molecule, halfway between the STT signs. The principal binding sites of the different compounds are marked by arrows. Key: Bezafibrate (BZF), ethacrynic acid (E), succinyl I Trp (STT), p-bromobenzyloxyacetic acid (CD) (29).

of narcotics, and enlarged organs from iron deposits if transfused often. Ulcerations often appear on the extremities, especially around the ankles.

Even though sickle cell anemia is at the top of the list for genetic disabilities, the small population of homozygous HbS individuals in the United States (estimated at 60,000) has placed sickle cell anemia drugs in the orphan drug category. Therefore the pharmaceutical industry has not mounted an intense campaign to discover a drug treatment. Drug discovery research is being conducted primarily in academic institutions.

One of the major reasons that a drug has not been found to prevent the polymerization process that underlies the disease is due to the large quantity of Hb found in blood. The human being has 5 mM Hb in red cells. A sickle cell patient with a 25% hematocrit in 4 L of blood would have a total of 5.0 mmole HbS (322.5 g). The amount of drug (MW 300) needed to interact on a 1 : 1 molar basis with Hbs would be 1.5 g. That Hb is a tetramer that has a twofold molecular symmetry indicates that a 2 : 1 drug·protein interaction will more than likely be required to get a maximum effect on the prevention of polymer formation. Even if interaction at only one site on the tetramer is needed to inhibit polymerization (e.g., along the twofold axis in the central water cavity of Hb), it is possible that 2–5 g of drug per day will be needed to initially load the red cells. Such high doses will probably be required since some of the drug will be lost by excretion, taken up by fat depots, bound by serum proteins, and metabolized. Even if one discovered a very selective and potent stereospecific inhibitor of HbS polymerization, treatment with such an agent would require it to be essentially nontoxic to be administered at such high doses over a lifetime.

Goodford and colleagues at Burroughs Wellcome in the U.K. have used the three-dimensional structure of hemoglobin to design aromatic aldehydes that might reverse the sickling process by shifting the Hb allosteric equilibrium toward the more soluble R (high-affinity) state (61). Since hemoglobin S polymerizes in the deoxy (T) state, such an agent would not act by directly inhibiting the polymer contact sites from interacting, but by exclusion of the oxygenated tetramers from the polymer.

Walder, Arnone, and colleagues at the University of Iowa have investigated the antisickling action of *bis*-halogenated aspirins and determined their binding sites via difference Fourier maps. Their agents do act as stereospecific inhibitors of gelation (62–64).

Our own efforts in designing potential therapeutic agents using the three-dimensional x-ray structure of a protein started in 1975. At that time it wasn't known that hemoglobin would bind so many different drugs in over a half dozen different sites.

We have used three different approaches in our search for active stereospecific inhibitors of HbS gelation. Common to these approaches is the use of information, obtained by x-ray crystallographic techniques, on Hb structure and binding of small molecules to Hb.

The first approach (65,66) involved the design, synthesis, and testing of agents that would bind to the surface of Hb near the mutation donor or acceptor sites. The binding sites used for modeling were modeled from the x-ray structures of HbA (67) and HbS (52–54) (Fig. 11). This approach enabled us to discover a series of very potent, noncovalently acting inhibitors, substituted anisic acids (66); however, recent solution studies performed in our laboratory indicate nonspecific binding (68).

The second approach employed the addition of a solubilizing polar chain to a known active but little soluble compound, *p*-bromobenzyl alcohol. This idea produced the more active, and more soluble, benzyloxy acids (69,70) (Fig. 12). Through the use of x-ray crystallographic techniques, the binding sites of the soluble compounds on Hb were located. In part, this structural information on the binding sites permitted us to design new

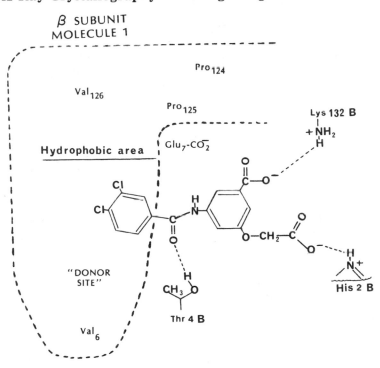

Figure 11 The proposed interaction of an anisic acid modeled to bind to hydrophilic and hydrophobic residues in the Val 6 mutation site (66).

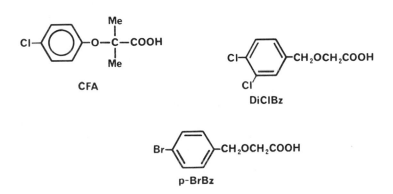

Figure 12 Dichlorobenzyloxyacetic acid (DiClBZ), *p*-bromobenzyloxyacetic acid (P-BrB₂), clofibric acid (CFA).

inhibitors with increased activity by adding appropriate hydrophobic moieties. The structurally similar phenoxy acids, such as the antilipidemic agent clofibric acid (Fig. 12), were also tested and found to be quite active (70).

The most exciting and fruitful approach has employed the use of x-ray structural information derived from difference electron density maps of weakly active antigelling agents. Stereochemical information on binding of these compounds to Hb and HbCO permitted us to select or design increasingly active analogs. The noncovalently (70) and covalently (71) acting phenoxy acids discussed above were discovered using this approach. The initial antigelling test we employ is run under anaerobic conditions. Therefore we could infer that the molecules inhibited gelation by a stereochemical mechanism and not by an allosteric modification of HbS to the more soluble oxy, (R) structure. It was also discovered that some of these agents (ethacrynic acid [ECA] and analogs) shift the allosteric mechanism toward the more soluble R structure. Therefore these compounds contain two antigelling mechanisms of action within the same molecule; stereospecific inhibition and allosteric modification toward the more soluble R structure (29, 71).

A third mechanism by which antigelling compounds can act is by increasing the red cell volume and decreasing the mean corpuscular hemoglobin concentrations (MCHC). Therefore the design of an agent that possesses the ability to act by all three mechanisms of action would produce a compound with ideal characteristics as an antisickling agent.

C. Hemoglobin and Antiischemic Drugs and Blood Storage

There are at present no antiischemic therapeutic agents available for treatment of stroke and related ischemic diseases. Since the delivery of oxygen to tissue is regulated by the allosteric properties of Hb, new allosteric inhibitors as potential antiischemic drugs have drawn attention. In this respect hemoglobin crystallography has contributed to the drug discovery process. Another role for the design of allosteric modulators involves the search for compounds that decrease oxygen affinity and improve the oxygen delivery characteristics of stored human blood. The following studies represent work being conducted in these areas.

Beddel, Goodford, and colleagues were the first to use the x-ray structure of Hb to develop agents that would decrease Hb affinity for oxygen and produce a right shift in the oxygen equilibrium curve (72,73). They designed a series of compounds that would bind to the natural allosteric effector (DPG) site.

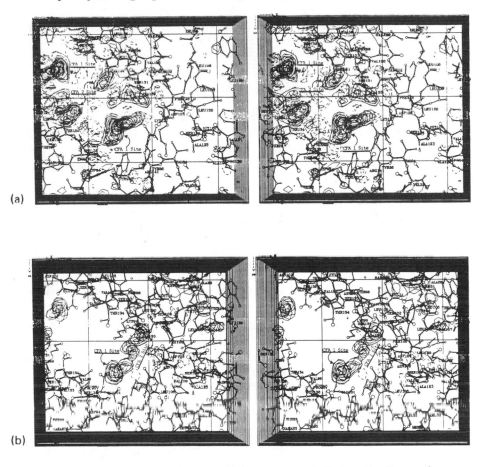

Figure 13 (a) Stereo diagram of the high-occupancy clofibric acids sites on deoxy Hb. CFA sites 1 and 2 are located around the molecular twofold axis (70). (b) Stereo diagram of bezafibrate bound to deoxy Hb. Notice that the top half of bezafibrate binds at the clofibric acid 1 site (70).

Klotz et al. (74–76) and Walder and Arnone and colleagues (62,63) have also studied diaspirin derivatives that bind and cross-link the DPG site and Lys 99 α residues (64). Abraham et al. were the first to discover non-DPG allosteric modulation sites for right-shifting the oxygen equilibrium curve (see Fig. 13 for binding sites of the antilipidemic drug clofibrate) (69). Perutz and Poyart discovered a much stronger right-shifting agent, bezafibrate, another antilipidemic drug (134). The binding site of one BZF showed it to overlap a minor and major site of clofibric acid (see Fig. 13). Efforts are in progress to model this site to produce possible therapeutic agents for treating ischemic diseases and for increasing the storage life of blood. Recently, Lalezari et al. have reported one such potential therapeutic agent that surpasses bezafibrate in efficacy (133).

D. Hemoglobin as a Model Drug Receptor

Hemoglobin has been considered as playing the same role in the development of structural molecular biology as hydrogen played in the development of quantum mechanics. For example, Hb has served as the premier model system for studying allosteric theory and has even been suggested as a model to understand potential quaternary structure of gap junction signal transduction over distances of hundreds of amino acids (77). The antisickling studies have added another dimension to hemoglobin research; the use of Hb as a model drug receptor. The x-ray drug studies with Hb have produced a better understanding of general and specific molecular characteristics of small-molecule–large-molecule interactions.

Hb has a number of binding pockets for a variety of small organic molecules. Figure 14 indicates the position and number of binding sites that we have observed for various agents bound to deoxy Hb.

It is worth noting that small changes in drug structure can result in binding to different and unrelated areas. Two closely related halogenated benzyloxy acids with similar activities bind to different sites when a bromo atom is replaced by a pair of adjacent chlorine atoms. QSAR failed to predict activity within the benzyloxy acids. This could be easily explained after the x-ray, and solution binding studies showed different binding sites for structurally related compounds.

One of the more striking structure-function comparisons we have seen in our studies was the great difference in activities between BZF and a compound we designed to interact (described above) at the mutation site, DG5, 5(p-chlorobenzamido)-α-carboxy-m-anisic acid (66). Both BZF and DG5 are p-chlorobenzamidophenoxy acids (Fig. 15). Whereas DG5 is a very active noncovalently acting compound, BZF is pro-gelling.

The binding of hydrophobic tails of drugs into hydrophobic pockets not exposed to the surface was another surprise. For example, the binding of p-bromobenzyl alcohol requires the movement of Trp 14α to gain access to that site. The detection of a pocket for binding p-bromobenzyloxyacetic acid in the interior of the α chains in a position hitherto believed to be filled by close-packed side chains of the globin (69) was unexpected. Searching for hidden or buried cavities that might bind hydrophobic moieties of drugs, as found in Hb, is a challenge to individuals who develop software for drug modeling studies.

The x-ray binding studies that elucidated the hidden hydrophobic cavities in Hb also gave rise to the idea that in vivo, Hb can transport hydrocarbons,

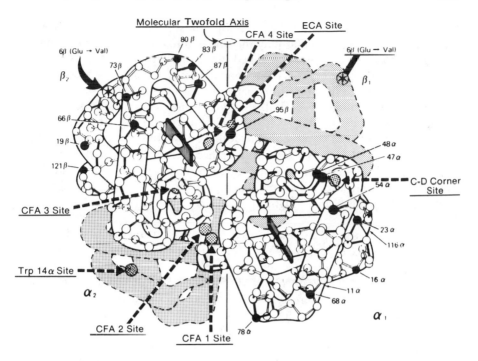

Figure 14 The binding sites of various drugs on deoxy hemoglobin; CFA binds to four sites, two with high occupancy (1 and 2) and two with low occupancy (3 and 4); one BZF molecule binds across CFA sites 1 and 3. p BrBz binds to the C-D corner, and ECA to CYS 93β. DiClBZ binds under the Trp 14α residue.

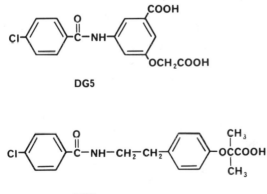

DG5

BZF

Figure 15 Dichloroanisic acid antigelling agent (DG5) and the progelling BZF.

hydrophobic halogenated aromatic compounds, and small hydrophobic molecules in general, as well as play the role of a toxin scavenger in animals and man. Taft et al. have developed an equation for correlating and predicting solubility of organic compounds in several types of solvents (78). They discovered that the predictions generated by this equation do not match the observed solubilities of most alkanes, alkylbenzenes, and chlorobenzenes in blood. Our findings that such hydrophobic compounds are needed to crystallize HbCO and are subsequently found in hydrophobic pockets on Hb was proposed as a reason for the variance between the predicted and observed solubilities (79,80). Likewise, three unrelated proteins that fold in a similar way that encloses a hydrophobic region between two crossed sections of antiparallel β sheets are thought to transport insoluble biological materials (81).

Detailed analyses of the interactions of the various drugs mentioned above demonstrated some expected general observations on bonding forces, as well as illustrated some unexpected, unusual close contacts between hydrophobic or polar atoms (29). The results show that the compounds seek out niches in the protein where the stereochemistry of binding is determined by the available Van der Waals space and, within that space, by a tendency to maximize electrostatic interactions. These range from strong hydrogen bonds to weakly polar interactions between halogens and aromatic quadrupoles. Another large part of the binding energy is due to hydrophobic effects.

A study of the nature of interactions between the drugs and protein revealed some unexpected features. We expected to find aromatic moieties of drugs or the peptides to form $\pi-\pi$ interactions with aromatic rings of the globin but found none of these. The dominant aromatic interactions that were found illustrated the hydrogens of one aromatic ring to interact with the π electrons of the other aromatic ring in herringbone fashion (29,82). Some unusual and to our knowledge heretofore unreported interactions were observed in the BZF structure. An amide hydrogen of Asn 108β is in close contact and centers the halogenated aromatic ring of BZF. The aliphatic side chain of Lys 99α is in contact with the flat face of BZF's amide group. The latter interaction supports a possible charge delocalization of the quaternary ammonium ion of Lys to the aliphatic side chain, as suggested by QSAR studies (83,84). Other Lys methylene residues interact with oxygen atoms in Hb (83). It will be of interest to see if the latter two types of interactions appear in other drug-binding studies.

V. CONCLUSIONS

The medicinal chemists' dream has been to rationally design therapeutic agents from the known stereochemistry of the receptor site. The development of x-ray crystallographic methods since the latter half of this century has brought this dream closer to reality. In 1974 the following ideas concerning the role of x-ray crystallography in drug design were put forward (1):

It is reasonable to assume then that the future of large molecule crystallography in medical chemistry may well be of monumental proportions. The reactivity of the receptor certainly lies in the nature of the environment and position of various amino acid residues. When the structured knowledge of the binding capabilities of the active site residues to specify groups on the agonist or antagonists becomes known, it should lead to proposals for syntheses of very specific agents with a high probability of biological action. Combined with what is known about transport of drugs through a Hansch-type analysis, etc., it is feasible that the drugs of the future will be tailor-made in this fashion. Certainly, and unfortunately, however, this day is not as close as one would like. The x-ray technique for large molecules, crystallization techniques, isolation techniques of biological systems, mechanism studies of active sites and synthetic talents have not been extensively intertwined because of the existing barriers between vastly different sciences.

Since that time, interdisciplinary scientists have broken down a number of the walls between the different disciplines. Today it is not unusual to see individuals who can, with their own hands, synthesize organic heavy-atom derivatives, grow crystals, solve x-ray structures of the hardest magnitude, clone genes, and talk rationally, in mechanistic terms, about substrate specificity. However, the best rational design by modeling from the surface of known receptors determined from x-ray analysis will not prevent the compound from bypassing the oxidative enzymes in the liver, or deter it from being taken up by fat depots or serum proteins, or keep it out of the urine, or stop it from having neurotoxicity. Will we do any better with the rational design of new agents based on the structural knowledge of the receptor than with older methods? The score as of this writing is that one drug, captopril, has made it to the market place, and a few others appear to be on their way. The hope for the success of any new agents will rest in the rational design of compounds with sufficient specificity to circumvent or greatly reduce the distribution, toxicity, and metabolism problems mentioned above.

What is to be expected in the future with regard to developments in the x-ray field that will influence drug design? Crystallography is moving in two directions: macro and mini. The solution of larger and more complex systems will continue to provide drug designers with atomic details that promote imaginative approaches to drug design. The most recent and truly amazing development in data collection indicates that a whole set of protein data may be acquired in a second or less using Laue photographs (85). Such short analysis times may soon provide structural features at near atomic resolutions of the movements involved in native and substrate bound proteins. On the opposite end of the kilodalton scale, detailed crystallographic analyses of the electron charge distribution in small molecules will permit the assignment of electrostatic potentials to atoms that could aid in the understanding of drug receptor interactions and how side chains pack in proteins. The addition to the understanding of packing, with a better understanding of water interactions in maintaining secondary and tertiary structure, may solve the protein folding problem. If that happens, then the nature of any receptor might be deduced from the genome, and x-ray crystallography will take a back seat to the dynamic computational and spectral methods of analyses of molecules. Until that day, however, crystallography will continue to have a dominant role in rational drug design.

REFERENCES

1. Abraham, D. J., The potential role of single crystal x-ray diffraction in medicinal chemistry. *Intra-Sc. Chem. Rep. 8*:1–9 (1974).
2. Pauling, L., Lecture presented at the International Congress of X-ray Crystallography at Stonybrook, N.Y. (Aug. 1973).
3. McPherson, A., *Preparation and Analysis of Protein Crystals.* John Wiley and Sons, New York (1982).
4. Feigelson, R. S., ed., Protein crystal growth. In *Proceedings of the First International Conference on Protein Crystal Growth*, Stanford University, Stanford, Calif., August 14–16, 1985. North Holland, Amsterdam (1986).
5. Abraham, D. J., and J. Sutcliffe, Unpublished results.
6. Luo, M., G. Vreind, G. Kamer, I. Minor, E. Arnold, M. G. Rossmann, U. Boege, D. G. Scraba, G. M. Duke, and A. C. Palmenberg, The atomic structure of mengo virus at 3.0 Å resolution. *Science 235*:182–191 (1987).
7. Green, D. W., V. M. Ingram, and M. F. Perutz, The structure of haemoglobin. IV. Sign determination by the isomorphous replacement method. *Proc. R. Soc. A225*:287–307 (1954).
8. Blow, D. M., and M. G. Rossmann, The single isomorphous replacement method. *Acta Cryst. 14*:1195–1202 (1961).
9. Wang, B.-C., Resolution of phase ambiguity in macromolecular crystallography. In *Diffraction Methods for Biological Macromolecules*, Vol. B115 of *Methods in Enzymology*. Academic Press, New York, pp. 90–112 (1985).
10. Rossmann, M. G., and D. M. Blow, The detection of sub-units within the crystallographic asymmetric unit. *Acta Cryst. 15*:24–34 (1962).
11. Woolfson, M. M., *Direct Methods in Crystallography.* Oxford University Press, New York (1961).
12. Karle, J., The determination of phase angles. In *Advances in Structure Research by Diffraction Methods*, Vol. 1, R. Brill and B. Mason, eds. Wiley-Interscience, New York, pp. 55–89 (1964).

13. Sobell, H. M., S. C. Jain, T. D. Sakore, and C. E. Nordman, Stereochemistry of actinomycin-DNA binding. *Nature New Biol. 231*:200–205 (1971).

14. Richmond, T. J., J. T. Finch, B. Rushton, D. Rhodes, and A. Klug, Structure of the nucleosome core particle at 7 Å resolution. *Nature 311*:532–537 (1984).

15. Deisenhofer, J., O. Epp, K. Miki, R. Huber, and H. Michel, Structure of the protein subunits in the photosynthetic reaction center of *Rhodopseudomonas viridis* at 3 Å resolution. *Nature 318*:618–624 (1985).

16. Colman, P. M., W. G. Laver, J. N. Varghese, A. T. Baker, P. A. Tulloch, G. M. Air, and R. G. Webster, Three-dimensional structure of a complex of antibody with influenza virus neuraminidase. *Nature 326*:358–362 (1987).

17. Hendrickson, W. A., and J. H. Konnert, Stereochemically restrained crystallographic least squares refinement of macromolecule structures. In *Biomolecular Structure, Conformation, Function, and Evolution*, Vol. 1, R. Srinivasan, ed. Pergamon Press, New York, pp. 41–57 (1981).

18. Konnert, J. R., A restrained-parameter structure-factor least-squares refinement procedure for large asymmetric units. *Acta Cryst. A32*:614–617 (1976).

19. James, M. N. G., and A. R. Sielecki, Structure and refinement of penicillopepsin at 1.8 Å resolution. *J. Mol. Biol. 163*:299–361 (1983).

20. Kuntz, I. D., Macromolecular Docking—The Design of Lead Compounds, Talk-2; Sheridan, R., New Methods in Drug Design (Talk 4); Wipke, T. and M. Hahn, AIMB Analogy and Intelligence in Model Building (Talk 8) *Drug Information Association Meeting*, Feb. 23–25, 1987, Hilton Head, S. C., contact Audio Transcripts, Alexander, VA 22314 (1987).

21. Wipke, W. T., and M. A. Hahn, Analogic and intelligence in model building. In *Applications of Artificial Intelligence in Chemistry*, ACS Symposium Series 306, T. Pierce and D. Hohne, eds., pp. 136–146 (1986).

22. Lotter, H., and A. Liptak, The configuration of isomers of methyl 4-0-acetyl-2,3-0(1-phenylethylidene)-α-L-rhamnopyranosides. *Z. Naturforsch. 36b*:997–999 (1981).

23. Lotter, H., H. Wagner, A. A. Saleh, G. A. Cordell, and N. R. Farnsworth, Potential anticancer agents. XI. X-ray structure determination of acantholide. *Z. Naturforsch. 34c*:677–682 (1979).

24. Duax, W. L., and D. A. Norton, *Atlas of Steroid Structures*, Vol. 1. Plenum Press, New York (1975).

25. Griffin, J. F., W. L. Duax, and C. M. Weeks, *Atlas of Steroid Structures*, Vol. 2. Plenum Press, New York (1984).

26. Duax, W. L., C. M. Weeks, and D. C. Rohrer, Crystal structures of steroids. In *Topics in Stereochemistry*, Vol. 9, N. L. Allinger and E. L. Eliel, eds. Wiley-Interscience, New York, pp. 271–383 (1976).

27. Prusiner, P., T. Brennan, and M. Sundaralingam, Crystal structure and molecular conformation of formycin monohydrates. Possible origin of the anomalous circular dichroic spectra in formycin mono- and polynucleotides. *Biochemistry 12*:1196–1202 (1973).

28. Abola, J. E., M. J. Sims, D. J. Abraham, A. F. Lewis, and L. Townsend, Molecular structure and conformation of the nucleoside antibiotic derivative 2-methylformycin with a c-glycosidic bond. *J. Med. Chem. 17*:62–65 (1974).

29. Perutz, M. F., G. Fermi D. J. Abraham, C. Poyart, and E. Bursaux, Hemoglobin as a receptor of drugs and peptides: X-ray studies of the stereochemistry of binding, *J. Am. Chem. Soc. 108*:1064–1078 (1986).

30. Hegde, R., P. Sawzik, R. McClure, and D. J. Abraham, Unpublished results.

31. Duax, W. L., and C. M. Weeks, Molecular basis of estrogenicity: X-ray crystallographic studies. In *Estrogens in the Environment*. Elsevier, New York, pp. 11–31 (1980).

32. Duax, W. L., J. F. Griffin, D. C. Rohrer, C. M. Weeks, and R. H. Ebright, Steroid hormone action interpreted from x-ray crystallographic studies. In *Biochemical Actions of Hormones*, Vol. XI. Academic Press, New York, pp. 187–206 (1984).

33. Motoc, I., R. A. Dammkoehler, and G. R. Marshall, Three-dimensional structure-activity relationships and biological receptor mapping. In *Mathematics and Computational Concepts in Chemistry*, N. Trinajstic, ed. Horwood, Chichester, U.K., pp. 221–251 (1986).

34. Marshall, G. R., Computer-aided drug design. *Annu. Rev. Pharmacol. Toxicol. 27*:193–213 (1987).

35. Kopka, M. L., C. Yoon, D. Goodsell, P. Pjura, and R. E. Dickerson, Binding of an antitumor drug to DNA: Netropsin and C–G–C–G–A–A–T–T–BrC–G–C–G. *J. Mol. Biol. 183*:553–563 (1985).

36. Dickerson, R. E., P. Pjura, M. L. Kopka, D. Goodsell, and C. Yoon, Crystallography in molecular biology. In *Proceedings of the NATO Advanced Study Institute and EMBO Lecture Course*, Bischenberg, Alsace, France, Sept. 12–21, 1985, NATO ASI Series, D. Moras, ed. Plenum Press, New York (1985).

37. Berman, H. M., S. Neidle, C. Zimmer, and H. Thrum, Netropsin, a DNA-binding oligopeptide: Structural and binding studies. *Biochim. Biophys. Acta 561*:124–131 (1979).

38. McClarin, J. A., C. A. Frederick, B.-C. Wang, P. Greene, H. W. Boyer, J. Grable, and J. M. Rosenberg, Structure of the DNA-Eco RI endonuclease recognition complex at 3 Å resolution. *Science 234*:1526–1541 (1986).

39. Quigley, G. J., G. Ughetto, G. A. van der Marel, J. H. van Boom, A, H.-J. Wang, and A. Rich, Non-Watson-Crick G. C and A. T base pairs in a DNA-antibiotic complex. *Science 232*:1255–1258 (1986).

40. Ughetto, Y. G., A. H.-J. Wang, G. J. Quigley, G. A. van der Marel, J. H. van Boom, and A. Rich, A comparison of the structure of echinomycin and triostin A complexed to a DNA fragment. *Nucleic Acids Res. 13*:2305–2323 (1985.

41. Wang, A. H.-J., G. Ughetto, G. J. Quigley, and A. Rich, Interactions of quinoxaline antibiotic and DNA: The molecular structure of a triostin A-d(GCGTACGC) complex. *J. Biomol. Struct. Dyn. 4*(3):319–342 (1986).

42. Wang, A. H.-J., G. Ughetto, G. A. Quigley, T. Hakoshima, G. A. van der Marel, J. H. van Boom, and A. Rich, The molecular structure of a DNA-triostin A complex. *Science 225*: 1115–1121 (1984).

43. Wang, A. H.-J., G. Ughetto, G. J. Quigley, and A. Rich, Interactions between an anthracycline antibiotic and DNA: Molecular structure of daunomycin complexed to d(CpGpTpApCpG) at 1.2 Å resolution. *Biochemistry 26*:1152–1163 (1987).

44. Fujii, S., A. H.-J. Wang, G. J. Quigley, H. Westerink, G. van der Marel, J. H. van Boom, and A. Rich. The octamers d(CGCGCGCG) and d(CGCATGCG) crystallize as Z-DNA in the same hexagonal lattice. *Biopolymers 24*:243–250 (1985).

45. Kelly, J. A., O. Dideberg, P. Charlier, J. P. Wery, M. Libert, P. C. Moews, J. R. Knox, C. Duez, C. L. Fraipont, B. Joris, J. Dusart, J. M. Frere, and J. M. Ghuysen, On the origin of bacterial resistence to penicillin: Comparison of a β-lactamase and a penicillin target. *Science 231*:1429–1431 (1986).

46. Knox, J. R., J. A. Kelley, P. C. Moews, H. Zhao, J. Moring, J. K. M. Rao, and J. Boyington, Crystallography of penicillin binding enzymes; in Three-dimensional structure and drug action. Tokyo Univ. of Tokyo Press (I. Itaka and A. Itai, ed. 1987.

47. Knox, J. R., J. A. Kelly, and O. Dideberg, Cell wall synthesizing enzymes and penicillinase: Crystallography to the aid of microbiology. Presented at 44th Pittsburgh Diffraction Conference, Abstract 1.1 (Oct. 29–31, 1986).

48. Ealick, S. E., M. Carson, S. V. L. Narayana, J. Fillers, S. Rowland, W. J. Cook, and C. E. Bugg, Inhibitor design by protein crystallography: Studies with human purine nucleoside phosphorylase. Presented at 44th Pittsburgh Diffraction Conference, Abstract 4.3 (Oct. 29–31, 1986).

49. Brunger, A. T., R. L. Campbell, G. M. Clore, A. M. Gronenborn, M. Karplus, G. A. Petsko, and M. M. Teeter, Solution of a protein crystal structure with a model obtained from NMR interproton distance restraints. *Science 235*:1049–1052 (1987).

50. Pauling, L., H. A. Itano, S. J. Singer, and I. C. Wells, Sickle cell anemia, a molecular disease. *Science 110*.543–548 (1949).

51. Ingram, V. M., A specific chemical difference between the globin of normal human and sickle cell anemia hemaglobin. *Nature 178*:792 (1956)

52. Wishner, B. C., K. B. Ward, E. E. Lattman, and W. E. Love, Crystal structure of sickle cell deoxyhemoglobin at 5 Å resolution. *J. Mol. Biol. 98*:179–194 (1975).

53. Padlan, E. A., and W. E. Love, Refined crystal structure of deoxyhemoglobin S. II. Molecular interactions in the crystal. *J. Biol. Chem. 260*:8280–8291 (1985).

54. Padlan, E. A., and W. E. Love, Refined crystal structure of deoxyhemoglobin S. I. Restrained least-squares refinement at 3.0 Å resolution. *J. Biol. Chem. 260*:8272–8279 (1985).

55. Edelstein, S. J., and R. H. Crepeau, Oblique alignment of hemoglobin S fibers in sickled cells. *J. Mol. Biol. 134*:851–855 (1979).

56. Dykes, G. W., R. H. Crepeau, and S. J. Edelstein, Three-dimensional reconstruction of the 14-filament fibers of hemoglobin S. *J. Mol. Biol. 130*:451–472 (1979).

57. Edelstein, S. J., Molecular Topology in Crystals and Fibers of Hemoglobin S. *J. Mol. Biol. 150*:557–575 (1981).

58. Rosen, L. S., and B. Magdoff-Fairchild, Molecular packing in a second monoclinic crystal of deoxygenated sickle hemoglobin. *J. Mol. Biol. 157*:181–189 (1982).

59. Magdoff-Fairchild, B., and L. S. Rosen, A model of deoxygenated sickle ·

hemoglobin fibers derived from x-ray diffraction data. *Biophys. J. 37*:348a (1982).

60. Magdoff-Fairchild, B., and C. C. Chiu, X-ray diffraction studies of Fibers and crystals of deoxygenated sickle cell hemoglobin. *Proc. Natl. Acad. Sci. USA 76*:223–226 (1979).

61. Beddell, C. R., P. J. Goodford, G. Kneen, R. D. White, S. Wilkinson, and R. Wootton, Substituted benzaldehydes designed to increase the oxygen affinity of human haemoglobin and inhibit the sickling of sickled erythrocytes. *Br. J. Pharmacol 82*:397–407 (1984).

62. Walder, J. A., R. Y. Walder, and A. Arnone, Development of antisickling compounds that chemically modify hemoglobin S specifically within the 2,3-diphosphoglycerate binding site. *J. Mol. Biol. 141*:195–216 (1980).

63. Chatterjee, R., R. Y. Walder, A. Arnone, and J. A. Walder, Mechanism for the increase in solubility of deoxyhemoglobin S due to cross-linking the β chains between lysine-82β_1 and lysine-82β_2. *Biochemistry 21*:5901–5909 (1982).

64. Chatterjee, R., E. V. Welty, R. Y. Walder, S. L. Pruitt, P. H. Rogers, A. Arnone, and J. A. Walder, Isolation and characterization of a new hemoglobin derivative cross-linked between the α chains (lysine 99α_1 → lysine 99α_2.*J. Biol. Chem. 261*:9929–9937 (1986).

65. Abraham, D. J., M. Mokotoff, L. Sheh, and J. E. Simmons, The design, synthesis, and testing of potential antisickling agents. 2. Proline derivatives designed for the donor site. *J. Med. Chem. 26*:549–554 (1983).

66. Abraham, D. J., D. M. Gazze, P. E. Kennedy, and M. Mokotoff, Design, synthesis and testing of potential antisickling agents. 5. Disubstituted benzoic acids designed for the donor site and proline salicylates designed for the acceptor site. *J. Med. Chem. 27*:1549–1559 (1984).

67. Fermi, G., M. F. Perutz, B. Shaanan, and R. Fourme, The crystal structure of human deoxyhaemoglobin at 1.74Å resolution. *J. Mol. Biol. 175*:159–174 (1984).

68. Mehanna, A., Design, synthesis, biochemical and toxicological studies of potential antisickling agents. Ph.D. Thesis, University of Pittsburgh (1986).

69. Abraham, D. J., M. F. Perutz, and S. E. V. Phillips, Physiological and x-ray studies of potential antisickling agents. *Proc. Natl. Acad. Sci. USA 80*:324–328 (1983).

70. Abraham, D. J., P. E. Kennedy, A. S. Mehanna, D. Patwa, and F. L. Williams, Design, synthesis and testing of potential antisickling agents. 4. Structure-activity relationships of benzyloxy and phenoxy acids. *J. Med. Chem. 27*:967–978 (1984).

71. Kennedy, P. E., F. L. Williams, and D. J. Abraham, Design, synthesis, and testing of potential antisickling agents. 3. Ethyacrynic acid. *J. Med. Chem. 27*:103–105 (1984).

72. Beddell, C. R., P. J. Goodford, F. E. Norrington, S. Wilkinson, and R. Wootton, Compounds designed to fit a site of known structure in human haemoglobin. *Br. J. Pharmacol 57*:201–209 (1976).

73. Brown, F. F., and P. J. Goodford, The interaction of some bis-arylhydroxysulphonic acids with a site of known structure in human haemoglobin. *Br. J. Pharmacol. 60*:337–341 (1977).

74. Klotz, I. M., D. N. Haney, and L. C. King, Rational approaches to chemotherapy: Antisickling agents. *Science 213*:724–731 (1981).

75. Walder, J. A., R. H. Zaugg, R. S. Iwaoka, W. G. Watkin, and I. M. Klotz, Alternative aspirins as antisickling agents: Acetyl-3, 5-dibromosalicylic acid. *Proc. Natl. Acad. Sci. USA 74*:5499–5503 (1977).

76. Walder, J. A., R. H. Zaugg, R. Y. Walder, J. M. Steele, and I. M. Klotz, Diaspirins that cross-link β chains of hemoglobin: bis(3,5-dibromosalicyl) succinate and bis(3,5-dibromosalicyl) fumarate. *Biochemistry 18*:4265–4270 (1979).

77. Racker, E., Structure, function and assembly of membrane proteins. *Science 235*:959–961 (1987).

78. Taft, R. W., M. H. Abraham, R. M. Doherty, and M. J. Kamlet, The molecular properties governing solubilities of organic nonelectrolytes in water. *Nature 313*:384–386 (1985).

79. Kamlet, M. J., D. J. Abraham, R. M. Doherty, R. W. Taft, and M. H. Abraham, Solubility properties in polymers and biological media. 6. An equation for correlation and predictions of solubilities of liquid organic nonelectrolytes in blood. *J. Pharm. Sci. 75*:350–355 (1986).

80. Kamlet, M. J., R. M. Doherty, R. W. Taft, M. H. Abraham, G. D. Veith, and D. J. Abraham, Solubility properties in polymers and biological media. 8. An analysis of the factors that influence toxicities of organic nonelectrolytes to the golden orfe fish (*Leuciscus idus melanotus*). *Environ. Sci. Technol. 21*:149–155 (1987).

81. Blundell, T. L., B. L. Sibanda, M. J. E. Sternberg, and J. M. Thornton, Knowledge-based prediction of protein structures and the design of novel molecules. *Nature 326*:347–352 (1987).

82. Burley, S. K., and G. A. Petsko, Aromatic-aromatic interaction: A mechanism of protein structure stabilization. *Science 229*:23–28 (1985)

83. Abraham, D. J., and A. J. Leo, Extension of the fragment method to calculate amino acid zwitterion and side chain partition coefficients. *Proteins: Struct. Funct. Genet. 2*: 130–152 (1987).

84. Hansch, C., and A. J. Leo, *Substituent Constants for Correlation Analysis in Chemistry and Biology.* John Wiley and Sons, New York (1979).

85. Hajdu, J., P. A. Machin, J. W. Campbell, T. J. Greenhough, I. J. Clifton, S. Zurek, S. Grover, L. N. Johnson, and M. Elder, Millisecond x-ray diffraction and the first electron density map from Laue photographs of a protein crystal. *Nature 329*:178–181 (1987).

86. Hogle, J. M., M. Chow, and D. J. Filman, Three-dimensional structure of poliovirus at 2.9 Å resolution. *Science 229*:1358–1365 (1985).

87. Rossmann, M., E. Arnold, J. W. Erickson, E. A. Frankenberger, J. P. Griffith, H.-J. Hecht, J. E. Johnson, G. Kamer, M. Luo, A. G. Mosser, R. R. Rueckert, B. Sherry, and G. Vriend, Structure of a human common cold virus and functional relationship to other picornaviruses. *Nature. 317*:145–153 (1985).

88. Smith, T. J., M. J. Kremer, M. Luo, G. Vriend, E. Arnold, G. Kamer, M. G. Rossmann, M. A. McKinlay, G. D. Diana, and M. J. Otto, The site of attachment in human rhinovirus 14 for antiviral agents that inhibit uncoating. *Science 233*:1286–1293 (1986).

89. Kopka, M. L., A. V. Fratini, H. R. Drew, and R. E. Dickerson, Ordered water structure around a B-DNA dodecamer: A quantitative study. *J. Mol. Biol.* *163*:129–146 (1983).

90. Finch, J. T., R. S. Brown, D. Rhodes, T. Richmond, B. Rushton, L. C. Lutter, and A. Klug, X-ray diffraction study of a new crystal form of the nucleosome core showing higher resolution. *J. Mol. Biol.* *145*:757–769 (1981).

91. Richmond, T. J., J. T. Finch, B. Rushton, D. Rhodes, and A. Klug, Structure of the nucleosome core particle at 7 Å resolution. *Nature* *311*:532–537 (1984).

92. Dewan, J. C., Binding of the antitumor drug cis-[PtCl(NH3)2] to crystalline tRNAPhe at 6-Å resolution. *J. Am. Chem. Soc.* *106*:7239–7244 (1984).

93. Deisenhofer, J., O. Epp, K. Miki, R. Huber, and H. Michel, X-ray structure analysis of a membrane protein complex: Electron density map at 3 Å resolution and a model of the chromophoses of the photosynthetic reaction center from *Rhodopseudomonas viridis*. *J. Mol. Biol.* *180*:385–398 (1984).

94. Ealick, S. E., T. J. Greenhough, Y. S. Babu, D. C. Carter, W. J. Cook, C. E. Bugg, S. A. Rule, J. Habash, J. R. Helliwell, J. D. Stoeckler, S. F. Chen, and R. E. Parks Jr., Three-dimensional structure of human erythrocytic purine nucleoside phosphorylase. *Ann. N.Y. Acad. Sci.* *451*:311–312 (1985).

95. Stockler, J. D., S. E. Ealick, C. E. Bugg, and R. E. Parks Jr., Design of purine nucleoside phosphorylase inhibitors. *Fed. Proc.* *25*:2773–2778 (1986).

96. Babu, Y. S., J. S. Sack, T. J. Greenhough, C. E. Bugg, A. R. Means, and W. J. Cook, Three-dimensional structure of calmodulin. *Nature* *315*:37–40 (1985).

97. Navia, M. A., J. P. Springer, M. Poe, J. Boger, and K. Hoogsteen, Preliminary x-ray crystallographic data on mouse submaxillary gland renin and renin inhibitors complexes. *J. Biol. Chem.* *259*:12714–12717 (1984).

98. Foundling, S. I., J. Cooper, F. E. Watson, A. Cleassby, L. H. Pearl, B. L. Sibanda, A. Hemmings, S. P. Wood, T. L. Blundell, M. J. Valler, C. G. Norey, J. Kay, J. Boger, B. M. Dunn, B. J. Leckie, D. M. Jones, B. Atrash, A. Hallett, and M. Szelke, High resolution x-ray analyses of renin inhibitor-aspartic proteinase complexes. *Nature* *327*:349–352 (1987).

99. Sibanda, B. L., T. Blundell, P. M. Hobart, M. Fogliano, J. S. Bindra, B. W. Dominy, and J. M. Chirgwin, Computer graphics modelling of human renin: Specificity, catalytic activity and intron-exon junctions. *FEBS Lett.* *174*:102–111 (1984).

100. Hardy, L. W., J. S. Finer-Moore, W. R. Montfort, M. O. Jones, D. V. Santi, and R. M. Stroud, Atomic structure of thymidylate synthase: Target for rational drug design. *Science* *235*:448–455 (1987).

101. Matthews, D. A., J. T. Bolin, J. M. Burridge, D. J. Filman, K. W. Volz, B. T. Kaufman, C. R. Bedell, J. N. Champness, D. K. Stammers, and J. Kraut, Refined crystal structures of *Escherichia coli* and chicken liver dihydrofolate reductase containing bound trimethoprim. *J. Biol. Chem.* *260*:381–391 (1985).

102. Bolin, J. T., D. J. Filman, D. A. Matthews, R. C. Hamlin, and J. Kraut, Crystal structures of *Escherichia coli* and *Lactobacillus casei* dihydrofolate reductase refined at 1.7 Å resolution. *J. Biol. Chem.* *257*:13650–13662 (1982).

103. Filman, D. J., J. T. Bolin, D. A. Matthews, and J. Kraut, Crystal structures of *Escherichia coli* and *Lactobacillus casei* dihydrofolate reductase refined at 1.7 Å resolution. II. Environment of bound NADPH and implications for catalysis. *J. Biol. Chem.* *257*:13663–13672 (1982).

104. Volz, K. W., D. A. Matthews, R. A. Alden, S. T. Freer, C. Hansch, B. T. Kaufman, and J. Kraut, Crystal structure of avian dihydrofolate reductase containing phenyltriazine and NADPH. *J. Biol. Chem.* 257:2528–2536 (1982).
105. Matthews, D. A., J. T. Bolin, J. M. Burridge, D. J. Filman, K. W. Volz, and J. Kraut, Dihydrofolate reductase: The stereochemistry of inhibitor selectivity. *J. Biol. Chem.* 260:392–399 (1985).
106. Sawyer, L., D. M. Shotton, J. W. Campbell, P. L. Wendell, H. Muirhead, and H. C. Watson, The atomic structure of crystalline porcine pancreatic elastase at 2.5 Å resolution: Comparisons with the structure of α-chymotrypsin. *J. Mol. Biol.* 118:137–208 (1978).
107. Loebermann, H., R. Tokuoka, J. Deisenhofer, and R. Huber, Human α_1-proteinase inhibitor: Crystal structure analysis of two crystal modifications, molecular model and preliminary analysis of the implications for function. *J. Mol. Biol.* 177:531–557 (1984).
108. Hughes, D. L., L. C. Sieker, J. Bieth, and J.-L. Dimicoli, Crystallographic study of the binding of a trifluoroacetyl dipeptide anilide inhibitor with elastase. *J. Mol. Biol.* 162:645–658 (1982).
109. Bott, R., E. Subramanian, and D. R. Davies, Three-dimensional structure of the complex of the *Rhizopus chinensis* carboxyl proteinase and pepstatin at 2.5-Å resolution. *Biochemistry* 21:6956–6962 (1982).
110. Subramanian, E., I. D. A. Swan, M. Liu, D. R. Davies, J. A. Jenkins, I. J. Tickle, and T. L. Blundell, Homology among acid proteases: Comparison of crystal structures at 3 Å resolution of acid proteases from *Rhizopus chinensis* and *Endothia parasitica*. *Proc. Natl. Acad. Sci. USA* 74:556–559 (1977).
111. McPhalen, C. A., H. P. Schnebli, and M. N. G. James, Crystal and molecular structure of the inhibitor eglin from leeches in complex with subtilisin Carlsberg, *FEBS Lett.* 188:55–58 (1985).
112. Bode, W., E. Papamokos, D. Musil, U. Seemueller, and H. Fritz, Refined 1.2 Å crystal structure of the complex formed between subtilisin Carlsberg and the inhibitor eglin c. Molecular structure of eglin and its detailed interaction with subtilisin. *EMBO J.* 5:813–818 (1986).
113. Holmes, M. A., and B. W. Matthews, Structure of thermolysin refined at 1.6 Å resolution. *J. Mol. Biol.* 160:623–639 (1982).
114. Tronrud, D. E., H. M. Holden, and B. W. Matthews, Structures of two thermolysin-inhibitor complexes that differ by a single hydrogen bond. *Science* 235:571–574 (1987).
115. Kester, W. R., and B. W. Matthews, Crystallographic study of the binding of depeptide inhibitors to thermolysin: Implications for the mechanism of catalysis. *Biochemistry* 16:2506–2516 (1977).
116. Hangauer, D. G., A. F. Monzingo, and B. W. Matthews, An interactive computer graphics study of thermolysin-catalyzed peptide cleavage and inhibition by N-carboxymethyl dipeptides. *Biochemistry* 23:5730–5741 (1984).
117. Monzingo, A. F., and B. W. Matthews, Structure of a mercaptan-thermolysin complex illustrates mode of inhibition of zinc proteases by substrate-analogue mercaptans. *Biochemistry* 21:3390–3394 (1982).
118. Monzingo, A. F., and B. W. Matthews, Binding of N-carboxymethyl dipeptide inhibitors to thermolysin determined by x-ray crystallography: A novel class of transition-state analogues for zinc peptidases. *Biochemistry* 23:5724–5729 (1984).

119. Herzberg, O., and M. N. G. James, Structure of the calcium regulatory muscle protein troponin-C at 2.8 Å resolution. *Nature 313*:653–659 (1985).

120. Gariepy, J., and R. S. Hodges, Localization of a trifluoperazine binding site on troponin C. *Biochemistry 22*:1586–1594 (1983).

121. Rees, D. C., and W. N. Lipscomb, Refined crystal structure of the potato inhibitor complex of carboxypeptidase A at 2.5 Å resolution. *J. Mol. Biol. 160*:475–498 (1982).

122. Rees, D. C., and W. N. Lipscomb, Crystallographic studies on apocarboxypeptidase A and the complex with glycyl-L-tyrosine. *Proc. Natl. Acad. Sci. USA 80*:7151–7154 (1983).

123. Cushman, D. W., H. S. Cheung, E. F. Sabo, and M. A. Ondetti, Design of potent competitive inhibitors of angiotensin-converting enzyme. Carboxyalkanoyl and mercaptoalkanoyl amino acids. *Biochemistry 16*(25):5484–5491 (1977).

124. Dijkstra, B. W., K. H. Kalk, J. Drenth, G. H. De Haas, M. R. Egmond, and A. J. Slotboom, Role of the N-terminus in the interaction of pancreatic phospholipase A2 with aggregated substrates. Properties and crystal structure of transaminated phospholipase A2. *Biochemistry 23*:2759–2766 (1984).

125. Brunie, S., J. Bolin, D. Gewirth, and P. B. Sigler, The refined crystal structure of dimeric phospholipase A2 at 2.5CA: Access to a shielded catalytic center. *J. Biol. Chem. 260*:9742–9749 (1985).

126. Dijkstra, B. W., G. J. H. van Nes, K. H. Kalk, N. P. Brandenburg, W. G. J. Hol, and J. Drenth, The structure of bovine pancreatic prophospholipase A2 at 3.0 Å resolution. *Acta Cryst. B38*:793–799 (1982).

127. Dijkstra, B. W., K. H. Kalk, W. G. J. Hol, and J. Drenth, Structure of bovine pancreatic phospholipase A2 at 1.7 Å resolution. *J. Mol. Biol. 147*:97–123 (1981).

128. Dijkstra, B. W., R. Renetseder, K. H. Kalk, W. G. J. Hol, and J. Drenth, Structure of porcine pancreatic phospholipase A2 at 2.6 Å resolution and comparison with bovine phospholipase A2. *J. Mol. Biol. 168*:163–179 (1983).

129. Rees, D. C., M. Lewis, and W. N. Lipscomb, Refined crystal structure of carboxypeptidase A at 1.54 Å resolution. *J. Mol. Biol. 168*:367–387 (1983).

130. Dickerson, R. E., H. R. Drew, M. L. Kopka, and P. Pjura, The importance of hydrogen bonding in stabilizing DNA and RNA-drug complexes. Presented at *43d Pittsburgh Diffraction Conference* (Nov. 6–8, 1985).

131. deVos, A. M., L. Tong, M. V. Milburn, P. M. Matias, J. Janoarik, S. Noguchi, S. Nishimura, K. Miura, E. Ohtsuka, and S.H. Kim, Three-dimensional structure of an oncogenic protein: Catalytic domain of human c-H-ras P^{21}. *Science 239*:888–893 (1988).

132. Swartzendruber, J. K., and N. D. Jones, Apocalypse: An automated protein crystallization system III; Jones, N. D., Crystalplate: The new ACA Protein Crystallization Plate, American Crystalographic Association Meeting (Abstracts), Philadelphia, PA, June 26–July 1, 1988.

133. Lalezari, I., S. Rahbar, P. Lalezari, G. Fermi, and M. F. Perutz, L.R.16, a compound with potent effects on the oxygen affinity of hemoglobin, on blood cholesterol and on low density lipoprotein. *Proc. Natl. Acad. Sci. USA 85*:6117–6121 (1988).

134. Perutz, M. F., and C. Poyart, Bezafibrate lowers oxygen affinity of haemoglobin. *Lancet 2*:881–888 (1983).

5

Approaches to Drug Design Using Nuclear Magnetic Resonance Spectroscopy

Stephen W. Fesik
Abbott Laboratories, Abbott Park, Illinois

I. INTRODUCTION

Nuclear magnetic resonance (NMR) is a powerful spectroscopic technique that can yield detailed structural and dynamic information on molecules in solution. Consequently, NMR has proved to be a valuable tool in pharmaceutical research. In addition to its importance as an analytical method to elucidate the primary structures of chemically synthesized compounds and isolated natural products, NMR can provide information on the three-dimensional structures of small molecules in solution, high-molecular-weight complexes, and the details of enzyme mechanisms that can be used to aid in drug design. Some of the recent advances in NMR that have allowed this information to be obtained include the availability of high magnetic fields; improved software, probe design, and electronics; more versatile pulse programmers; and perhaps most importantly, the development of two-dimensional NMR techniques.

In this chapter, some of the recently developed NMR methods for studying the conformational properties of molecules in solution, small molecule–large molecule interactions, and enzyme reactions will be described as well as some of the exciting possibilities on how this structural information may be utilized for the design of drugs. The goal is to acquaint the reader with some of the more modern NMR methods that can yield structural information that may be applied to drug design. Detailed descriptions on the physical and experimental aspects of the individual NMR methods will not be presented here, as these can be found in the original papers cited within the chapter.

II. CONFORMATIONAL ANALYSIS

It has long been realized that the interaction of a drug with its target site depends not only on the presence of the chemical entities involved in the interaction but on the proper spatial positioning of these functional groups as determined by the drug's conformation. Knowledge of the conformation of a drug when bound to the active site could be of great help in designing improved pharmaceutical agents. For example, this information could be used in the design of rigid analogs that restrict the molecule in the bioactive conformation. Because of a decrease in entropy upon binding, this new analog may exhibit a higher affinity for the receptor or, when related subclasses of receptors/enzymes exist, a higher selectivity for its particular target site. In addition, the conformational information could be used to design new compounds that are drastically different in their structural framework and therefore in their physical properties. These types of changes are especially important in the design of peptide analogs in which peptide bond replacements are sought to increase metabolic stability and oral activity.

Ideally, one would like to determine the three-dimensional structure of a drug when bound to its biological site of action. However, in many cases, the drug's target site is a membrane-bound protein or a biomacromolecule that is not amenable for study by high-resolution NMR techniques, nor is it usually available in quantities sufficient for the NMR experiments. In lieu of studying the conformation of a drug when bound to its active site, the conformational properties of drug molecules in solution by themselves may be examined using NMR methods. Indeed, many investigations (for examples see Refs. 1– 10) have focused on the conformational analysis of drug molecules in solution in an attempt to understand the conformational requirements for biological activity.

In the next few parts of this section, modern one- and two-dimensional NMR methods for studying the conformations of molecules in solution will be described as well as the computational methods used to generate three-dimensional structures that are consistent with the NMR data. In addition, applications and limitations of these methods toward the design of new pharmaceutical agents will be presented.

A. Chemical Shift Assignments

1. Proton NMR

To obtain three-dimensional structures by NMR, the individual NMR signals must first be associated with a particular nucleus in the molecule; in other words, the NMR spectrum must be assigned. Typically, the first step in assigning a proton NMR spectrum is to identify those protons that are scalar (through-bond) coupled to one another (i.e., those that belong to the same spin system). These individual spin systems are composed of protons that are generally connected by no more than three bonds, since proton-proton couplings are typically very small or absent for protons separated by more than three bonds.

The protons belonging to the same spin systems can be identified by a variety of two-dimensional scalar correlation experiments, each having its own particular advantage (for a review of the basic principles of 2-D NMR and the advantages of different 2-D NMR experiments, see Refs. 11–16). An example of one of these experiments (double quantum filtered correlation spectroscopy; DQF COSY) (17,18) is shown in Figure 1. From an analysis of the locations of the cross-peaks (signals that have different frequencies in the two dimensions), the scalar (through-bond) coupled protons are identified as illustrated (Fig. 1) for the leucine residue of a cyclic hexapeptide LHRH antagonist [1] (structure shown in Fig. 2).

Other two-dimensional correlation experiments that are useful in identifying scalar coupled protons have also been described. These experiments complement the basic COSY experiment. For example, correlation experiments have been designed to simplify the analysis of 2-D NMR contour maps (e.g., multiple quantum filters) (18,19), eliminate unwanted diagonal peaks (e.g., multiple quantum NMR experiments) (20–24), or produce additional correlations used in resolving ambiguities in the assignments—e.g., relayed correlation (25–29) and total correlation spectroscopy (TOCSY) (30).

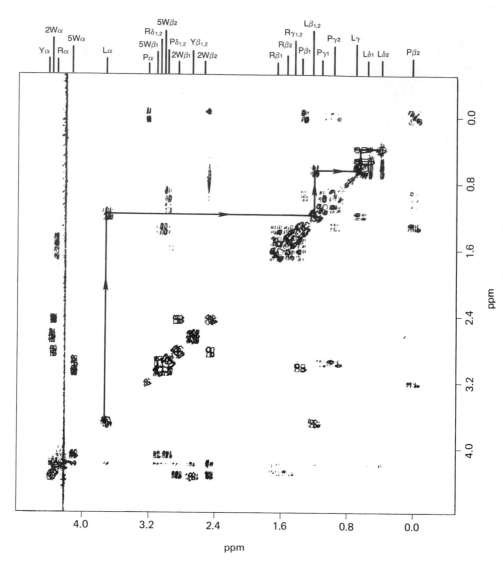

Figure 1 Contour plot of a two-dimensional double-quantum filtered COSY experiment of a cyclic hexapeptide LHRH antagonist [1] acquired in DMSO–d6/D$_2$O (66/34). The solid lines connect the cross-peaks corresponding to the protons of the leucine residue and illustrate how the scalar coupled protons are correlated.

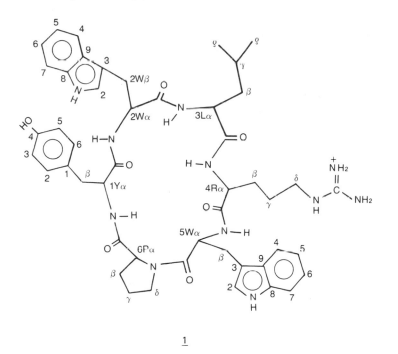

<u>1</u>

Figure 2 Chemical structure of a cyclic hexapeptide that has been shown to act as an LHRH antagonist.

An example of a TOCSY, or homonuclear Hartmann-Hahn (HOHAHA) experiment (31,32) as it is sometimes called, is shown in Figure 3. In this experiment, net coherence transfer (scalar coupling information) between all members of the spin systems can be obtained while retaining the possibility of near absorption line shapes (important for higher sensitivity and better resolution). Thus, unlike in the COSY experiment, in which only directly coupled protons can be identified, additional cross-peaks (Fig. 3; e.g., R$\alpha \rightarrow \gamma$, δ; L$\alpha \rightarrow \gamma$, δ; P$\alpha \rightarrow \gamma$, δ) are present in the 2-D HOHAHA spectra of the cyclic LHRH antagonist that are not observed in the 2-D double quantum filtered COSY spectra (cf. Fig. 1). These additional cross-peaks can be very helpful in resolving assignment ambiguities due to spectral overlap. Futhermore, these spectra have the advantage of being nearly absorptive (see slices displayed at the top of the contour map).

Three-dimensional NMR experiments have also been recently described (33–35) to identify scalar coupled protons. Analogous to the comparison of 2-D with 1-D NMR, 3-D NMR spectroscopy allows an increase in resolution

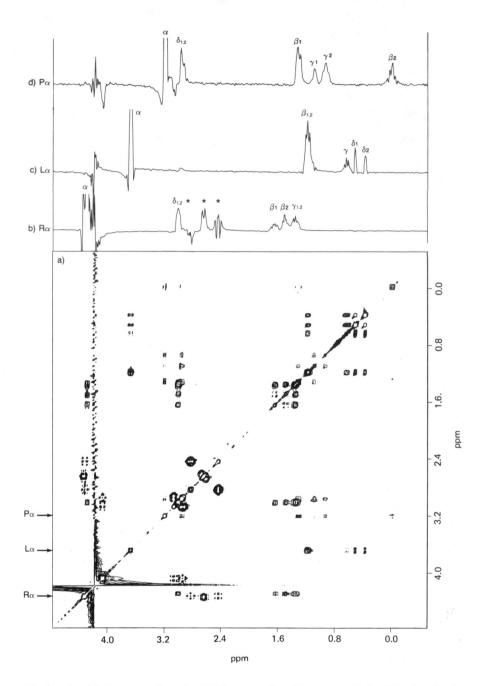

Figure 3 (a) Contour plot of a 2-D homonuclear Hartmann-Hahn experiment of [1] in DMSO−d6/D₂O (66/34). Note the additional cross-peaks observed in this spectrum compared to the double-quantum filtered COSY spectrum (Fig. 1). (b−d) Slices along ω2 extracted from the homonuclear Hartmann-Hahn experiment at the

138

compared to 2-D NMR by separating the chemical shift and scalar/dipolar connectivity information such as that obtained from correlation spectroscopy (COSY) or nuclear Overhauser effect spectroscopy (NOESY) along a third axis. Indeed, homonuclear 3-D NMR experiments (e.g., COSY–COSY, NOESY–COSY) have been reported (33,34) which provide additional resolving power as demonstrated from the proton NMR spectra of a nonapeptide (34). Another approach for the simplification of homonuclear 2-D NMR spectra is heteronuclear 3-D NMR spectroscopy (35). In these experiments, conventional 2-D NMR spectra (COSY, NOESY) are simplified by editing along the third axis with respect to the different heteronuclear frequencies. Because of the lack of correlation between proton and heteronuclear (e.g., ^{15}N) chemical shifts, spectral overlap may be resolved, allowing even complicated spectra to be interpreted.

After identifying the scalar coupled protons, the next step in a typical assignment procedure (e.g., 36,37) is to spatially connect the scalar coupled networks. For this purpose, the nuclear Overhauser effect (NOE) can be used to identify the protons that are close in space (38). Figure 4A depicts a contour map of a 2-D NOE experiment of the cyclic hexapeptide [1] in DMSO–d6/H$_2$O (66/34). By tracing the location of the NH→αCH cross-peaks as shown in Figure 4B, the individual amino acid spin systems can be connected, completing the proton NMR assignments.

2. Carbon-13 NMR

Once either the proton or carbon-13 NMR signals have been assigned, the unassigned NMR resonances (^1H or ^{13}C) can be identified using a two dimensional one-bond heteronuclear scalar correlation experiment. Several variations of this experiment have been described in which the carbon-13 NMR signals are detected (11,39–45). However, the most sensitive way of performing heteronuclear shift correlation experiments is by the detection of the protons (40–45). An example of a proton detected one-bond heteronuclear shift correlation spectrum of [1] is shown in Figure 5. As illustrated for tyrosine, the protonated ^{13}C NMR resonances are assigned by correlating the ^{13}C NMR signals to the assigned proton NMR signals. Heteronuclear relay experiments (45–48) have also proved to be useful to assign protonated

α-proton frequency of (b) arginine, (c) leucine, and (d) proline. As described in the text, the signals are nearly absorptive, which has several advantages over experiments (e.g., relayed COSY) with mixed phase/line shapes that are typically processed in the absolute value mode. Some additional signals (*) are observed in the slice (b) at the arginine α-proton frequency which correspond to overlapping signals of tyrosine and 2-tryptophan.

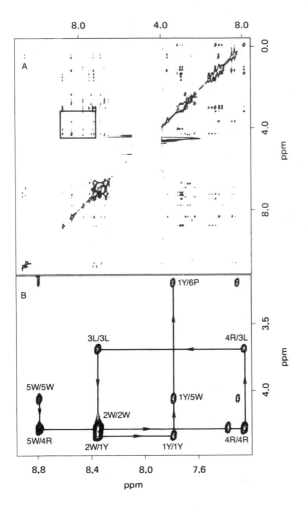

Figure 4 A. Contour plot of an absorption mode 2-D NOE experiment of [1] in DMSO–d6/H$_2$O (66/34) acquired using a mixing time of 100 msec. The large H$_2$O signal was suppressed by selective irradiation during the delay between scans and mixing time. B. Expansion of the NH/αCH region (boxed-in portion) of the 2-D NOE spectrum shown in A. The cross-peaks corresponding to the NH/αCH dipolar connectivities within the same amino acid and between adjacent residues are traced by solid lines. Note the cross-peak (1Y/5W) corresponding to a NOE between the tyrosine NH and 5-tryptophan αCH, supporting a defined conformation (*cis*-peptide bond between proline and 5-tryptophan).

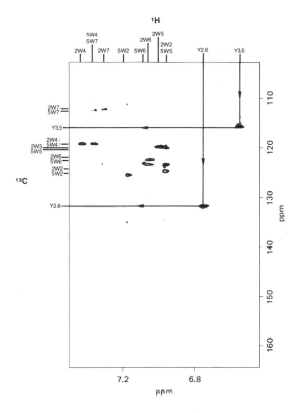

Figure 5 The aromatic region of a proton-detected one-bond $^1H\,^{13}C$ correlation map of **1**. As illustrated for the tyrosine residue (solid lines), the location of the cross-peaks identifies the frequencies of the carbon ($\omega1$) and directly attached proton ($\omega2$). The proton and carbon assignments are indicated in the figure.

^{13}C NMR spectra. In these experiments, the ^{13}C NMR resonances are assigned from correlations between the carbons and protons attached to adjacent ^{13}C nuclei.

To assign the nonprotonated carbon-13 NMR signals and confirm the protonated carbon assignments, long-range $^1H–^{13}C$ correlation experiments (49–52) may be used. Analogous to the one-bond heteronuclear shift correlation experiments, the proton-detected versions of these experiments (51,52) offer the highest sensitivity and are the methods of choice. Figure 6 depicts the aromatic region of a proton-detected multiple-bond heteronuclear correlation map of **1**. As illustrated in the figure, the 2-tryptophan-8 carbon (2W8) (solid lines) and the non-protonated 1,4-tyrosine carbon ro

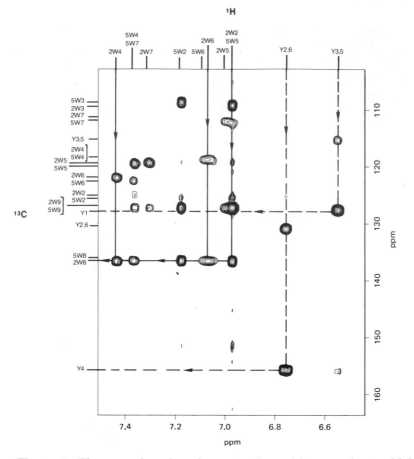

Figure 6 The aromatic region of a proton-detected heteronuclear multiple bond correlation map of [1]. As illustrated for tyrosine (dashed lines) and 2-tryptophan (solid lines), the cross-peaks connect the proton ($\omega2$) and carbon ($\omega1$) frequencies of those coupled nuclei that are separated by two or three bonds. Although one-bond ^{1}H–^{13}C correlations were suppressed in the experiment, some cross-peaks corresponding to these correlations were detected (e.g., tyrosine 2,6).

sonances (dashed lines) could be easily assigned through their three-bond coupling to protons 2W4, 2W6, 2W2, and Y2,6, Y3,5, respectively. The long-range ^{1}H–^{13}C correlations observed in this experiment can also be used to connect the individual proton NMR spin systems. As previously described (50), this may be accomplished in peptides through the detection of long-range ^{1}H–^{13}C scalar correlations between the carbonyl carbon resonances of one amino acid and the protons of the adjacent residue.

B. NMR Parameters Describing Conformations

1. Chemical Shifts

After assigning the proton and carbon-13 NMR signals, the next step is to extract the important NMR parameters from the spectra which define the three-dimensional structure. One of these parameters, chemical shifts, is obtained directly from the assignments. Large variations in chemical shifts have been interpreted in terms of the proximity of the nucleus to aromatic rings (53–55). However, ring current shifts (53–55) are generally difficult to interpret owing to the dependence of the shifts on other contributions besides the distance between the proton/carbon and aromatic ring and therefore should only be used as confirmatory evidence for a structure determined by other means.

2. J-Coupling

Another NMR parameter that has been used to provide structural information is vicinal spin-spin coupling constants. Three-bond $^1H-^1H$ and $^1H-^{13}C$ J-couplings can provide information on dihedral angles through a semiempirical relationship originally described by Karplus (56):

$$^3J(\theta) = A\cos^2\theta - B\cos\theta + C$$

The coefficients (A, B, and C) depend, among other factors, on the electronegativities of the substituents. In practice, the coefficients that are used are those derived from the measured vicinal coupling constants of rigid, low-molecular-weight compounds (for a review see Bystrov, 57) or those experimentally observed for small proteins (58).

To obtain the proton-proton vicinal coupling constants from the NMR spectra, the difference in frequency between the component lines of a multiplet are analyzed and, in many cases, may simply be extracted from one-dimensional proton NMR spectra. However, when severe overlap of the NMR signals is present, it may be difficult to extract the coupling information in this manner. In these cases, various one- (59,60) and two-dimensional NMR experiments (61–66) may be of help. For example, from an analysis of the cross-peaks from a high-resolution phase-sensitive COSY data set shown in Figure 7 of atrial natriuretic factor, the $^3J_{NH-\alpha CH}$ couplings for all of the amino acid residues were obtained.

For larger spin systems, the COSY cross-peaks are not as easy to interpret owing to their complexity, and other approaches are required to obtain the J values. These include (1) different methods of processing the COSY data (taking the sums and differences of appropriately phased cross and diagonal peaks) (62); (2) COSY experiments with soft pulses (66); and (3) exclusive correlation spectroscopy (E.COSY) (63,64) in which the coherence transfers

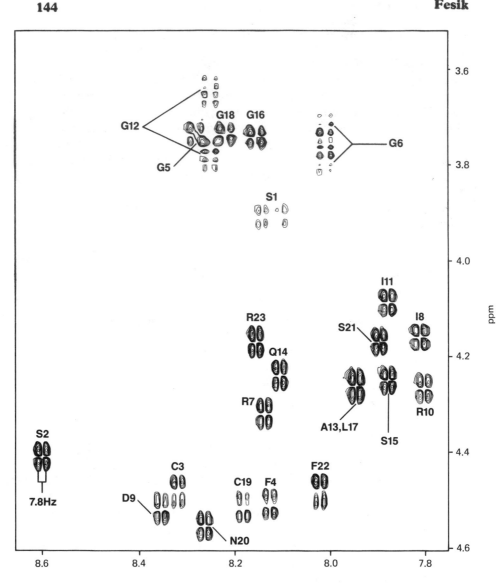

Figure 7   Contour plot of the NH(ω2)/αCH(ω1) region of a high-resolution phase-sensitive COSY experiment of ANF(5–27). The vicinal spin-spin coupling constants ($^3J_{NH-\alpha CH}$) are obtained by measuring the difference in frequency between the positive and negative contours of the individual cross peaks. [Source: Fesik et al. (110).]

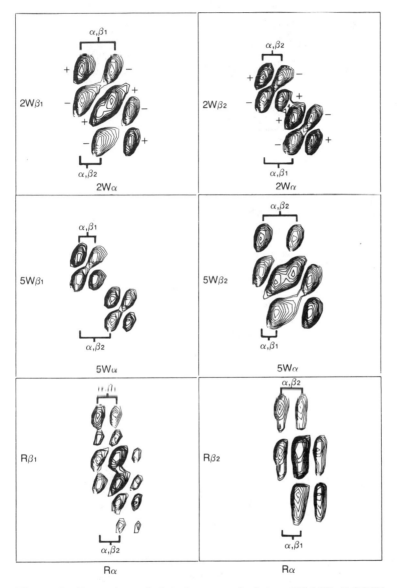

Figure 8 Expansions of selected cross-peaks from a 500-MHz E.COSY spectrum of
[1] in DMSO–d6/D$_2$O (66/34). Both positive and negative contours are plotted.
From the cross-peak simplication achieved in this experiment, coupling constants can
more easily be extracted.

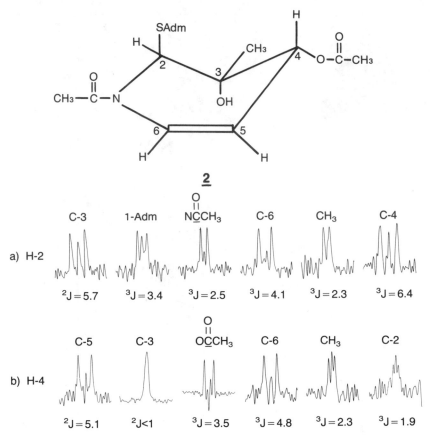

Figure 9 Slices taken along $\omega 1$ from a selective long-range heteronuclear 2-D J-resolved spectrum of [2]. Long-range $^1H-^{13}C$ couplings are observed between the carbons indicated at the top of the $\omega 1$ plots (20 Hz) and the protons (a) H-2 and (b) H-4 that were inverted with a selective 180° pulse. From an analysis of the data (e.g., J-couplings of H-2/1-Adm, H-4/O(C = O)CH$_3$, H-2/C-4), the location and stereochemistry of the substituents were determined (69).

are restricted exclusively to connected transitions. As illustrated in the E.COSY spectra of Figure 8, the cross-peak fine structure is simplified compared to COSY cross-peaks, allowing vicinal proton-proton coupling constants to be readily extracted.

Three-bond $^1H-^{13}C$ coupling constants can also provide information on dihedral angles (57) and therefore have proved to be useful in structural elucidation and in conformational studies (68–71). These data may be extracted from an analysis of ^{13}C NMR spectra acquired with selective proton decoupling or from heteronuclear 2D J-resolved experiments using a selective 180° proton pulse (72,73). As shown in Figure 9, in the selective 2-D J-resolved experiment, long-range $^1H-^{13}C$ coupling is only observed between the carbons and the proton that was selectively inverted. This feature greatly facilitates the identification and extraction of the three-bond $^1H-^{13}C$ coupling constants. As illustrated in the spectra shown in Figure 9, the heteronuclear coupling constants were easily extracted and used to determine the structure of the substituted tetrahydropyridine [2] shown above the spectra (69).

Approaches to *qualitatively* measure three-bond $^1H-^{13}C$ coupling constants have also been proposed (51,70,71). Using the intensity of $^1H-^{13}C$ cross-peaks in ^{13}C or ^1H detected long-range heteronuclear correlation experiments, information on the relative size of the heteronuclear couplings was obtained and used in conformational studies (70,71). However, although the cross-peak intensities measured in these experiments may actually reflect the size of the $^1H-^{13}C$ coupling in some cases, the cross-peak intensity is also a function of the passive coupling that can lead to erroneous interpretations. Nevertheless, when appropriately applied, these methods can be a valuable aid in conformational investigations.

3. Nuclear Overhauser Effect

Perhaps the most important and widely used NMR parameter to define three-dimensional structures is the nuclear Overhauser effect (NOE). The NOE is a measure of the dipole-dipole relaxation between spins that are close in space. The magnitude of the NOE is both a function of the proton-proton distance (r) and the correlation time (r_c) (a measure of mobility) as given by the expression:

$$NOE \; \alpha \; \frac{1}{r^6} \cdot f(\tau_c)$$

Because of the r^{-6} dependence, NOEs are very large for protons in close spatial proximity (2.0–3.0 Å) but rapidly become smaller as the distance is increased. Depending on the signal-to-noise ratio in the NOE experiment, NOEs corresponding to proton-proton distances up to 3.5–4.5 Å can typically be detected.

Although a qualitative interpretation of the NOE data is sufficient for assignment purposes, a more quantitative analysis of the NOEs is useful in conformational studies. For a quantitative evaluation of two-dimensional NOE data, a measure of the cross-peak volumes/intensities is required as well as a method to convert these measurements into proton-proton distances.

Several methods with varying degrees of complexity have been proposed (74–82) for quantifying NOE data in terms of proton-proton distances. In the complete relaxation rate matrix approach, the cross relaxation rate matrix, R, is obtained from a matrix of measured cross (76–80) and diagonal peak

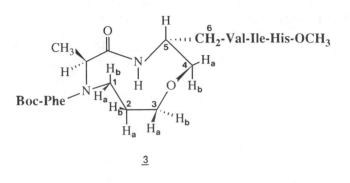

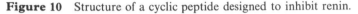

<u>3</u>

Figure 10   Structure of a cyclic peptide designed to inhibit renin.

volumes, $V(\tau_m)$, using the equation

$$V(\tau_m) = V° e^{-R\tau_m}$$

where $V°$ is the volume matrix of the cross and diagonal peaks at $\tau_m = 0$. The individual cross-relaxation rates, σ_{ij}, extracted from the relaxation rate matrix, R, are used to calculate proton-proton distances. Assuming that the dynamics of the internuclear vectors are similar, unknown distances, r_{ij}, are obtained from the cross-relaxation rates, σ, and a known distance, r_{kl}, using the equation

$$r_{ij} = \left[r_{kl}^6 \frac{\sigma_{kl}}{\sigma_{ij}} \right]^{1/6}$$

This method has the advantage of accounting for spin diffusion in the data analysis, resulting in a more accurate determination of proton-proton distances (83,84). In addition, NOEs obtained at longer mixing times may be analyzed where the sensitivity is higher, allowing additional long-range proton-proton distances to be interpreted. The disadvantage with this method is that many peak volumes are required that are difficult to obtain, especially for the diagonal peaks. Nevertheless, provided that some of these limitations can be overcome, this method can be very effective (84) as illustrated in the conformational analysis of a cyclic peptide (Fig. 10, [**3**]). Figure 11 depicts a two-dimensional NOE spectrum of [**3**] from which the cross- and diagonal peak volumes were extracted. Proton-proton distances were calculated from a multispin analysis of the measured volumes obtained from a series of two-dimensional NOE data sets acquired with different mixing times. In Figure 12, representative examples of the NOE data are shown, including simulations based on the relaxation matrix obtained from the measured cross- and diagonal peak volumes. By obtaining many accurate

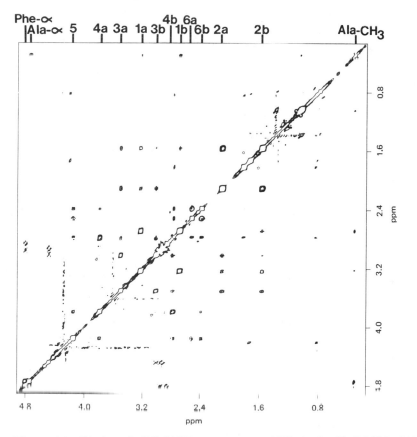

Figure 11 Portion of a 2-D NOE contour map of [3] obtained in DMSO–d6/D₂O (66/34). Assignments are given at the top of the plot. [Source: Fesik et al. (84).]

proton-proton distances from a quantitative analysis of two-dimensional NOE data, three-dimensional structures of the constrained cyclic peptide were obtained and used, in part, to explain the compound's inability to inhibit human renin (85) as described in Chapter 8 (86).

A much simpler approach for calculating unknown proton-proton distances, r_{ij}, from two-dimensional NOE data can be applied (75) using the expression:

$$r_{ij} = \left[r_{kl}^6 \frac{I_{kl}}{I_{ij}} \right]^{1/6}$$

in which r_{kl} is a known distance and I_{kl} and I_{ij} are cross-peak volumes or intensities. In addition to the assumption that the correlation times for the different parts of the molecule are the same, this equation assumes that the

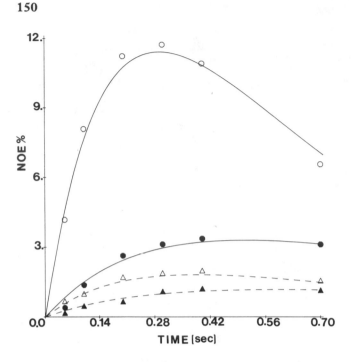

Figure 12   Experimental 2-D NOE data [(○) 2a−2b; (●) 4b−6b; (△) 2a−3b; (▲) 4a−6a] compared to multispin simulations based on the relation matrix obtained from the measured cross-peak and diagonal peak volumes. [Source: Fesik et al. (84).]

cross-peak volumes/intensities are proportional to the cross-relaxation rates. This assumption will only hold true at short mixing times where spin-diffusion and other relaxation effects are negligible. Therefore, in these studies, short mixing times must be employed. Unfortunately, NOEs observed under these conditions are low in intensity, especially for protons separated by longer distances, which are often the most important in defining molecular structure. On the other hand, this method has the advantage of only requiring the cross-peak intensities (diagonal peak intensities are not required) and, because of the r^{-6} dependence on the NOE, can be a reasonably accurate method for calculating proton-proton distances.

   In addition to the methods used to calculate proton-proton distances from NOE data, an important consideration is the manner in which the NOE data are collected. For example, in addition to cross-peaks arising from NOEs, two-dimensional NOE spectra may contain additional peaks originating from the coherent transfer of magnetization (J-peaks) (87−89). Fortunately, modifications of the basic two-dimensional NOE experiment have been described (87−89) that can suppress these unwanted peaks.

Another problem that can occur in the collection of two-dimensional NOE data is the absence of NOE cross-peaks despite the close proximity of protons. This can occur when the reciprocal of the spectrometer frequency is close to the correlation time, τ_c (90,91). To overcome some of these limitations, experimental approaches [rotating frame NOE (CAMEL-SPIN/ROESY) (90–94), alterations of solvent viscosities (95–99)] have been devised.

Other useful variations of the basic two-dimensional NOE experiment have been proposed for resolving some of the overlap in two-dimensional NOE spectra. Two-dimensional NOE experiments have been designed to suppress diagonal peaks (100,101), transfer NOE cross-peaks from crowded to sparse spectral regions (102), and simplify NOE spectra by filtering out all NOEs except those arising from a proton attached to a heteronuclear label using isotope filtering (103–109). Heteronuclear three-dimensional experiments have also been devised in which 2-D NOE spectra are edited in a third dimension with respect to the heteronuclear frequencies (35).

An example (109) of the utility of the isotope-filtering techniques for simplifying two-dimensional NOE spectra is illustrated in the conformational analysis of atrial natriuretic factor (ANF) (7–23) [**4**] in sodium dodecyl sulfate (SDS-d25) micelles (109) aimed at elucidating the conformational requirements associated with the natriuretic, diuretic, and vasorelaxant activities of these compounds (67,109,110).

```
        10              15              20

C-F  G  G  R  I  D-R-I-G-A-Q-S  G  L  G -C
    |_____|
```

4

SDS was used in these studies to approximate an anisotropic, amphophilic environment such as that found in biological membranes (111).

As shown in Figure 13A, from the conventional two-dimensional NOE experiment, many NOEs could not be interpreted unambiguously because of the overlap of the Q18/G20, G10/R11, and A17/L21 NH signals. However, in the $\omega 2$ isotope-filtered two-dimensional NOE experiment (Fig. 13B) of trilabeled [^{15}N-G10, A17, G20] ANF (7-23), the two-dimensional NOE spectrum is markedly simplified, and those ambiguities can be resolved. For example, as shown in Figure 13B, NOEs are only observed along $\omega 1$ between the protons attached to the ^{15}N-labeled nuclei (G10, A17, G20) and the protons in close proximity to these nuclei within the rest of the molecule. Thus, these NOEs can now be differentiated from NOEs arising from overlapping R11, Q18, and L21 NH protons. Also, by a suitable manipulation of the data, NOEs involving G10, A17, and G20 NH protons can be

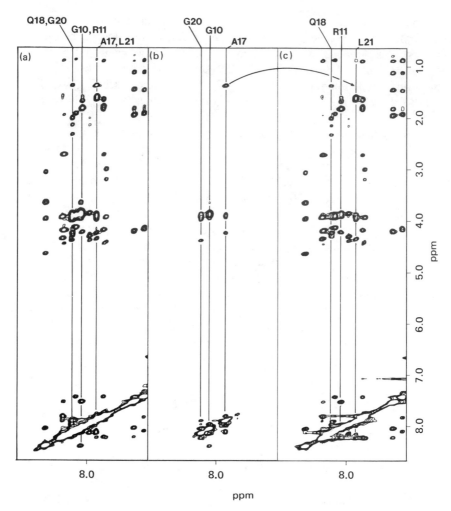

Figure 13 Two-dimensional NOE contour plots of a 10-mM solution of (^{15}N–G10, A17, G20) ANF(7–23) [3] in SDS-d25 micelles (200 mM). A. Conventional 2-D NOE spectrum acquired with ^{15}N decoupling during t_1 and t_2. B, C. $\omega 2$ isotope-filtered 2-D NOE spectra. NOE cross-peaks are observed between protons (B) attached to isotopically labeled (^{15}N) nuclei and all other protons or (C) between protons that are *not* attached to a labeled heteronucleus and the other protons. As illustrated by the arrow for the missing A17NH/A17CH$_3$ NOE, NOEs involving the amide protons attached to ^{15}N labels are absent from the isotope-filtered 2-D NOE spectrum in C. [Source: Fesik et al. (109).]

eliminated, allowing the NOE information arising from the NH protons of Q18, R11, and L21 to be unambiguously obtained (Fig. 13C) (109).

Unlike the conformational averaging observed in our previous NMR studies of ANF analogs in bulk solvent (67,110), the NMR data (NOEs, J-coupling) of ANF (7-23) in SDS micelles was indicative of a more ordered three-dimensional structure composed of three defined loops (112,113).

C. Molecular Modeling

In order to interpret the NMR-derived structural data (proton-proton distances, dihedral angles), computational methods are useful in generating three-dimensional structures. Although hand-held models could be used in the analysis, there are several advantages of computer-generated models. These include the capabilities of (1) evaluating the energetics of the system, (2) obtaining proton-proton distances and dihedral angles more accurately, (3) creating structures that are less biased by user interaction, and (4) having the ability to overlap multiple structures.

Several methods have been proposed (83,84,114–123) for incorporating NMR data into computer-generated structures. These methods, which play an important part in the interpretation and evaluation of the NMR data, are briefly described in the following parts of this section.

1. Interactive Model Building

One method of fitting structures to NMR data is through the manual rotation about the covalent bonds, satisfying one distance constraint at a time. Using this method, however, it is generally difficult to maintain all of the distance constraints simultaneously, especially for larger systems. In addition, besides being tedious and time-consuming, the method is heavily biased by user interactions, making it difficult to evaluate the uniqueness of the structures that are generated.

2. Distance Geometry

Another approach (84,113–118) to generate structures consistent with NMR data is by using a metric matrix or dihedral angle space distance geometry algorithm. For the metric matrix methods (115,119), an $n \times n$ matrix is generated for a molecule with n atoms that contains all possible interatomic distances. The known distances defined by the covalent bonding are input directly, and the experimentally determined distances (e.g., from NOE data) are input in the form of upper and lower bounds. For the remaining interatomic distances, upper and lower bounds are chosen on the basis of the geometry and size of the molecule. After randomly picking distances within the boundary conditions, an initial cartesian coordinate set is generated from the $n \times n$ matrix through an embedding procedure (119).

This initial set of coordinates is then optimized by minimizing the difference in the interatomic distances of the computer-generated structure compared to distances within the chosen upper and lower bounds.

In the dihedral angle distance geometry algorithm (114), initial conformations of a peptide are randomly chosen and folded by varying dihedral angles. The target function used for convergence is varied to include only short-range distance constraints in the initial stages of the calculation and gradually widened to include the long-range distance constraints. These methods have played an important role in generating protein structures consistent with NMR data.

Figure 14 depicts several conformations of a cyclic peptide [3] generated from a distance geometry algorithm using NMR data as constraints (84). As shown, the structures generated had similar well-defined conformations for the macrocyclic ring but, owing to an insufficient amount of NMR data, the noncyclic portion of the peptide could not be defined. These results point to some of the advantages and disadvantages of distance geometry. A key advantage is that the structures are generated automatically and are unbiased by user interaction. Thus, structures may be found by this approach that may not have been considered otherwise, and information on the ability of the NMR data to define the structure for different parts of the molecule may be obtained. The disadvantage of the structures obtained from distance geometry is that the energetics of the bonded and nonbonded interactions are not taken into account. Consequently, the structures that are generated may be energetically unfavorable. These limitations can be overcome when distance geometry is combined with other methods that consider the energetics of the system.

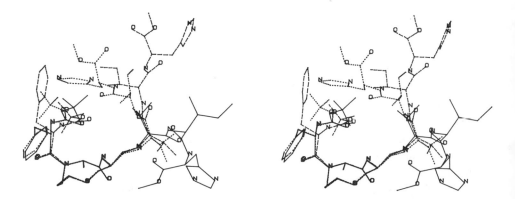

Figure 14 Stereoview of representative structures of [3] generated from distance geometry followed by energy minimization. [Source: Fesik et al. (84).]

(a)

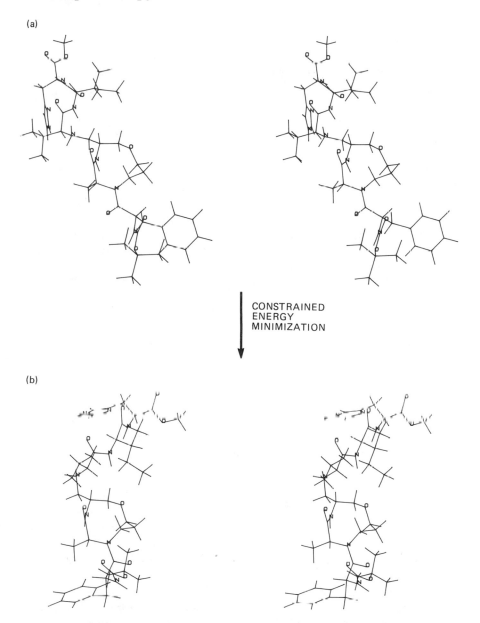

CONSTRAINED
ENERGY
MINIMIZATION

(b)

Figure 15 (a) Stereoview of [3] that was inconsistent with the NMR data (*trans* Phe–Ala peptide bond). (b) Structure consistent with the NMR data that was generated by constrained energy minimization. [Source: Fesik et al (84).]

3. Constrained Energy Minimization

Another approach, constrained or restrained energy minimization (83,84,120), employs an energy minimization routine with a force field containing an extra term of the form, $K(r - ro)^2$, to constrain the interproton distances (r) of the structure to the experimentally determined distances (ro). In some cases, this method is sufficient to create structures that are consistent with NMR data. For example (84), as shown in Figure 15, using a starting structure of [3] inconsistent with the NMR data (*trans*-Phe-Ala peptide bond), constrained energy minimization was successful in producing a structure with a *cis*-Phe-Ala peptide bond that agreed with the NMR results. However, in general, owing to the inability of overcoming local energy minima, constrained energy minimization is expected and has been shown (120) to have poor convergence properties. Therefore, constrained energy minimization is most effectively applied when the starting structure that is used as input is close to the optimum structure, such as those structures obtained from distance geometry.

4. Constrained Molecular Dynamics

A more convergent method to refine structures on the basis of NMR data is constrained molecular dynamics (84,117,118,120–123). Using this approach, molecular dynamics calculations (124) are performed using a modified potential energy function such as that used in constrained energy minimization. Compared to constrained energy minimization, constrained molecular dynamics can more easily overcome energy barriers between local minima and is therefore less sensitive to starting structure. However, for large molecules in which enormous energy barriers must be crossed to produce structural changes, interactive manipulation of the structure may be required (121) in combination with constrained molecular dynamics to get out of deep energy wells.

D. Applications and Limitations

How can the conformational information determined by NMR for molecules in solution be applied to drug design? As mentioned previously, knowledge of the "bioactive" conformation could be used to design rigid analogs with increased affinity and/or higher selectivity for a particular biological target as well as to design compounds that contain the important functional groups held together in the correct spatial orientation by a more metabolically resistant framework. However, it is well known that the conformation of a drug in solution is often highly dependent on its environment and is not necessarily the same as the bioactive conformation. In fact, for most molecules, several conformations with only very small energy differences exist in solution, and, in these cases, very little can be learned from conformational studies to aid in the design of new molecules. On the other hand, if conformational restrictions can be introduced without significant alteration in the biological activity, the solution conformation as determined from NMR is likely to be similar to the bioactive conformation and can be used to propose new analogs. In addition, the solution conformation of the new synthetic restricted molecules may be examined using NMR and compared to the template from which they were designed. In this way, the contributions to biological activity from conformation may be separated from the requirements of the particular chemical entities needed for interaction with the biological target. Thus, provided an active rigid analog can be found, a better understanding of structure-activity relationships can be gained.

Examples of this approach in the design of conformationally constrained opioid peptides (125) and peptide inhibitors of cholate uptake by hepatocytes (126) are described in Chapters 11 and 12, respectively. In both examples, NMR spectroscopy was employed to determine the solution conformations of conformationally restricted peptides. As described in the individual chapters, this information was helpful in the design of peptide analogs with increased biological activity (125) or improved receptor selectivity (126).

III. SMALL MOLECULE–
LARGE MOLECULE INTERACTIONS

In principle, NMR studies on drug/active site complexes could provide additional and more useful structural information than can be obtained from conformational investigations of drug molecules by themselves. In studies of drugs interacting with their target site, the "bioactive" conformation is *not* determined on the basis of the assumed similarities between it and the solution conformation, but is obtained directly. Therefore, these studies do not require conformationally restricted, biologically active lead compounds (which are generally not available). In contrast to conformational studies of drug molecules by themselves, compounds that are relatively flexible in solution may be used, since they are likely to adopt a preferred conformation upon interaction with their target site. In addition to the conformation of the bound drug, structural information may be obtained from these studies with regard to new potential binding sites in close proximity to the bound drug. This information may help in designing compounds that possess additional functional groups for interaction with new areas of the target.

Unfortunately, as mentioned previously, the biomacromolecules that function as drug target sites are not generally available in sufficient quantity or purity, nor are they usually amenable for study by high-resolution NMR techniques owing to the large number and increased line width of the resonances. Recently, however, technological advances have been made that allow for the isolation and preparation of large quantities of biomacromolecules. In addition, new NMR methods have been developed for studies of large systems. These new developments will be described as well as experimental approaches that employ small models for a drug's active site that are more amenable to study by conventional high-resolution NMR techniques.

A. Small Molecular Complexes

Provided that a small (MW < 10,000), realistic model for a drug's target can be found, the conformation of a bound drug as well as the relative spatial orientation of the functional groups necessary for binding may be determined. The NMR methods that can be used to obtain structural information on small molecular complexes are those that were described earlier in this chapter. The proton NMR signals are assigned by identifying the scalar and dipolar coupled protons, and the relevant conformational parameters (J-coupling, NOEs) for the complex are extracted and analyzed. In addition to intramolecular NOEs, which define the conformation of the ligand and macromolecule, intermolecular NOEs are obtained that are important to define those protons of the ligand that are in close proximity to the protons of the target biomacromolecule.

An example of the power of this approach is illustrated in the NMR studies of drug-DNA interactions (127–132). Detailed structures of drugs bound to small fragments of DNA have been elucidated using NMR spectroscopy (131,132). From these studies, the bound conformation of the drug as well as the binding mode (intercalator, minor groove, etc.) and chemical groups of the drug that interact with DNA are deduced. For example, in a ^1H and ^{31}P NMR study of a chromomycin/d(ATGCAT)$_2$ complex (132), the bound conformation of the DNA duplex (a right-handed B conformation with distortions at the TCG region) and the orientation of chromomycin in the active site (major groove near the TG region) was elucidated.

Another example in which NMR has been used to define the interactions of a drug with a model "receptor" is in the study of the glycopeptide antibiotics bound to models for the bacterial cell wall (83,133–138). The glycopeptide antibiotics act by binding specifically to cell wall precursors ending in D-alanyl-D-alanine. Di- and tripeptide models (Ac–D–Ala–D–Ala and Ac$_2$–Lys–D–Ala–D–Ala) of cell wall precursors have been shown (133–136) to be suitable models for the glycopeptide's site of action. NMR studies of glycopeptide/peptide complexes have yielded detailed structures

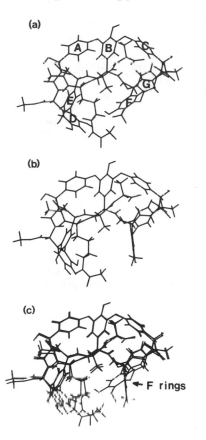

(a)

(b)

(c)

← F rings

Figure 16 Structures (a and b) of the ristocetin aglycone/Ac$_2$–Lys–D–Ala–D–Ala complex obtained after energy minimization of two structures selected from a molecular dynamics trajectory. The NOE data suggest that both structures, which differ in F-ring conformations (c), are present in solution. [Source: Fesik et al. (83).]

(83,135–138) which have been used in an attempt to design analogs that retain the binding affinity to peptide precursors ending in D-alanyl-D-alanine with additional advantages (e.g., oral activity, activity against gram-negative bacteria) compared to the naturally occurring glycopeptide antibiotics (16).

Figure 16 depicts a set of computer-generated structures of a glycopeptide: Ac$_2$–Lys–D–Ala–D–Ala complex that were consistent with the proton-proton distances obtained from a quantitative evaluation of several 2-D NOE data sets. As previously described (83), the NMR data were best explained by considering an average between two structures with different F-ring conformations (Fig. 16C) which were selected from a short molecular dynamics trajectory. From the structural information obtained in these (83) and other NMR studies of glycopeptide: peptide complexes (135–138) as well as from conformational studies of glycopeptides in solution, important structural features for binding were obtained. Attempts have been made to utilize this information in the design of smaller analogs of the glycopeptide antibiotics with potentially greater clinical utility. Unfortunately, however, the synthesis of substituted diphenyl ethers is difficult, and, to date, no biologically active small analog has been identified.

B. Large Molecular Complexes—Weakly Bound Ligands

A severe limitation of NMR studies on the interactions of drugs with receptor mimics is the lack of suitable small active-site models. Typically, drug target sites are larger than MW 10,000 and are difficult to study by conventional proton NMR experiments owing to the severe overlap and increased line width of the NMR signals. For weakly bound ligands, however, experimental approaches originally described by Feeney and co-workers (139) have been developed to study large molecular complexes, thus providing the groundwork for NMR studies on many more pharmacologically relevant biological systems. In principle, the approach involves the transfer of cross-relaxation (NOE) information between two bound ligand protons to the more easily observed free or averaged resonances of the ligand by chemical exchange (139–142). Unlike the ligand, the biomacromolecule to which it binds is generally in the slow tumbling limit (i.e., $\omega\tau_C \gg 1$). Consequently, NOEs observed between protons of the bound ligand appear as negative NOEs and can be used to define the bound conformation of the ligand. Indeed, for molecules with the proper exchange rate, the conformations of ligands bound to proteins (143–148), phospholipids (149), and nucleic acids (150) have been determined.

An application of the transferred NOE experiment is illustrated for the study of the conformation of cytidine triphosphate (CTP) when bound to CMP–KDO synthetase. This bacterial enzyme catalyzes the synthesis of the activated precursor (CMP–KDO) from CTP (Fig. 17) that is required for the incorporation of 3-deoxy-D-mannooctulosonic acid (KDO) into lipopolysaccharide (151). Figure 18B depicts part of an NMR spectrum of a CTP/CMP–KDO synthetase (20/1) mixture. As shown in the spectrum, the signals corresponding to the ligand are relative sharp compared to the protein, but broader than the signals of free CTP. When the C6 proton of CTP was irradiated in a transferred NOE experiment (Fig. 18A), NOEs were observed between H6 and H5 and between H6 and the 2' proton of the ribose ring.

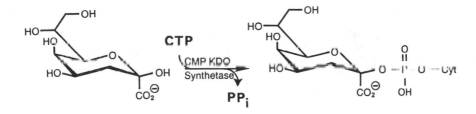

Figure 17 The reaction catalyzed by CMP *KDO synthetase.*

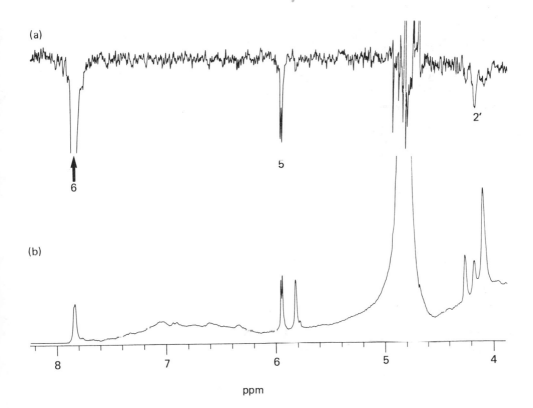

Figure 18 (a) One dimensional transferred NOE difference spectrum of a cytidine triphosphate/CMP*KDO synthetase* complex (20/1) in which the 6-proton of CTP was irridiated. The NOE observed between the 6 and 2' proton is indicative of a 2'-endo-anti conformation. (b) Conventional 1-D spectrum of the same sample shown for comparison.

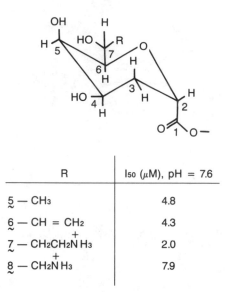

R	I_{50} (μM), pH = 7.6
$\underset{\sim}{5}$ — CH₃	4.8
$\underset{\sim}{6}$ — CH = CH₂	4.3
$\underset{\sim}{7}$ — CH₂CH₂$\overset{+}{N}$H₃	2.0
$\underset{\sim}{8}$ — CH₂$\overset{+}{N}$H₃	7.9

Figure 19 Structures of CMPKDO synthetase inhibitors studied by 2-D transferred NOE experiments and their inhibitory potencies (I_{50}).

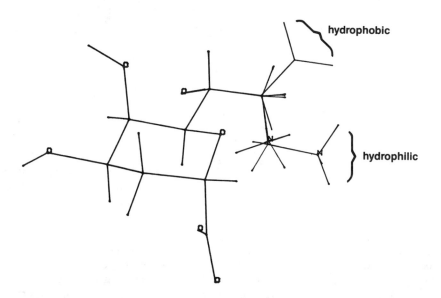

Figure 20 Molecular models of the enzyme-bound conformations of the inhibitors
shown in Figure 19 based on the results from 2-D transferred NOE experiments.

These results are consistent with a C(2′)-endo-anticonformation for CTP when bound to CMP–KDO synthetase.

As mentioned previously, knowledge of the conformation of a bound ligand could be extremely useful to design analogs that mimic this structure. In addition, since it is possible for different molecules to bind to the target site in different conformations, the conformation of a bound ligand may aid in the understanding of structure-activity relationships. Toward this goal, from an analysis of two-dimensional transferred NOE experiments, the bound conformations of a series of CMP-KDO synthetase inhibitors (structures shown in Fig. 19) were determined. The bound conformation of the sugar ring was found to be the same for all of the inhibitors studied; however, the side-chain conformation differed for the inhibitors depending on the hydrophobicity of the side chain (Fig. 19). As will be described elsewhere, these results were used to propose the location of a hydrophobic and hydrophilic binding site (Fig. 20) on the enzyme.

C. Large Molecular Complexes—Tightly Bound Ligands

Although the transferred NOE experiment has been effective in the conformational determinations of bound ligands, a limitation of this experiment is that only weakly bound ligands can be studied. Ideally, one would like to obtain structural information on the compounds with the highest affinity, typically $K_a \geqslant 10^7$. Early attempts to study tightly bound ligands involved the analysis of heteronuclear chemical shifts of isotopically labeled (^{13}C, ^{15}N) ligands in the presence and absence of biomacromolecules. Unfortunately, however, heteronuclear chemical shifts depend on many factors and are therefore usually very difficult to interpret.

In principle, a more fruitful approach would be to utilize the proton-proton distance information that could be obtained from NOE experiments. However, for large systems it is difficult to selectively irradiate the proton of interest and to assign the observed NOEs. Strategies to solve these problems have recently been proposed that could potentially be very valuable in the study of large molecular complexes (47,103–109,112,152–159). These experiments involve the selective observation of protons that are attached to an isotopically labeled nucleus (152,153) as well as their scalar (47,159) or dipolar coupled partners (103–109). These experiments can provide the same detailed structural information and high sensitivity typical of proton NMR experiments with selectivity achieved by editing through the isotope labels.

An example of the type of structural information that can be obtained from isotope-edited proton NMR experiments is illustrated in an NMR study of a pepsin inhibitor [9] (Fig. 21) bound to pepsin (112,160–162). Figure 22 depicts (1) a ^{15}N-decoupled and (2) a ^{15}N-coupled isotope-edited proton

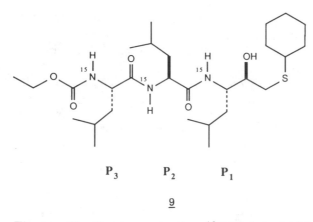

$$\underline{9}$$

Figure 21 Structure of the ^{15}N-labeled inhibitor of porcine pepsin ($IC_{50} = 1.7 \times 10^{-7}$ M) used in the isotope-edited proton NMR experiments.

NMR spectrum of the pepsin/inhibitor complex (1 mM) in H_2O/D_2O (9/1) compared to a conventional proton NMR spectrum of the complex (Fig. 22C). Only those NMR signals corresponding to protons of **9** (Fig. 21) that are attached to ^{15}N are observed in the isotope-filtered experiment (160). As shown in Figure 23, the ability to selectively observe the amide protons of the bound ligand allowed the NH exchange rates of the bound inhibitor to be measured from a series of ^{15}N isotope-filtered proton NMR spectra acquired at various times after preparation of the complex in D_2O (160). As judged by the rate of disappearance of the NH signals, which were assigned from experiments using singly labeled inhibitors, the NH exchange rates for the different sites were found to be very different and followed the relative order $P_3 > P_2 > P_1$. These results were explained by the relative solvent accessibility for the different amide protons of the bound inhibitor (160). Currently, it is being examined whether the observed differences in NH exchange rate can also be correlated to the structural requirements of the P_1-P_3 NH groups of the inhibitor for hydrogen bonding to porcine pepsin.

Isotope-filtered proton NMR experiments have also been used to simplify 2-D NOE spectra (103–109,112,161,162). An example of an isotope-filtered 2-D NOE experiment of the pepsin/inhibitor [**9**] complex is shown in Figure 24. NOEs were observed (112,161,162) along $\omega 1$ between the protons attached to the ^{15}N-labeled nuclei of the ligand and the protons in close proximity to these nuclei within the inhibitor and pepsin. NOE cross-peaks were assigned from additional experiments using ^{15}N-labeled inhibitors with per-deuterated residues. From an analysis of these NOEs and those observed in ^{13}C-isotope-edited 2-D NOE spectra of ^{13}C-labeled inhibitors bound to

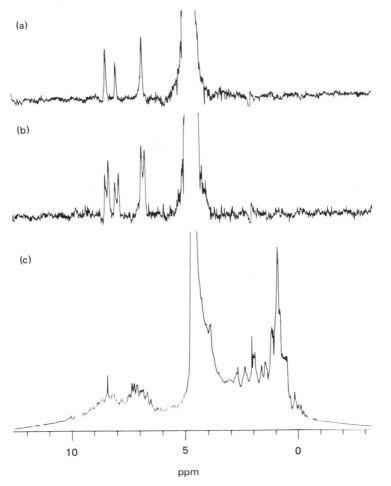

Figure 22 Proton NMR spectra of a H_2O/D_2O (9/1) solution (1 mM) of [9] bound to porcine pepsin (a) ^{15}N-decoupled isotope-edited, (b) ^{15}N-coupled isotope-edited, and (c) conventional proton NMR spectra. [Source: Fesik et al. (160).]

pepsin, the backbone and side-chain conformations of the P_2 and P_3 leucine residues were determined (161).

Isotope-edited 2-D NOE experiments can also be used to elucidate the structure of the active site (161). NOEs observed between the protons of the inhibitor [9] and enzyme identify those protons of the enzyme that are close to the protons of the inhibitor. Although it may be difficult to unambiguously assign these inhibitor/enzyme NOEs, even unassigned NOEs can be of value

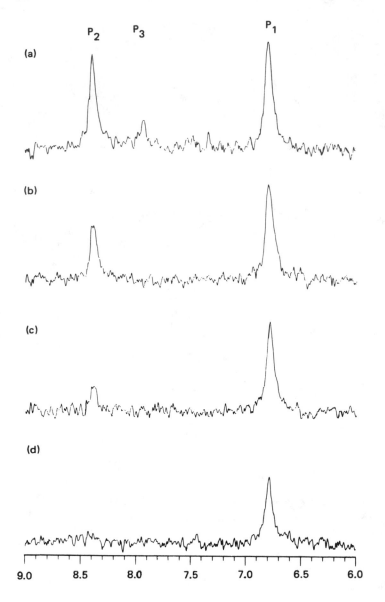

Figure 23 Isotope-edited proton NMR spectra (40°C) acquired at (A) 20, (B) 90, (C) 283, and (D) 1200 min after the preparation of a D$_2$O solution of the pepsin/inhibitor [9] complex. The ^{15}NH assignments of the inhibitor shown at the top of the spectra were made from isotope-edited proton NMR spectra of singly labeled inhibitors. [Source: Fesik et al. (160).]

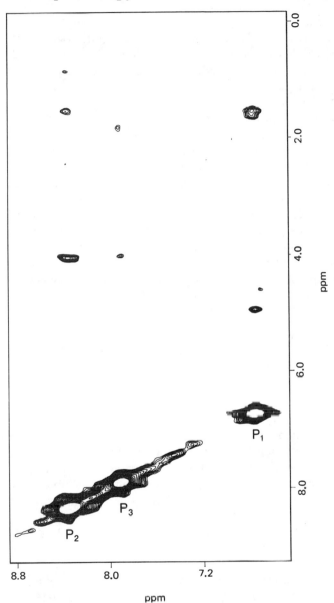

Figure 24 Contour plot of an isotope-filtered 2-D NOE experiment of a 1-mM pepsin/inhibitor [8] complex acquired at 500 MHz using a mixing time of 30 msec. The cross-peaks indicate NOEs between the protons of the bound inhibitor that are bonded to ^{15}N and the other protons of the inhibitor and pepsin. [Source: Fesik et al. (112).]

to test whether different inhibitors are binding to the same site on the enzyme as evidenced by the observation of the same NOEs. In addition, the NOE data may be combined with structural information from other sources such as x-ray crystallography or model building. In these cases, as recently demonstrated for a pepsin/inhibitor complex (161), the structure of the active site may be characterized in detail.

The structural information that is obtained from isotope-edited NMR studies of enzyme/inhibitor complexes could be extremely helpful in the design of improved inhibitors. For example, the NH exchange rates of bound peptide enzyme inhibitors could be used to determine which amides are important for interacting with the enzyme, suggesting which of the individual amides could be modified without altering the binding affinity of the inhibitor. Knowledge of the bound conformation of an enzyme inhibitor could suggest compounds to be synthesized that contain very different and potentially more suitable structural frameworks (e.g., peptidomimetics) which hold the important functional groups of the inhibitor in the orientation determined by the conformation of the bound inhibitor. Finally, the active-site structure could be used to design compounds that fit better into the active site. Indeed, isotope-edited proton NMR experiments can provide useful structural information on inhibitors bound to enzymes or soluble receptors and show great promise for aiding in the design of improved pharmaceutical agents (162).

IV. ENZYME REACTIONS

In addition to providing conformational information on enzyme-bound ligands and identifying amino acid residues in enzyme active sites, NMR has been used to measure the kinetics, stereochemistry, and mechanisms of enzymatic reactions (163) using a variety of NMR parameters (e.g., relaxation measurements, paramagnetic effects, isotope-induced chemical shifts). Thus, NMR is also a useful tool to study enzymatic reactions and the effects of drugs on these reactions which, in turn, could aid in the design of more potent enzyme inhibitors. An example in which even relatively simple NMR experiments (164,165) provided structural information that helped to design a series of enzyme inhibitors is presented below.

Although it has been known for sometime that CMP–KDO synthetase (MW $\sim$ 30,000) catalyzes the reaction shown in Figure 17 (151), the stereochemical and mechanistic details of the reaction were unknown. Information about this reaction was sought from NMR to aid in the development of CMP–KDO synthetase inhibitors which could be of clinical utility as antibiotics against gram-negative bacteria. This approach seemed reasonable, since CMP–KDO is required for the biosynthesis of lipopolysac-

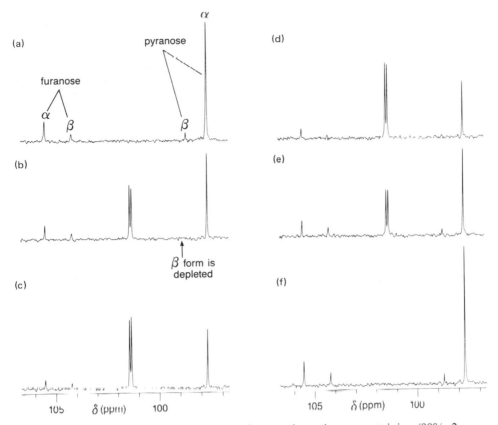

Figure 25 Carbon-13 NMR spectra of a reaction mixture containing (90%, 2-^{13}C)KDO at various times after the addition of CMP–KDO synthetase. Spectrum (a) was taken prior to the addition of enzyme and shows the chemical shifts of the anomeric carbons (C-2) of the four major KDO forms in solution. The times from enzyme addition to the middle of data acquisition were 34, 44, 69, 169, and 369 min for spectra (b–f), respectively. [Source: Kohlbrenner and Fesik (164).]

charide, an important component of the outer membrane of gram-negative bacteria, and is unique to bacterial cells.

Figure 25 shows a series of proton-decoupled ^{13}C NMR spectra taken at different intervals after the addition of CMP–KDO synthetase to a reaction mixture that contained (90%, 2-^{13}C)KDO and other reactants necessary for the formation of CMP–KDO (164). Spectrum (a) was taken prior to the addition of enzyme and shows only the anomeric region of the ^{13}C spectrum where the four major resonances of the two furanose and two pyranose

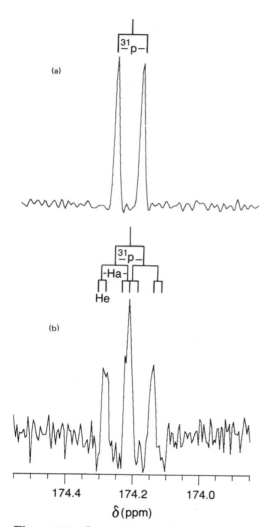

Figure 26 Comparison of the proton-decoupled (a) and proton-coupled (b) ^{13}C NMR spectra of CMP-[1-^{13}C]KDO. [Source: Kohlbrenner and Fesik (164).]

anomers of KDO are found. As shown in spectra (b–d) after the addition of CMP-KDO synthetase, a decrease in the steady-state level of the β-pyranose is observed. These results indicate that the β-pyranose form of KDO, the least populated form in solution, is the actual substrate for the reaction (164).

To determine whether CMP–KDO formation occurs with retention or inversion of configuration at the anomeric center of KDO, long-range [1]H–[13]C couplings between the protons at C-3 and carbon-1 of the KDO were obtained (164). Figure 26A is a proton-decoupled ^{13}C spectrum showing the C-1 resonance of the KDO in CMP-[1-^{13}C]KDO. The 6.9-Hz splitting is due to the 3-bond coupling with the phosphoryl group. In the proton-coupled ^{13}C spectrum of this same resonance (Fig. 26B), the signal is further split, because of additional couplings of 5.7 and 0.9 Hz. These data reflect a diaxial relation between C-1 and H-3$_a$ of the KDO in CMP–KDO and indicate that CMP–KDO has a β-pyranoside structure. CMP–KDO formation thus occurs with retention of configuration at the anomeric center of KDO (164).

Using ^{31}P and ^{13}C NMR, the retention of ^{18}O during CMP–KDO formation was also demonstrated (165). Figure 27 shows a series of ^{13}C NMR

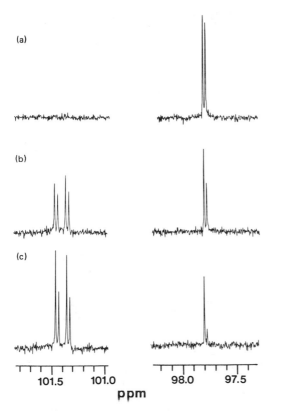

Figure 27 Carbon-13 NMR spectra of CMP–KDO formed in the presence of [90% 2-^{13}C, 50% ^{18}O]KDO at (a) 0, (b) 8.5, and (c) 25 min after the addition of CMP–KDO synthetase. Spectra shown on the left and right are those regions of the spectra for the C-2 resonance of KDO and the C-2 resonance of KDO in CMP–KDO, respectively. Note that the 50% ^{18}O label (spectrum a) is retained in the product CMP–KDO (spectrum b). [Source: Kohlbrenner et al. (165).]

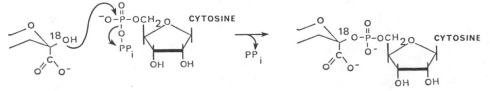

Figure 28 Nucleophilic displacement mechanism postulated for CMP–KDO formation suggested by the NMR experiments. [Source: Kohlbrenner et al. (165).]

spectra of a reaction mixture containing 90% (2-^{13}C, ^{18}O)KDO. As indicated by the relative intensities of the α-pyranose peaks (spectrum a), the KDO pool contained approximately 50% ^{18}O at the anomeric position just prior to starting the reaction. Upon addition of CMP–KDO synthetase, two sets of doublets appeared corresponding to ^{18}O- and ^{16}O-labeled CMP-KDO. These results demonstrate that ^{18}O is retained in the bridge position between CMP and KDO, which suggests that the reaction occurs by a nucleophilic displacement of the pyrophosphoryl group of CTP by the anomeric hydroxyl of KDO (Fig. 28).

On the basis of these NMR results, inhibitors of CMP-KDO synthetase were designed that were locked in the active β-pyranose form (166). In addition, since the mechanism of the reaction was found to involve a nucleophilic displacement by the anomeric hydroxyl of KDO, this hydroxyl group was removed in the analogs so that the inhibitors could no longer act as substrates. These compounds (see Fig. 19) were found to be inhibitors of CMP–KDO synthetase (166).

V.   CONCLUSIONS AND FUTURE PERSPECTIVES

As illustrated in this chapter, at the present time, NMR spectroscopy can provide detailed information on the conformational properties of small molecules in solution, the structure of large molecular complexes, and enzyme reaction mechanisms. It is expected that future developments in NMR and other fields will contribute to even further progress in the ability of NMR to provide useful information toward the design of drugs. Some of these new developments which are expected in the near future include (1) the availability of large quantities of enzymes and drug receptors through improved expression systems and cloning technology; (2) the availability of isotopically labeled (^{13}C, ^{15}N, ^{2}H) inhibitors, enzymes, and soluble receptors suitable for NMR studies by chemical synthesis and biosynthetic means; (3) improvements in NMR techniques, especially those designed for NMR studies of large systems; and (4) the availability of increased magnetic-field strengths at a low cost due to the recently demonstrated improvements in superconducting materials. These developments should vastly increase our capability to study the three-dimensional structures of enzyme-bound ligands, enzyme active sites, and soluble drug-receptor complexes. In addition, improvements in solid-state NMR techniques (167–169) and NMR imaging (170) (topics not covered in this chapter) should allow structural studies of drugs bound to membrane-bound receptors and the physiological effects of drugs to be examined, respectively. Clearly, the future holds even more exciting prospects for the use of NMR spectroscopy in the rational design of new pharmaceutical agents.

ACKNOWLEDGMENTS

I thank Jay Luly and Nwe BaMaung for the synthesis of the isotopically labeled pepsin inhibitors, Todd Rockway for the ^{15}N-labeled ANF analog, V. Sarin and F. Haviv for the synthesis of the LHRH antagonist, and T. J. O'Donnell and Giorgio Bolis for their efforts in molecular modeling. I also thank Bill Kohlbrenner, who collaborated with me on the KDO work presented in this chapter; Tom Perun for his support and encouragement; and my NMR colleagues at Abbott, especially Robert Gampe Jr., Ed Olejniczak, Erik Zuiderweg, Steve Spanton, and Dave Whittern.

REFERENCES

1. Zetta, L., and F. Cabassi, 270 MHz ^{1}H nuclear magnetic resonance study of met-enkephalin in solvent mixtures, Conformational transition from dimethyl-sulphoxide to water. *Eur. J. Biochem. 122*:215–222 (1982).

2. Mirau, P. A., and R. H. Shafer, High-resolution proton nuclear magnetic resonance analysis of conformational properties of biosynthetic actinomycin analogues. *Biochemistry 21*:2622–2626 (1982).

3. Hruby, V. J., and H. I. Mosberg, Conformational and dynamic considerations in peptide structure-function studies. *Peptides 3*:329–336 (1982).

4. Kessler, H., Conformation and biological activity of cyclic peptides. *Angew. Chem. Int. Ed. Engl. 21*:512–523 (1982).

5. De Jong, A. P., S. W. Fesik, and A. Makriyannis, Conformational requirements for norepinephrine uptake inhibition by phenethylamines in brain synaptosomes. Effects of α-alkyl substitution. *J. Med. Chem. 25*:1438–1441 (1982).

6. Fesik, S. W., I. M. Armitage, G. A. Ellestad, and W. J. McGahren, Nuclear magnetic resonance studies on the antibiotic avoparcin. Conformational properties in relation to antibacterial activity. *Mol. Pharmacol. 25*:275–280 (1984).

7. Mammi, N. J., M. Hassan, and M. Goodman, Conformational analysis of a cyclic enkephalin analogue by ^{1}H NMR and computer simulations. *J. Am Chem. Soc. 107*:4008–4013 (1985).

8. Fournié-Zaluski, M. C., J. Belleney, B. Lux, C. Durieux, D. Gerard, G. Gacel, B. Maigret, and B. P. Roques, Conformational analysis of cholecystokinin CCK_{26-33} and related fragments by ^1H NMR spectroscopy, fluorescence-transfer measurements, and calculations. *Biochemistry* 25:3778–3787 (1986).

9. Kessler, H., M. Klein, A. Miller, K. Wagner, J. W. Bats, K. Ziegler, and M. Frimmer, Conformational prerequisites for the in vitro inhibition of cholate uptake in hepatocytes by cyclic analogues of antamanide and somatostatin. *Angew. Chem. Int. Ed. Engl.* 25:997–999 (1986).

10. Baniak, E. L. III, J. E. Rivier, R. S. Struthers, A. T. Hagler, and L. M. Gierasch, Nuclear magnetic resonance analysis and conformational characterization of a cyclic decapeptide antagonist of gonadotropin-releasing hormone. *Biochemistry* 26:2642–2656 (1987).

11. Bax, A., *Two-Dimensional Nuclear Magnetic Resonance in Liquids*. Delft University Press, Delft, Holland (1982).

12. Wüthrich, K., *NMR of Proteins and Nucleic Acids*. John Wiley and Sons, New York (1986).

13. Ernst, R. R., G. Bodenhausen, and A. Wokaun, *Principles of Nuclear Magnetic Resonance in One and Two-Dimensions*. Clarendon Press, Oxford, U.K. (1987).

14. Morris, G. A., Modern NMR techniques for structure elucidation. *Magn. Reson. Chem.* 24:371–403 (1986).

15. Kessler, H., W. Bermel, A. Müller, and K. H. Pook, Modern nuclear magnetic resonance spectroscopy of peptides, in *The Peptides*, Vol. 7. Academic Press, New York, pp. 437–473 (1985).

16. Fesik, S. W., The use of current two-dimensional NMR methods in drug research. The structure of a drug-active site complex, in *New Methods in Drug Research*, Vol. 3, A. Makriyannis, ed. J. R. Prous Science, Barcelona (in press).

17. Rance, M., O. W. Sørensen, G. Bodenhausen, G. Wagner, R. R. Ernst, and K. Wüthrich, Improved spectral resolution in COSY ^1H NMR spectra of proteins via double quantum filtering. *Biochem. Biophys. Res. Commun.* 117:479–485 (1983).

18. Piantini, U., O. W. Sørensen, and R. R. Ernst, Multiple quantum filters for elucidating NMR coupling networks. *J. Am. Chem. Soc.* 104:6800–6801 (1982).

19. Shaka, A. J., and R. Freeman, Simplification of NMR spectra by filtration through multiple-quantum coherence. *J. Magn. Reson.* 51:169–173 (1983).

20. Braunschweiler, L., G. Bodenhausen, and R. R. Ernst, Analysis of networks of coupled spins by multiple quantum NMR. *Mol. Physics* 48:535–560 (1983).

21. Mareci, T. H., and R. Freeman, Mapping proton-proton coupling via double quantum coherence. *J. Magn. Reson.* 51:531–535 (1983).

22. Wagner, G., and E. R. P. Zuiderweg, Two-dimensional double quantum ^1H NMR spectroscopy of proteins. *Biochem. Biophys. Res. Commun.* 113:854–860 (1983).

23. Fesik, S. W., T. J. Perun, and A. M. Thomas, ^1H assignments of glycopeptide antibiotics by double quantum NMR and relayed correlation spectroscopy. *Magn. Reson. Chem.* 23:645–648 (1985).

24. Dalvitt, C., M. Rance, and P. E. Wright, Differentiation of direct and remote connectivities in phase-sensitive double-quantum spectra of proteins by variat-

ion of the multiple-quantum excitation period. *J. Magn. Reson.* 69:356–361 (1986).

25. Eich, G., G. Bodenhausen, and R. R. Ernst, Exploring nuclear spin systems by relayed magnetization transfer. *J. Am. Chem. Soc.* 104:3731–3732 (1982).

26. Bax, A., and G. Drobny, Optimization of two-dimensional homonuclear relayed coherence transfer NMR spectroscopy. *J. Magn. Reson.* 61:306–320 (1985).

27. Wagner, G., Two-dimensional relayed coherence transfer spectroscopy of a protein. *J. Magn. Reson.* 55:151–156 (1983).

28. King, G., and P. E. Wright, Application of two-dimensional relayed coherence transfer experiments to ¹H NMR studies of macromolecules. *J. Magn. Reson.* 54:328–332 (1983).

29. Chazin, W. J., and K. Wüthrich, Optimization of homonuclear relayed coherence transfer experiments with proteins in H₂O solution. *J. Magn. Reson.* 72:358–363 (1987).

30. Braunschweiler L., and R. R. Ernst, Coherence transfer by isotropic mixing: Application to proton correlation spectroscopy. *J. Magn. Reson.* 53:521–528 (1983).

31. Davis, D. G., and A. Bax, Assignment of complex ¹H NMR spectra via two-dimensional homonuclear Hartmann-Hahn spectroscopy. *J. Am. Chem. Soc.* 107:2820–2821 (1985).

32. Bax, A., and D G. Davis, MLEV-17 based two-dimensional homonuclear magnetization transfer spectroscopy. *J. Magn. Reson.* 65:355–360 (1985).

33. Griesinger, C. O. W. Sørensen, and R. R. Ernst, A practical approach to three-dimensional NMR spectroscopy. *J. Magn. Reson.* 73:574–579 (1987).

34. Griesinger, C., O. W. Sørensen, and R. R. Ernst, Novel three-dimensional NMR techniques for studies of peptides and biological macromolecules. *J. Am. Chem. Soc.* 109:7227–7228 (1987).

35. Fesik, S. W., and E. R. P. Zuiderweg, Heteronuclear three-dimensional NMR spectroscopy. A strategy for the simplification of homonuclear two-dimensional NMR spectra. *J. Magn. Reson.* 78:588–593 (1988).

36. Wagner, G., A. Kumar, and K. Wüthrich, Systematic application of two-dimensional ¹H nuclear magnetic resonance techniques for studies of proteins. 2. Combined use of correlated spectroscopy and nuclear Overhauser spectroscopy for sequential assignments of backbone resonances and elucidation of polypeptide secondary structures. *Eur. J. Biochem.* 114:375–384 (1981).

37. Summers, M. F., L. G. Marzilli, and A. Bax, Complete ¹H and ¹³C assignments of coenzyme B₁₂ through the use of new two-dimensional NMR experiments. *J. Am. Chem. Soc.* 108:4285–4294 (1986).

38. Noggle, J. H., and R. E. Schirmer, *The Nuclear Overhauser Effect. Chemical Applications.* Academic Press, New York (1971).

39. Bax, A., and G. A. Morris, An Improved method for heteronuclear chemical shift correlation by two-dimensional NMR, *J. Magn. Reson.* 42:501–505 (1981).

40. Bax, A., Broadband homonuclear decoupling in heteronuclear shift correlation NMR spectroscopy. *J. Magn. Reson.* 53: 517–520 (1983).

41. Bax, A., R. H. Griffey, and B. L. Hawkins, Correlation of proton and nitrogen-15 chemical shifts by multiple quantum NMR. *J. Magn. Reson. 55*:301–315 (1983).

42. Müller, L., Sensitivity enhanced detection of weak nuclei using heteronuclear multiple quantum coherence· *J. Am. Chem. Soc. !01*:4481–4484 (1979).

43. Bax, A., and S. Subramanian, Sensitivity-enhanced two-dimensional heteronuclear shift correlation NMR spectroscopy. *J. Magn. Reson. 67*:565–569 (1986).

44. Wagner, G., and D. Brühwiler, Toward the complete assignment of the carbon nuclear magnetic resonance spectrum of the basic pancreatic trypsin inhibitor. *Biochemistry 25*:5839–5843 (1986).

45. Brühwiler, D., and G. Wagner, Selective excitation of ^1H resonances coupled to ^{13}C. Hetero COSY and relay experiments with ^1H detection for a protein. *J. Magn. Reson. 69*:546–551 (1986).

46. Bolton, P. H., Assignments and structural information via relayed coherence transfer spectroscopy. *J. Magn. Reson. 48*:336–340 (1982).

47. Bolton, P. H., Heteronuclear relay transfer spectroscopy with proton detection. *J. Magn. Reson. 62*:143–146 (1985).

48. Lerner, L., and A. Bax, Sensitivity-enhanced two-dimensional heteronuclear relayed coherence transfer NMR spectroscopy. *J. Magn. Reson. 69*:375–380 (1986).

49. Bodenhausen, G., and R. Freeman, Correlation of chemical shifts of protons and carbon-13. *J. Am. Chem. Soc. 100*:320–321 (1978).

50. Kessler, H., C. Griesinger, J. Zarbock, and H. R. Loosli, Assignment of carbonyl carbons and sequence analysis in peptides by heteronuclear shift correlation via small coupling constants with broadband decoupling in t_1 (COLOC). *J. Magn. Reson. 57*:331–336 (1984).

51. Bax, A., and M. F. Summers, ^1H and ^{13}C assignments from sensitivity-enhanced detection of heteronuclear multiple-bond connectivity by 2D multiple quantum NMR. *J. Am. Chem. Soc. 108*:2093–2094 (1986).

52. Bermel, W., C. Griesinger, H. Kessler, and K. Wagner, Assignment of carbonyl groups and sequence analysis in peptides by inverse correlation using long-range couplings. *Magn. Reson. Chem. 25*:325–326 (1987).

53. Perkins, S. J., and K. Wüthrich, Ring current effects in the conformation dependent NMR chemical shifts of aliphatic protons in the basic pancreatic trypsin inhibitor. *Biochim. Biophys. Acta 576*:409–423 (1979).

54. Redfield, C., J. C. Hoch, and C. M. Dobson, Chemical shifts of aromatic protons in protein NMR spectra. *FEBS Lett. 159*:132–136 (1983).

55. Weiss, M. A., and J. C. Hoch, Interpretation of ring-current shifts in proteins: Application of phase λ repressor. *J. Magn. Reson. 72*:324–333 (1987).

56. Karplus, M., Contact electron-spin coupling of nuclear magnetic moments. *J. Phys. Chem. 30*:11–15 (1959).

57. Bystrov, V. F., Spin-spin coupling and the conformational states of peptide systems. *Prog. NMR Spectrosc. 10*:41–81 (1976).

58. Pardi, A., M. Billeter, and K. Wüthrich, Calibration of the angular dependence of the amide proton-Cα proton coupling constants, $^3J_{HN\alpha}$ in a globular protein. Use of $^3J_{HN\alpha}$ for identification of helical secondary structure. *J. Mol. Biol. 180*:741–751 (1984).

59. Subramanian, S., and A. Bax, Generation of pure phase NMR subspectra for measurement of homonuclear coupling constants. *J. Magn. Reson.* 71:325–330 (1987).

60. Kessler, H., H. Oschkinat, and C. Griesinger, Transformation of homonuclear two-dimensional NMR techniques into one-dimensional techniques using gaussian pulses. *J. Magn. Reson.* 70:106–133 (1986).

61. Marion, D., and K. Wüthrich, Application of phase sensitive two-dimensional correlated spectroscopy (COSY) for measurements of $^1H-^1H$ spin-spin coupling constants in proteins. *Biochem. Biophys. Res. Commun.* 113:967–974 (1983).

62. Oschkinat, H., and R. Freeman, Fine structure in two-dimensional NMR correlation spectroscopy. *J. Magn. Reson.* 60:164–169 (1984).

63. Griesinger, C., O. W. Sørensen, and R. R. Ernst, Two-dimensional correlation of connected NMR transitions. *J. Am. Chem. Soc.* 107:6394–6396 (1985).

64. Griesinger, C., O. W. Sørensen, and R. R. Ernst, Correlation of connected transitions by two-dimensional NMR spectroscopy. *J. Chem. Phys.* 85:6837–6852 (1986).

65. Mueller, L., P.E.COSY, a simple alternative to E.COSY. *J. Magn. Reson.* 72:191–196 (1987).

66. Brüschweiler, R., J. C. Madsen, C. Griesinger, O. W. Sørensen, and R. R. Ernst, Two-dimensional NMR spectroscopy with soft pulses. *J. Magn. Reson.* 73:380–385 (1987).

67. Gampe, R. T. Jr., P. J. Connolly, T. Rockway, and S. W. Fesik, Two-dimensional NMR studies of [Pro-10] atrial natriuretic factor [7–23]. *Biopolymers* 27:313–321 (1988).

68. Seto, H., K. Furihata, N. Otake, Y. Itoh, S. Takahaski, T. Haneishi, and M. Ohuchi, Application of long-range J C–H resolved 2D spectroscopy (LRJR) in structural elucidation of natural products. The structure of oxirapentyn. *Tetrahedron Lett.* 25:337–340 (1984).

69. Prachayasittikul, S., J. M. Kokosa, L. Bauer, and S. W. Fesik, Tetrahydropyridines from 3-picoline 1-oxide and tert-butyl and 1-adamantyl mercaptans in acetic anhydride. Structure elucidation by long-range 2D J(C-H) resolved NMR spectroscopy. *J. Org. Chem.* 50:997–1001 (1985).

70. Bax, A., L. G. Marzilli, and M. F. Summers, New insights into the solution behavior of cobalamins. Studies of the base-off form of coenzyme B_{12} using modern two-dimensional NMR methods. *J. Am. Chem. Soc.* 109:566–574 (1987).

71. Kessler, H., C. Griesinger, and K. Wagner, Peptide conformations 42. Conformation of side chains in peptides using heteronuclear coupling constants obtained by two-dimensional NMR spectroscopy. *J. Am. Chem. Soc.* 109:6927–6933 (1987).

72. Bax, A., and R. Freeman, Long-range proton carbon 13 NMR spin coupling constants. *J. Am. Chem. Soc.* 104:1099–1100 (1982).

73. Bax, A., Determination of heteronuclear coupling constants via semiselective two-dimensional J spectroscopy. *J. Magn. Reson.* 52:330–334 (1983).

74. Kumar, A., G. Wagner, R. R. Ernst, and K. Wüthrich, Buildup rates of the nuclear Overhauser effect measured by two-dimensional proton magnetic

resonance spectroscopy: Implications for studies of protein conformation. *J. Am. Chem. Soc. 103*:3654–3658 (1981).

75. Macura, S., and R. R. Ernst, Elucidation of cross relaxation in liquids by two-dimensional NMR spectroscopy. *Mol. Phys. 41*:95–117 (1980).

76. Bodenhausen, G., and R. R. Ernst, Direct determination of rate constants of slow dynamic processes by two-dimensional "accordion" spectroscopy in nuclear magnetic resonance. *J. Am. Chem. Soc. 104*:1304–1309 (1982).

77. Keepers, J. W., and T. L. James, A theoretical study of distance determinations from NMR. Two-dimensional nuclear Overhauser effect spectra. *J. Magn. Reson. 57*:404–426 (1984).

78. Olejniczak, E. T., R. T. Gampe Jr., and S. W. Fesik, Accounting for spin diffusion in the analysis of 2D NOE data. *J. Magn. Reson. 67*:28–41 (1986).

79. Mirau, P. A., and F. A. Bovey, 2D NMR analysis of the conformational and dynamic properties of α-helical poly (γ-benzyl L-glutamate). *J. Am. Chem. Soc. 108*:5130–5134 (1986).

80. Macura, S., B. T. Farmer II, and L. R. Brown, An improved method for the determination of cross-relaxation rates from NOE data. *J. Magn. Reson. 70*:493–499 (1986).

81. Davis, D. G., A novel method for determining internuclear distances and correlation times from NMR cross-relaxation rates. *J. Am. Chem. Soc. 109*:3471–3472 (1987).

82. Hyberts, S. G., W. Marki, and G. Wagner, Stereospecific assignments of side-chain protons and characterization of torsion angles in Elgin C. *Eur. J. Biochem. 164*:625–635 (1987).

83. Fesik, S. W., T. J. O'Donnell, R. T. Gampe Jr., and E. T. Olejniczak, Determining the structure of a glycopeptide–Ac$_2$–Lys–D–Ala–D–Ala complex using NMR parameters and molecular modeling. *J. Am. Chem. Soc. 108*:3165–3170 (1986).

84. Fesik, S. W., G. Bolis, H. L. Sham, and E. T. Olejniczak, Structure refinement of a cyclic peptide from two-dimensional NMR data and molecular modeling. *Biochemistry 26*:1851–1859 (1987).

85. Sham, H. L., G. Bolis, H. Stein, S. W. Fesik, P. Marcotte, J. J. Plattner, C. Rempel, and J. Greer, Renin inhibitors: Design and synthesis of a new class of conformationally restricted analogs of angiotensinogen. *J. Med. Chem. 31*:284–295 (1988).

86. Bolis, G., and J. Greer, The role of computer-aided molecular modeling in the design of novel inhibitors of renin, in *Computer-Aided Drug Design*, T. Perun and C. Propst, eds. Marcel Dekker, New York, Ch. 8 (1989).

87. Macura, S., K. Wüthrich, and R. R. Ernst, The relevance of J cross-peaks in two-dimensional NOE experiments of macromolecules. *J. Magn. Reson. 47*:351–357 (1982).

88. Macura, S., K. Wüthrich, and R. R. Ernst, Separation and suppression of coherent transfer effects in two-dimensional NOE and chemical exchange spectroscopy. *J. Magn. Reson. 46*:269–282 (1982).

89. Rance, M., G. Bodenhausen, G. Wagner, K. Wüthrich, and R. R. Ernst, A systematic approach to the suppression of J cross-peaks in 2D exchange and 2D NOE spectroscopy. *J. Magn. Reson. 62*:497–510 (1985).

90. Bothner-By, A. A., R. L. Stephens, J. Lee, C. D. Warren, and R. W. Jeanloz, Structure determination of a tetrasaccharide: Transient nuclear Overhauser effects in the rotating frame. *J. Am. Chem. Soc. 106*:811–813 (1984).

91. Bax, A., and D. G. Davis, Practical aspects of two-dimensional transverse NOE spectroscopy. *J. Magn. Reson. 63*:207–213 (1985).

92. Neuhaus, D., and J. Keeler, "False" transverse NOE enhancements in CAMELSPIN spectra. *J. Magn. Reson. 68*:568–574 (1986).

93. Farmer, B. T. II, S. Macura, and L. R. Brown, Relay artifacts in ROESY spectra. *J. Magn. Reson. 72*:347–352 (1987).

94. Kessler, H., C. Griesinger, R. Kerssebaum, K. Wagner, and R. R. Ernst, Separation of cross-relaxation and J cross-peaks in 2D rotating-frame NMR spectroscopy. *J. Am. Chem. Soc. 109*:607–609 (1987).

95. Szevernyi, N. M., A. A. Bothner-By, and R. Bittner, Kinetics of spin diffusion in the protons of brucine-d_2 in solution in deuteriophosphoric acid. *J. Phys. Chem. 84*:2880–2883 (1980).

96. Williamson, M. P., and D. H. Williams, Manipulation of the nuclear Overhauser effect by the use of a viscous solvent: The solution conformation of the antibiotic echinomycin. *J. C. S. Chem. Commun.* 165–166 (1981).

97. Neuhaus, D., H. S. Rzepa, R. N. Sheppard, and I. R. C. Bick, Assignment of the structure of dihydrodapnine diacetate by nuclear Overhauser effect difference spectroscopy. *Tetrahedron Lett. 22*:2933–2936 (1981).

98. Gierasch, L. M., A. L. Rockwell, K. F. Thompson, and M. S. Briggs, Conformation function relationships in hydrophobic peptides: Interior turns and signal sequences. *Biopolymers 24*:117–135 (1985).

99. Fesik, S. W., and E. T. Olejniczak, Increased NOEs for small molecules using mixed solvents. *Magn. Reson. Chem. 25*:1046–1048 (1987).

100. Bodenhausen, G., and R. R. Ernst, Two-dimensional exchange difference spectroscopy: Applications to indirect observation of quadrupolar relaxation. *Mol. Phys. 47*:319–328 (1982).

101. Harbison, G. S., J. Feigon, D. J. Ruben, J. Herzfeld, and R. G. Griffen, Diagonal peak suppression in 2D-NOE spectra. *J. Am. Chem. Soc. 107*:5567–5569 (1985).

102. Wagner, G., Two-dimensional relayed coherence transfer–NOE spectroscopy. *J. Magn. Reson. 57*:497–505 (1984).

103. Griffey, R. H., M. A. Jarema, S. Kunz, P. R. Rosevear, and A. G. Redfield, Isotopic-label-directed observation of the nuclear Overhauser effect in poorly resolved proton NMR spectra. *J. Am. Chem. Soc. 107*:711–712 (1985).

104. Griffey, R. H., and A. G. Redfield, Identification of isotope-labeled resonances in two-dimensional proton-proton correlation and exchange spectroscopy with gated heteronuclear decoupling. *J. Magn. Reson. 65*:344–347 (1985).

105. Otting, G., H. Senn, G. Wagner, and K. Wüthrich, Editing of 2D ^{1}H NMR spectra using X half-filters. Combined use with residue-selective ^{15}N labeling of proteins. *J. Magn. Reson. 70*:500–505 (1986).

106. Senn, H., G. Otting, and K. Wüthrich, Protein structure and interactions by combined use of sequential NMR assignments and isotope labeling. *J. Am. Chem. Soc. 109*:1090–1092 (1987).

107. Bax, A., and M. A. Weiss, Simplification of two-dimensional NOE spectra of proteins by ^{13}C labeling. *J. Magn. Reson. 71*:571–575 (1987).

108. Rance, M., P. E. Wright, B. A. Messerle, and L. D. Field, Site-selective observation of nuclear Overhauser effects in proteins via isotopic labeling. *J. Am. Chem. Soc. 109*:1591–1593 (1987).

109. Fesik, S. W., R. T. Gampe Jr., and T. W. Rockway, Application of isotope-filtered 2D NOE experiments in the conformational analysis of atrial natriuretic factor (7-23). *J. Magn. Reson. 74*:366–371 (1987).

110. Fesik, S. W., W. H. Holleman, and T. J. Perun, Two-dimensional ^{1}H NMR studies of rat atrial natriuretic factor (1–23). *Biochem. Biophys. Res. Commun. 131*:517–523 (1985).

111. Gierasch, L. M., J. E. Lacy, K. F. Thompson, A. L. Rockwell, and P. I. Watnick, Conformations of model peptides in membrane-mimetic environments. *Biophys. J. 37*:275–284 (1982).

112. Fesik, S. W., R. T. Gampe Jr., E. T. Olejniczak, J. R. Luly, H. H. Stein, and T. W. Rockway, Isotope-filtered proton NMR experiments for the conformational determination of peptides in solution and bound to biomacromolecules. *Proc. Tenth Am. Peptide Symp. 57–59* (1988).

113. Olejniczak, E. T., R. T. Gampe Jr., T. W. Rockway, and S. W. Fesik, NMR study of the solution conformation of rat atrial natriuretic factor (7–23) in SDS micelles. *Biochemistry* (in press).

114. Braun, W., and N. Go, Calculation of protein conformations by proton-proton distance constraints. A new efficient algorithm. *J. Mol. Biol. 186*:611–626 (1985).

115. Havel, T. F., and K. Wüthrich, An evaluation of the combined use of nuclear magnetic resonance and distance geometry for the determination of protein conformations in solution. *J. Mol. Biol. 182*:281–294 (1985).

116. Williamson, M. P., T. F. Havel, and K. Wüthrich, Solution conformation of proteinase inhibitor IIa from bull seminal plasma by ^{1}H nuclear magnetic resonance and distance geometry. *J. Mol. Biol. 182*:295–315 (1985).

117. Clore, G. M., D. K. Sukumaran, M. Nilges, and A. M. Gronenborn, Three-dimensional structure of phoratoxin in solution: Combined use of nuclear magnetic resonance, distance geometry, and restrained molecular dynamics. *Biochemistry 26*:1732–1745 (1987).

118. Clore, G. M., M. Nilges, A. T. Brünger, M. Karplus, and A. M. Gronenborn, A comparison of the restrained molecular dynamics and distance geometry methods for determining three-dimensional structures of proteins on the basis of interproton distances. *FEBS Lett. 213*:269–277 (1987).

119. Crippen, G. M., *Distance Geometry and Conformational Calculations.* John Wiley and Sons, New York (1981).

120. Clore, G. M., A. M. Gronenborn, A. T. Brünger, and M. Karplus, Solution conformation of a heptadecapeptide comprising the DNA binding helix F of the cyclic AMP receptor protein of *Escherichia coli:* Combined use of ^{1}H nuclear magnetic resonance and restrained molecular dynamics. *J. Mol. Biol. 186*:435–455 (1985).

121. Zuiderweg, E. R. P., R. M. Scheek, R. Boelens, W. F. van Gunsteren, and R. Kaptein, Determination of protein structures from nuclear magnetic resonance data using a restrained molecular dynamic approach: The lac repressor DNA binding domain. *Biochimie 67*:707–716 (1985).

122. Kaptein, R., E. R. P. Zuiderweg, R. M. Scheek, R. Boelens, and W. F. van Gunsteren, A protein structure from nuclear magnetic resonance data. Lac repressor headpiece. *J. Mol. Biol. 182*:179–181 (1985).

123. Clore, G. M., A. T. Brunger, M. Karplus, and A. M. Gronenborn, Application of molecular dynamics with interproton distance restraints to three-dimensional protein structure determination. A model study of crambin. *J. Mol. Biol. 191*:523–551 (1986).

124. Karplus, M., and J. A. McCammon, Dynamics of proteins: Elements and function. *Annu. Rev. Biochem. 53*:263–300 (1983).

125. Hruby, V. J., and B. M. Pettitt, Conformation-biological activity relationships for receptor selective, conformationally constrained opioid peptides, in *Computer-Aided Drug Design*, T. Perun and C. Propst, eds. Marcel Dekker, New York, Ch. 11 (1989).

126. Kessler, H., A. Haupt, and M. Will, Design of conformationally restricted cyclopeptides for the inhibition of cholate uptake of hepatocytes, in *computer-Aided Drug Design*, T. Perun and C. Propst, eds. Marcel Dekker, New York, Ch. 12 (1989).

127. Feigon, J., W. A. Denny, W. Leupin, and D. R. Kearns, Interactions of antitumor drugs with natural DNA: ^{1}H NMR study of binding mode and kinetics. *J. Med. Chem. 27*:450–465 (1984).

128. Graves, D. E., C. Pattaroni, B. S. Krishnan, J. M. Ostrander, L. H. Hurley, and T. R. Krugh, The reaction of anthramycin with DNA. Proton and carbon nuclear magnetic resonance studies on the structure of the anthramycin-DNA adduct. *J. Biol. Chem. 259*:8202–8209 (1984).

129. Brown, S. C., K. Mullis, C. Levenson, and R. H. Shafer, Aqueous solution structure of an intercalated actinomycin D-dATGCAT complex by two-dimensional and one-dimensional proton NMR. *Biochemistry 23*:403–408 (1984).

130. Wilson, W. D., R. L. Jones, G. Zon, E. V. Scott, D. L. Banville, and L. G. Marzilli, Actinomycin D binding to oligonucleotides with 5'd (GCGC)3 sequences. Definitive ^{1}H and ^{31}P NMR evidence for two distinct d(GC) 1:1 adducts and for adjacent site binding in a unique 2:1 adduct. *J. Am. Chem. Soc. 108*:7113–7114 (1986).

131. Leupin, W., W. J. Chazin, S. Hyberts, W. A. Denny, and K. Wüthrich, NMR studies of the complex between the decadeoxynucleotide d-(GCATTAATGC)$_2$ and a minor-groove-binding drug, *Biochemistry 25*:5902–5910 (1986).

132. Keniry, M. A., S. C. Brown, E. Berman, and R. H. Shafer, NMR studies on the interaction of chromomycin A$_3$ with small DNA duplexes I. *Biochemistry 26*:1058–1067 (1987).

133. Brown, J. P., J. Feeney, and A. S. V. Burgen, A nuclear magnetic resonance study of the interaction between vancomycin and acetyl-D-alanyl-D-alanine in aqueous solution. *Mol. Pharmacol. 11*:119–125 (1975).

134. Convert, O., A. Bongini, and J. Feeney, A ^{1}H nuclear magnetic resonance study of the interactions of vancomycin with N-acetyl-D-alanyl-D-alanine and related peptides. *J. C. S. Perkin II* 1262–1270 (1980).

135. Kalman, J. R., and D. H. Williams, An NMR study of the interaction between the antibiotic ristocetin A and a cell wall peptide analogue. Negative nuclear

Overhauser effects in the investigation of drug binding sites. *J. Am. Chem Soc.* *102*:906–912 (1980).

136. Williams, D. H., M. P. Williamson, D. W. Butcher, and S. J. Hammond, Detailed binding sites of the antibiotics vancomycin and ristocetin A. Determination of intermolecular distances in antibiotic/substrate complexes by use of the time-dependent NOE. *J. Am. Chem. Soc.* *105*:1332–1339 (1983).

137. Fesik, S. W., I. M. Armitage, G. A. Ellestad, and W. J. McGahren, Nuclear magnetic resonance studies on the interaction of avoparcin with model receptors of bacterial cell walls. *Mol. Pharmacol.* *25*:281–286 (1984).

138. Williamson, M. P., and D. H. Williams, ^{1}H NMR studies of the structure of ristocetin A and of its complexes with bacterial cell wall analogues in aqueous solution. *J. Chem. Soc. Perkin Trans.* *I*;949–956 (1985).

139. Albrand, J. P., B. Birdsall, J. Feeney, G. C. K. Roberts, and A. S. V. Burgen, The use of transferred nuclear Overhauser effects in the study of the conformations of small molecules bound to proteins. *Int. J. Biol. Macromol.* *1*:37–41 (1979).

140. Clore, G. M., G. C. K. Roberts, A. Gronenborn, B. Birdsall, and J. Feeney, Transfer-of-saturation NMR studies of protein-ligand complexes. Three-site exchange. *J. Magn. Reson.* *45*:151–161 (1981).

141. Clore, G. M., and A. M. Gronenborn, Theory and applications of the transferred nuclear Overhauser effect to the study of the conformations of small ligands bound to proteins. *J. Magn. Reson.* *48*:402–417 (1982).

142. Clore, G. M., and A. M. Gronenborn, Theory of the time dependent transferred nuclear Overhauser effect: Applications to structural analysis of ligand-protein complexes in solution. *J. Magn. Reson.* *53*:423–442 (1983).

143. Levy, H. R., A. Ejchart, and G. C. Levy, Conformations of nicotinamide coenzymes bound to dehydrogenases determined by transferred nuclear Overhauser effects. *Biochemistry* *22*:2792–2796 (1983).

144. Gronenborn, A. M., G. M. Clore, M. Brunori, B. Giardina, G. Falcioni, and M. Perutz, Stereochemistry of ATP and GTP bound to fish haemoglobins. A transferred nuclear Overhauser enhancement ^{31}P-nuclear magnetic resonance, oxygen equilibrium and molecular modelling study. *J. Mol. Biol.* *178*:731–742 (1984).

145. Clore, G. M., A. M. Gronenborn, J. Greipel, and G. Maass, Conformation of the DNA undecamer 5′d(A–A–G–T–G–T–G–A–T–A–T) bound to the single-stranded DNA binding protein of *Escherichia coli.* A time-dependent transferred nuclear Overhauser enhancement study. *J. Mol. Biol.* *187*:119–124 (1986).

146. Banerjee, A., H. R. Levy, G. C. Levy and W. W. C. Chan, Conformations of bound nucleoside triphosphate effectors in aspartate transcarbamylase. Evidence for the London-Schmidt model by transferred nuclear Overhauser effects. *Biochemistry* *24*:1593–1598 (1985).

147. Glasel, J. A., and P. N. Borer, NMR studies of flexible opiate conformations at monoclonal antibody binding sites. I. Transferred nuclear Overhauser effects show bound conformations. *Biochem. Biophys. Res. Commun.* *141*:1267–1273 (1986).

148. Clore, G. M., A. M. Gronenborn, G. Carlson, and E. F. Meyer, Stereochemistry of binding of the tetrapeptide acetyl–Pro–Ala–Pro–Tyr–NH₂ to porcine pancreatic elastase. Combined use of two-dimensional transferred nuclear Overhauser enhancement measurements, restrained molecular dynamics, x-ray crystallography and molecular modelling. *J. Mol. Biol. 190*:259–267 (1986).

149. Wakamatsu, K., A. Okada, T. Miyazawa, Y. Masui, S. Sakakibara, and T. Higashijima, Conformations of yeast α-mating factor and analog peptides as bound to phospholipid bilayer. Correlation of membrane-bound conformation with physiological activity. *Eur. J. Biochem. 163*:331–338 (1987).

150. Gronenborn, A. M., G. M. Clore, L. W. McLaughlin, E. Graeser, B. Lorber, and R. Giegé, Yeast tRNA^Asp: Codon and wobble codon-anticodon interactions. A transferred nuclear Overhauser enhancement study. *Eur. J. Biochem. 145*:359–364 (1984).

151. Ghalambor, M. A., and E. C. Heath, The enzymatic synthesis of cytidine monophospho-2-keto-3-deoxy-octonate. *Biochem. Biophys. Res. Commun. 10*:346–351 (1963).

152. Bendall, M. R., D. M. Doddrell, and D. T. Pegg, Editing of ¹³C NMR spectra. A pulse sequence for the generation of subspectra. *J. Am. Chem. Soc. 103*:4603–4605 (1981).

153. Freeman, R., T. H. Mareci, and G. A. Morris, Weak satellite signals in high-resolution NMR spectra: Separating the wheat from the chaff. *J. Magn. Reson. 42*:341–345 (1981).

154. Bendall, M. R., D. T. Pegg, D. M. Doddrell, and J. Field, NMR of protons coupled to ¹³C nuclei only. *J. Am. Chem. Soc. 103*:934–936 (1981).

155. Doddrell, D., D. H. Williams, D. G. Reid, K. Fox, and M. J. Waring, Application of a simple technique for the sole observation of NMR resonances of protons which are directly bonded to nitrogen. *J. Chem. Soc. Chem. Commun* 218–220 (1983).

156. Kingsley-Hickman, P. B., and K. Ugurbil, Selective observation of ¹H resonances from hydrogens directly bonded to ¹³C atoms. *J. Magn. Reson. 64*:339–342 (1985).

157. Griffey, R. H., A. G. Redfield, R. E. Loomis, and F. W. Dahlquist, Nuclear magnetic resonance observation and dynamics of specific amide protons in T4 lysozyme. *Biochemistry 24*:817–822 (1985).

158. Griffey, R. H., A. G. Redfield, L. P. McIntosh, T. G. Oas, and F. W. Dahlquist, Assignment of proton amide resonances of T4 lysozyme by ¹³C and ¹⁵N multiple isotopic labeling. *J. Am. Chem. Soc. 108*:6816–6817 (1986).

159. Wilde, J. A., P. H. Bolton, N. J. Stolowich, and J. A. Gerlt, A method for the observation of selected proton NMR resonances of proteins. *J. Magn. Reson. 68*:168–171 (1986).

160. Fesik, S. W., J. R. Luly, H. H. Stein, and N. BaMaung, Amide proton exchange rates of a bound pepsin inhibitor determined by isotope-edited proton NMR experiments. *Biochem. Biophys. Res. Commun. 147*:892–898 (1987).

161. Fesik, S. W., J. R. Luly, J. W. Erickson, and C. Abad-Zapatero, Isotope-edited proton NMR study on the structure of a pepsin/inhibitor complex. *Biochemistry* (in press).

162. Fesik, S. W., Isotope-edited NMR spectroscopy. *Nature 332*:865–866 (1988).
163. Mildvan, A. S., and D. C. Fry, NMR studies of the mechanism of enzyme action, in *Advances in Enzymology*, Vol. 59, A. Meister, ed. John Wiley and Sons, New York, pp. 241–313 (1987), and the references therein.
164. Kohlbrenner, W. E., and S. W. Fesik, Determination of the anomeric specificity of the *Escherichia coli* CTP:CMP-3-deoxy-D-manno-oculosonate cytidyl-transferase by ^{13}C NMR spectroscopy. *J. Biol. Chem. 260*:14695–14700 (1985).
165. Kohlbrenner, W. E., M. M. Nuss, and S. W. Fesik, ^{31}P and ^{13}C NMR studies of oxygen transfer during catalysis by 3-deoxy-D-manno-octulosonate cytidyl-transferase from *Escherichia coli. J. Biol. Chem. 262*:4534–4537 (1987).
166. Goldman, R., W. Kohlbrenner, P. Lartey, and A. Pernet, Antibacterial agents specifically inhibiting lipopolysaccharide synthesis. *Nature 329*:162–164 (1987).
167. Haeberlen, U., High resolution NMR in solids. Selective averaging, in *Advances in Magnetic Resonance*, Vol. 1, J. S. Waugh, Academic Press, New York (1976).
168. Mehring, M., *Principles of High Resolution NMR in Solids.* Springer-Verlag, New York (1983).
169. Fyfe, C. A., *Solid State NMR for Chemists.* C. F. C. Press, Guelph, Ontario, Canada (1983).
170. James, T. L., and A. R. Margulis (eds.), *Biomedical Magnetic Resonance.* Radiology Research and Education Foundation, San Francisco (1984).

6
Enzyme Kinetics in Drug Design: Implications of Multiple Forms of Enzyme on Substrate and Inhibitor Structure-Activity Correlations

Daniel H. Rich and Dexter B. Northrop
University of Wisconsin—Madison, Madison, Wisconsin

I. INTRODUCTION: EVIDENCE FOR MULTIPLE FORMS OF ENZYMES

The purpose of this article is to review the evidence for multiple forms of enzyme-substrate and enzyme-inhibitor complexes and to consider how these multiple forms can complicate our attempts to interpret structure-activity data and to design novel enzyme inhibitors. Recent studies of the physical properties of proteins, using a variety of spectroscopic and physical methods, have provided overwhelming evidence for the existence of multiple conformational forms of many enzymes. X-ray crystal structures of native enzymes and of the same enzyme with inhibitors bound in the active site clearly reveal altered protein conformations induced by the binding of the ligand (1). Nuclear magnetic resonance (NMR) measurements of proteins (2) have shown that individual amino acid residues are much more conformationally mobile than previously thought, and molecular dynamics simulations of protein conformational transitions (3) are consistent with the modern concept that proteins generally, and enzymes in particular, are dynamic species that equilibrate between many subtle and a few major conformational transitions. Catalysis itself often consists of multiple forms of enzyme complexes. Application of the multiple-isotope effect method of Hermes et al. (87) has given direct evidence that enzymatic reactions composed of multiple bond-breaking steps are often stepwise rather than concerted reaction processes (88). Multiple conformational forms of enzyme complexes can confound the interpretation of steady-state kinetic data. This is important to the design of enzyme inhibitors and other pharmaceutically useful agents, because steady-state kinetics provide the data to indicate how well an inhibitor will perform and also provide the "real numbers" to which theoretical calculations of enzyme inhibitor interactions must agree. Steady-state kinetics also provide information about the "comings and goings" of substrates and products and whether inhibitors are acting at one of these sites or at remote sites. Multiple forms of enzyme inhibitor complexes can also be revealed by the judicious application of kinetic methods. All of this information should be known, whenever possible, before molecular modeling is started.

Misinterpretation of steady-state kinetic data can obviously mislead the medicinal chemist and molecular modeler alike. Three mistakes are especially common: (a) the failure to explicitly state in both schematic and mathematical forms the enzyme mechanism being considered and tested; (b) the failure to obtain sufficient kinetic data to distinguish between alternate possible kinetic mechanisms; and (c), the tendency to assume that catalysis can be assigned to a single, dominant slow step in the reaction pathway, the so-called rate-limiting step. All three derive from a mental image of catalytic turnover that is too simplistic. Medicinal chemists who seek a defined goal of simply blocking specific enzymatic reactions have traditionally considered enzyme inhibition in terms of only a single form of enzyme, namely, free enzyme, the form to which a substrate analog will bind. On the other hand, enzyme kineticists investigating the intricacies of mechanisms of enzymatic catalysis sometimes encounter complex patterns of inhibition that show unusual dependencies on the distribution of forms of enzyme lying along the pathway of catalytic turnover. The latter are often subtle and consist largely of indirect evidence, with the understandable result that these more complex mechanisms have not had much impact on the imagery of medicinal chemistry or even of enzymology. But the results of the multiple-isotope effect method cited previously has radically changed that. Here is a clear and unambiguous method for distinguishing between stepwise and concerted catalytic processes that has suggested that concerted catalysis is relatively uncommon in enzymatic reactions. It says, in effect, that we should not necessarily push all of our arrows at once when formulating chemical mechanisms of enzymatic catalysis. This obviously could have far-reaching consequences when searching for transition state analog inhibitors. But in a larger sense, by shattering the traditional image of a single catalytic form of enzyme undergoing a single rate-limiting step, it opens the way for new images which include multiple forms of enzymes which have nothing to do with stepwise catalysis but may have a lot to do with inhibition.

In this article we will briefly review the development of the steady-state assumptions and equations that are operative to the study of the inhibitors today. We will propose a general scheme for an enzyme-catalyzed bond breaking (forward reaction) or bond synthesis (reverse reaction) transformation, which in the simplest case requires five enzyme-ligand forms. We will analyze the significance of multiple forms on V_{max} (k_{cat}), K_m, V/K, and K_i for enzyme reactions and show how increased interactions between enzyme and substrate affect these kinetic parameters. The special problems that arise with slow-binding and tight-binding enzyme inhibitors will be reviewed, and we will look at cases where detailed enzyme kinetic analyses altered preconceptions of how inhibitors bind to enzymes. Finally, we will outline a strategy for properly conducting kinetic analyses of enzyme catalyzed reactions.

II. DERIVATION OF A GENERAL MODEL FOR ENZYME–SUBSTRATE INTERACTION

A. Kinetic Evidence for Multiple Forms of Enzyme During Catalytic Turnover

The rate of an enzymatic reaction varies with changes in the concentration of substrate, usually as a hyperbolic function, according to the Michaelis-Menten equation:

$$v = \frac{V[S]}{K_m + [S]} \tag{1}$$

where V is the maximal velocity, $[S]$ the concentration of substrate, and K_m the Michaelis-Menten constant. The essence of the Michaelis-Menten hypothesis is that a second form of enzyme must exist to account for the saturation kinetics displayed by all enzymes. As illustrated in Scheme I, Michaelis and Menten (4) surmised that an enzyme and its substrate came together as a metastable complex, ES, prior to catalysis. They also surmised that catalysis was relatively slow compared to the formation of the complex, which was therefore in rapid equilibrium with free enzyme and substrate. As a result of this assumption, their Michaelis-Menten constant was equal to the dissociation constant describing that equilibrium, or $K_m = K_D = k_2/k_1$ of Scheme I. Similarly, their maximal velocity was identical to catalysis, or $V = k_3 x[E_t]$ (and often referred to as k_{cat}).

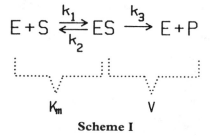

Scheme I

In 1925, Briggs and Haldane (5) showed that the rapid-equilibrium assumption was not necessary for the Michaelis-Menten equation and could be replaced by a steady-state assumption. All that is necessary to achieve this is that during the period of measurement of reaction velocities, the rate of formation of the Michaelis-Menten complex be balanced by its removal, which may include catalysis as well as dissociation. Thus, the Michaelis-Menten constant became more than a simple equilibrium constant; it became a kinetic constant, which in Scheme I is: $K_m = (k_2 + k_3)/k_1$

Nevertheless, in the more than half a century since the formulation of the steady-state hypothesis of enzyme kinetics, few investigators have come to terms with its implications. During the last quarter century, for example, the results of stopped-flow kinetics, nuclear magnetic resonance measurements, kinetic isotope effects, and other approaches have clearly shown the steady-state hypothesis to have widespread application to many enzymes. More importantly, the same studies have documented the existence of other complexes in addition to the initial Michaelis-Menten complex, and of additional chemical steps instead of the singular catalytic one. Thus, a more general illustration of an enzymatic turnover must contain multiple steps and multiple forms of enzyme, such as the mechanism shown in Scheme II.

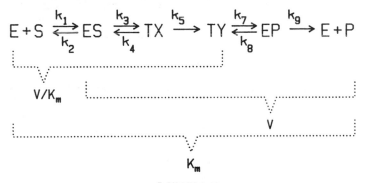

Scheme II

The sequence of steps in Scheme II represents an enzymatic reaction in which a conformational change (i.e., between E and T) is required before and after irreversible catalysis—fairly common propositions. The conformational changes are not restricted to the enzyme but are expressed on the substrate and product as well, indicated by X and Y, respectively. Thus, TX and TY represent intermediates on the substrate and product sides, respectively, of the transition state for bond cleavage or formation. As illustrated underneath the mechanism, the maximal velocity again represents the rate of conversion of the Michaelis-Mented complex to free enzyme and product, but there the similarity with Scheme I ends. Under the steady-state hypothesis, this velocity is no longer a direct measure of catalysis, but rather it becomes a complex function of all steps following the formation of the Michaelis-Menten complex [see Appendix 2, Eq. (13)].

To understand steady-state kinetics under nonsaturating conditions, a new concept has been introduced, that of V/K_m (or k_{cat}/K_m), which is an apparent first-order rate constant (at constant E_t) describing the coming together of free enzyme and substrate *in collisions committed to catalysis* (6). It includes all steps up to and including the first irreversible step. For "sticky" or highly committed substrates, V/K_m has the upper limit of a diffusion-controlled reaction, e.g., k_1. The term V/K_m is now accepted as a fundamental kinetic constant for an enzymatic reaction, despite its continued representation as a ratio of older terms (7). The Michaelis-Menten constant has become less useful, for as illustrated in Scheme II, it is derived from the ratio of V and V/K_m and is therefore more complex than either fundamental constant [see Eqs. (13–15) of Appendix 2]. It retains the dimensions of a dissociation constant, but it describes the steady-state equilibration between free enzyme and *all* of the other forms of enzyme present in a complete catalytic turnover.

In spite of the foregoing, people continue to try to express enzyme-catalyzed reactions as though only one step were kinetically significant. The most frequent expression of this attempt to simplify is the effort to identify the so-called "rate-limiting step" and thus again be able to address the maximal velocity as if it were a single catalytic rate constant. For example, if catalysis were presumed to be rate-limiting in Scheme II, one would expect the maximal velocity to become equivalent to $k_5[E_t]$, but rigorous rather than intuitive derivations of this and other rate equations show this not to be the case [see Eq. (16), Appendix 2].

The problem is, extension of the concept of a rate-limiting step from simple chemical reactions to the more complex enzymatic turnover has proceeded without a clear or accepted definition (8,9). Johnson (10) and Boyd (11) have shown that it is inappropriate to apply the concept to a series of reversible steps in chemical reactions; instead, the concept must be restricted to processes that are irreversible. Because these processes may consist of many discrete steps in an enzymatic reaction, Radika and Northrop (12) referred to them as reaction segments and formulated a replacement concept of "rate-limiting segments."

How rate-limiting each segment is can be shown to be proportional to the amount of enzyme participating in it during steady-state turnovers at saturating concentrations of substrates—which provides both a definition and a potential means of measurement. Thus, the mechanism of Scheme II consists of just two segments, the irreversible conversion of ES to TY (collectively referred to as the catalytic segment) and the irreversible conversion of TY to E + P (called a product release segment, irreversible under initial velocity conditions, because the concentration of P is zero). Working from experimental kinetic data rather than models or free energy diagrams, it is not possible to ascertain if an enzyme obeys a simpler scheme or if simpler definitions of K_m and V/K_m obtain.

The attempt to treat catalysis as an irreversible process has been rendered untenable for many enzymes, first by Nageswara Rao and Cohen (13) and by many others since, who have examined the equilibria between enzyme-bound substrates and products using nuclear magnetic resonance and have found

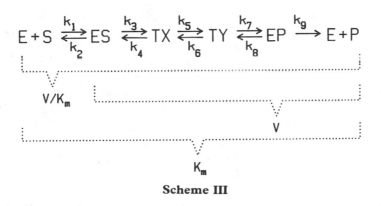

Scheme III

values near unity—even for enzymes catalyzing highly exothermic reactions. This finding is consistent with the image of enzymatic catalysis within the transition state as being composed solely of the movement of electrons, which ought to be freely reversible and also very fast. Given reversible catalysis, a more general mechanism is needed, such as that illustrated in Scheme III.

Predicting or interpreting correlations of V/K_m now becomes more difficult, because, as illustrated below the mechanism in Scheme III, V/K_m may extend beyond the catalytic step. In this example, V/K_m encompasses the complete enzymatic turnover, because a single product release is the only irreversible step. As an aid to visualizing the significance of highly reversible catalysis, the free-energy profiles shown in Figure 1 were constructed. These

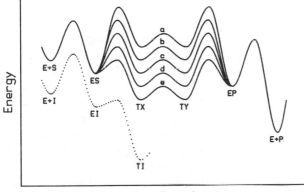

Figure 1   Free-energy profiles for reaction mechanism in Scheme III. The dotted line represents analogous finding of transition state analog inhibitors. See text for definitions of TX, TY, etc.

will be discussed in detail below, but for the moment, note that TX and TY are at equivalent energy levels and that the barrier between them is relatively small.

For the purpose of subsequent discussions of proteases and considerations of other hydrolytic enzymes, the reaction schemes need to be expanded to include the formation and release of two products. Two possibilities consistent with the features developed in Scheme III are presented in Scheme IV, in which a single product, P, is replaced with two products, designated P and Q. The first, mechanism IVa, is directly analogous to Scheme III in that product release steps follow the postcatalytic conformational change, and V/K_m resembles that of Scheme III. The second, mechanism IVb, allows for the possibility of release of one product prior to the postcatalytic conformational change. Because product release steps are effectively irreversible during initial velocity measurements, the second mechanism generates a V/K_m similar to that of Scheme II, in that both are insensitive to the second conformational change.

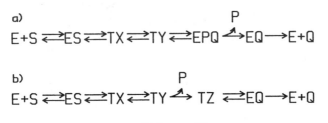

Scheme IV

B.   Structural Evidence for the General Mechanism

It is useful to show how the general reaction mechanisms depicted in Schemes III and IV translate to a physical model of an enzyme. For this purpose, we summarize some of the data obtained in recent years from multidisciplinary studies of aspartic proteinases that support the general mechanism given in Scheme IVa. James et al. (14) discovered that binding of a reaction pathway inhibitor to penicillopepsin was accompanied by the closing of a mobile portion of the enzyme, the so-called "flap" region consisting of residues 73–80, which entraps the inhibitor in the enzyme active site. Movement of related flaps has been found to occur for other aspartic proteinases during the binding of inhibitors (15) so that entrapment appears to be a characteristic of this enzyme class. These observations provide direct experimental evidence consistent with multiple enzyme-inhibitor complexes that support the existance of EI and TI, analogous to ES and TX (see Fig. 1). Since the inhibitor structures closely resemble the structure of a tetrahedral intermediate for the enzyme-catalyzed hydrolysis of substrate, it is reasonable to assume that this closure of the flap region also occurs during catalysis. We presume here that the closed flap complex with the transition-state analog inhibitor Iva–Val–Val–Sta–OEt (16,17) (7) closely approximates the geometries of the transition state form of enzyme (defined as T in Scheme IV) and the strained form of substrate (defined as X in Scheme IV). The flap region probably remains closed immediately after the substrate amide bond has been cleaved, because the product complex (TY) is the pre-transition-state complex for the corresponding reverse reaction—i.e., the peptide synthesis reaction. The enzyme is closed (hence T), and the two products are bound in a compressed fashion with the amine nitrogen and the carboxyl carbonyl group approaching covalent binding distances, because this complex is required for the reverse reaction to form peptides. The appearance of the EPQ complex follows the opening of the flap to permit departure of products that are now in the ground state. These can then dissociate from the native form of the enzyme. Both the formation of the ES and the EPQ complex from free enzyme and ground-state ligands are assumed to proceed at rates approaching diffusion limits (18).

The properties of the TX complex can be inferred from the crystal structures of aspartic proteinases in which the active site contains inhibitors clearly related to tetrahedral intermediates for amide bond hydrolysis. The best examples to date are the complexes between *R. chinensis* pepsin and pepstatin (19), penicillopepsin and Iva–Val–Val–Sta–OEt (14), endothiapepsin and methyleneamino inhibitors (15), and *R. chinensis* pepsin and a reduced amide bond isostere (20). In addition to visualizing the presumed resemblance of the tetrahedral inhibitors to the transition state for the hydrolytic reaction, the crystal structures also show that the environment about the catalytically essential aspartic acid carboxyl groups and the tetrahedral reaction center (–CHOH– or –CH$_2$NH–) is devoid of solvent. Thus, one of the long-suspected consequences (21) of binding of substrate to this type of enzyme is to desolvate the active site. Additionally, as the substrate binds to the enzyme, the normal geometry of the substrate amide bond is distorted into a twisted form more closely approximating the tetrahedral transition state; this process has been anticipated for some time 22–24).

The driving force to compensate for these energetically unfavorable processes comes from the precise alignment of hydrogen bonds between substrate and the enzyme (as visualized with the inhibitors), involving many of the residues found in the flap region, which are possible only when the flap region is closed tightly upon the substrate (or inhibitor). Hydrophobic interactions also stabilize the complex coincident with the formation of intact S_1, S_3, and S'_1 pockets, which are formed only when the flap closes upon the substrate (or inhibitor). The substrate side chains that project away from the enzyme cannot be expected to form strong hydrophobic interactions with the enzyme, but these side chains may indirectly stabilize the complex by forming a hydrophobic barrier that shields the active site and amide hydrogen bonds from re-solvation from bulk solvent.

Bond cleavage is presumed to be fast because the stressed form of the substrate is in close proximity to the enzyme catalytic groups; interconversion between substrate and products requires only rapid movement of electrons (which may or may not be concerted) and little atomic motion occurs other than that resulting from rehybridization of orbitals. Supporting this view are calculations that reactions that are normally slow in aqueous solution can be very fast in a desolvated environment (25), plus the model for the amide cleavage step proposed by Davies and co-workers (20), which suggests minimal motion of atoms during the cleavage step. Thus, consistent with the mechanisms described in Scheme IV, the barrier between TX and TY is probably low for aspartic proteinases (Fig. 1).

The foregoing model is presented to provide molecular correlates for each of the enzyme forms postulated in Schemes III and IV. Each of these forms has a structural correlate for aspartic proteinases. Other enzymes are known to follow analogous mechanistic schemes with multiple forms and rapid catalysis, so this may have a general application, but that remains to be established.

The kinetic properties of the enzymatic mechanism proposed in Schemes III and IV as expressed in structure-activity correlations are very difficult to envision because of the algebraic complexity of the kinetic parameters, but these can be evaluated with the aid of computer simulations and visualized through the application of free-energy diagrams (Fig. 1). The energy profile in Figure 1 was drawn by assuming reasonable rate constants, relative to each other, for each of the steps in the mechanism in Scheme III. Our energy diagrams differ from previous attempts in that we posit two types of transition states—those leading to the formation of the stressed enzyme-substrate complex, ES→TX (and similarly EPQ→TY for the corresponding reverse reaction); and one leading to bond rehybridization to form product side complexes (TX→TY), the cleavage step. In fact, these may very well merge, but the diagrams enable us to examine reasonable effects on binding without altering the activation barriers for the bond cleavage step itself, something that was not possible with previous models. We can now ask what might happen if a series of hydrophobic groups were added to the substrate at appropriate positions (i.e., no steric hindrance) such that the strained form of the enzyme-substrate complex (TX) would be stabilized. This is illustrated successively with curves B–F.

It seems reasonable also to assume that the enzyme-product complex (TY) will also be stabilized comparably. Using the same series of rate constants, the

Table 1 Relative Values[a] for V and V/K as a Function of the Free-Energy Level of Transition-State Conformers of Enzyme in Figure 1

Curve	V	V/K
a	5	47
b	39	329
c	120	810
d	80	949
e	14	966

[a]Values for rate constants in the top diagram in Figure 1 were: $k_1 = 1000$, $k_2 = 100$, $k_3 = 10$, $k_4 = 1000$, $k_5 = 100,000$, $k_6 = 100,000$, $k_7 = 1000$, $k_8 = 1$, $k_9 = 300$, and $k_{10} = 0.001$. To generate the series of diagrams, k_3 and k_8 were successively increased by 10-fold.

effects of this stabilization of the precleavage complex TX as expressed on the values of V/K and V were computed and are presented in Table 1. One of the exciting results of this simulation is that the energy diagrams successfully predict the effects that increased binding of substrates to enzyme could have on V/K and V. As the energy levels of TX and TY are lowered, because of the Hammond postulate (26) the barriers between the E and T forms of enzyme also decrease, and V/K approaches a limit of k_1, the diffusion-controlled rate constant for the bimolecular association reaction. This is, of course, what one often observes with increasingly efficient enzyme substrates.

However, the effect that increased substrate binding will have on V is even more interesting. As the energy level of TX is lowered owing to enhanced binding to the enzyme, V increases, but not continuously. The maximal velocity instead follows a biphasic function; as the precleavage forms of enzyme are stabilized, V increases up to a certain point, after which further stabilization leads to a decrease in V. One would expect, therefore, that a substrate that binds unusually favorably with the enzyme (low TX) should act initially as a very good inhibitor (i.e., its apparent K_m being the result of a small V divided by a maximal V/K_m), but such inhibition being short-lived owing to catalytic turnover. It is interesting that one form of the cynic's mnemonic "methyl, ethyl, propyl, futile" actually falls out of these simulations insofar as substrates are concerned. The effects on inhibitors will be described later.

C. Correlations of V/K_m with K_i of Transition-State Analog Inhibitors

The mechanism outlined in Scheme III provides a basis to consider the characteristics of transition-state analog inhibitors. The origin of this design of inhibitor began with Pauling (22), who had hypothesized that substrates were bound more tightly to enzymes in the transition state than in the Michaelis-Menten complex. Wolfenden (23) and Leinhard (24) extended the idea to inhibitors, suggesting that those with structures resembling the substrate in the transition state will bind more tightly than will analogs of the free substrate. Because transition states are by definition unstable, closely related structures, such as the so-called tetrahedral intermediate, are often sought instead. We propose that their structures will approach—insofar as chemically feasible—the stressed geometry of the substrate as it exists in TX. Because the transition state analog inhibitor does not undergo strain in forming the analogous complex, designated here as TI, this complex should lie at a lower relative energy level than TX; therefore the inhibitor should bind more tightly. Also, because the energy barrier separating TI from EI is relatively lower, the inhibitor is predicted to bind more quickly to enzyme than does substrate. Rates of inhibitor binding, and the fact that many bind more slowly rather than more quickly, will be discussed in Section II.

The problem with transition-state analog inhibitor design, however, is that such a stressed geometry in substrates is not amenable to direct structural determination, and kinetic data on inhibitors themselves provide no way to discriminate between those structural features that contribute to binding within the Michaelis-Menten form of an enzyme complex (which by analogy we will designate EI) and those that contribute to binding within TI. Several attempts have been made to find a kinetic means test to identify when an inhibitor mimics the stressed geometry rather than rely on structural inferences alone. The most significant approach was put forward by Westerik and Wolfenden (27) and Thompson (28) and was extended by Bartlett and Marlowe (29), who reasoned that because substrates *must* pass through the transition state, it followed that information about transition-state binding ought to come from comparisons of kinetic data on sets of alternative substrates rather than sets of inhibitors only or, more specifically, from comparisons of V/K_m. Their hypothesis was based on thermodynamic considerations for a single-step reaction and predicted a linear correlation between K/V and K_i. Implicit in this derivation are the assumptions that the rate-limiting step of the catalyzed reaction does not change over a series of closely related structures nor do the rates for the uncatalyzed reactions change from substrate to substrate. Bartlett and Marlowe (30) found a good correlation between logarithmic values of K_i and K_m/V for inhibitors and substrates of thermolysin, and no correlation between logarithmic values of K_i and K_m.

A general kinetic solution for correlating K_i with K_m/V for multistep catalytic reactions can be sought with the aid of Scheme III. We begin by defining K_T as the equilibrium constant for the interconversion between TX and ES; K_T therefore contains the contributions to binding that are unique to the transition state conformer of enzyme and is thus responsible for the special binding interactions of transition state analog inhibitors of the cleavage step. K_T cannot be factored from the full expression for V/K_m, so there is no basis to expect V/K_m to be proportional to K_T and thus to K_i under steady-state kinetic conditions. Instead, it is necessary to impose rapid-equilibrium conditions on the system in order to solve for equilibria. For example, if one assumes that a late rate constant such as k_9 were smaller than other rate constants, one finds [see Eq. (11) of Appendix 2]

$$V/K_m = \frac{k_9}{K_D K_T K_C K_{T'}} \tag{2}$$

where K_C and $K_{T'}$ are the equilibrium constants for the catalytic step and the second conformational change, respectively. K_D is the normal dissociation constant for ES. V/K_m is therefore inversely proportional to K_T and thus ought to be proportional to K_i. But V/K_m is also inversely proportional to $K_{T'}$. These ought to cancel each other out in the series of alternative substrates at least for a series of closely related analogs, because structural features that stabilize interactions between the substrate and the transition state conformer of the enzyme would also stabilize the same interactions between product and enzyme (e.g., k_7 and k_8 would change proportionately). Alternatively, catalysis itself is often assumed to be slow in order to establish rapid-equilibrium conditions, but as noted above, the cleavage step of the mechanism in Scheme III is presumed to be fast, leaving only the rates of conformational changes as candidates to impose rapid equilibration, and a high barrier preceding TX removes K_T from the kinetic expression. Thus, there would appear to be no general basis for the correlations between K_i and V/K_m for the full mechanism shown in Scheme III.

Nevertheless, despite the foregoing, excellent correlations between V/K_m and K_i have been observed for several enzymes (28,29). Most likely, this means that the rate data were obtained in such a way that the full mechanism (Scheme III) is not operative. Assuming that a conformation change in the enzyme does occur, a possible explanation is that the first of two products is released immediately after catalysis but before the reversal of the conformational change, as depicted in mechanism (b) of Scheme IV. This would intersperse an irreversible step prior to $K_{T'}$ and reduce V/K_m to the form obtained in Scheme II, which under rapid equilibrium conditions is [see Eq. (17), Appendix 2]:

$$V/K_m = \frac{k_5}{K_D K_T} \tag{3}$$

Thus, given irreversible catalysis, or an irreversible step immediately following catalysis, V/K_m can be inversely proportional to K_T. Consequently, for a
series of related structures (e.g., methyl-, ethyl-, propyl-, etc.) that contribute
to the binding of inhibitors with the transition state form of enzyme, the series
of inhibition constants should show a *linear* correlation with reciprocal
values of V/K_m for an analogous series of substrates. The K_m, on the other
hand, should not show other than a fortuitous correlation, given the same
restriction, because it retains a complex dependence upon a complete
enzymatic turnover [see Eq. (15), Appendix 2]. But given the added
restriction of the catalytic segment being rate-limiting, K_m reduces to [see Eq.
(18), Appendix 2]:

$$K_m = \frac{K_D K_T}{1 + K_T} \tag{4}$$

Thus, K_m becomes equal to the dissociation constant (K_D) when K_T is large,
in which case there would be little or no correlation with changes in the
inhibition constants due to transition state binding.

This analysis demonstrates that the utility of correlations between values
of K_I and V/K_m is limited to reactions governed by *both* restrictions, because
Eq. (3) also contains an inverse proportionality between V/K_m and K_D. To
eliminate significant contributions of binding with the Michaelis-Menten
form of enzyme, the *lack* of correlation with K_m is important and must be
demonstrated as was done by Bartlett and Marlowe (30). It should be noted
that the necessary restrictions are equivalent to the assumptions that
prevailed under the original Michaelis-Menten formulation, and these are
unlikely to obtain with natural substrates under physiological conditions.
But given synthetic substrates with poor turnovers or nonphysiological
structures, the conditions are readily obtainable. Kinetic studies of inhibitors
of serine proteases, for example, are likely to approach these conditions,
especially when highly reactive synthetic substrates (e.g., p-nitrophenyl esters
or aromatic amide derivatives) are used as substrates for ease in spectrophotometric assays. These compounds generate products that may readily
escape the active site before the enzyme reverts to the native conformer.
Other examples can no doubt be found in which either of the two products
might escape the active site quickly. Correlations are less likely to be found
when a conformational change, e.g., a "flap" opening, is *mandatory* for
product release. The latter was observed for a series of closely related
hydroxyethylene transition-state analog inhibitors of pepsin, for which K_I did
not correlate with V/K_m (31,32).

Examination of the trends shown in Figure 1 and Table 1 show that
another breakdown in the correlation between K_m/V and K_i is likely to occur,
even in the limited case just described, when V/K_m approaches diffusion

control; under these circumstances, the inhibitor can be *better* than anticipated on the basis of the substrate data! The reason for this is that changes in
the substrate structure that lead to tighter binding in TX will not greatly
increase V/K_m as it asymptotically approaches the diffusion-controlled limit,
but these same structural changes will continue to lead to tighter binding of
the corresponding inhibitor when steric hindrance is absent. Thus K_i
continues to decrease while V/K approaches a limit. Bartlett and Marlowe
have provided a clear example where inhibitors of thermolysin are better
than expected on the basis of the V/K_m vs. K_i correlations (30). As predicted
from the foregoing discussion and Figure 1, the breakdown in the correlation
between V/K and K_i occurs with inhibitors that are analogs of the best
substrates—those for which V/K_m approaches diffusion limits
$(10^6 \text{ M}^{-1} \text{ sec}^{-1})$.

In summary, successful correlations of V/K_m with K_i can be used to
support the hypothesis that an inhibitor is mimicking a transition state for an
enzyme-catalyzed bond formation or cleavage. Correlations are likely to fail
when V/K_m extends much beyond catalysis or when the substrates are too
good, even though the inhibitor is a good chemical analog of the transition
state in question.

III. SLOW-BINDING AND TIGHT-BINDING ENZYME INHIBITORS

A variety of potent enzyme inhibitors have been designed by preparing stable
synthetic analogs of reaction pathway intermediates, and it has been
observed that many of these inhibitors bind to the enzyme more slowly than
the corresponding substrates or classical competitive inhibitors. By 1986
nearly 40 examples of slow-binding inhibitors of various enzymes had been
described (33), and many more can be expected as new inhibitors of
therapeutically important enzymes are sought.

The slow onset of inhibition characteristic of these compounds is illustrated in Figure 2, in which the rate of the reaction shows a burst phase
when the reaction is initiated by adding enzyme to a solution of inhibitor and
substrate, or a lag phase when substrate is added to a preequilibrated
solution of enzyme and inhibitor. Morrison (34) developed a general
theoretical framework for analyzing the kinetics of slow- and tight-binding
enzyme inhibitors. Kinetic solutions for three general cases where inhibition
involves slow binding to enzyme or multiple conformations of native enzyme
or inhibitor separately (Scheme Va–c) or of enzyme-inhibitor complexes
(Scheme VI) were proposed. Many low-molecular-weight, tight-binding
inhibitors appear to follow the kinetic mechanism shown in Scheme VI (33),
although this can be difficult to establish (4,30). In this discussion we will call

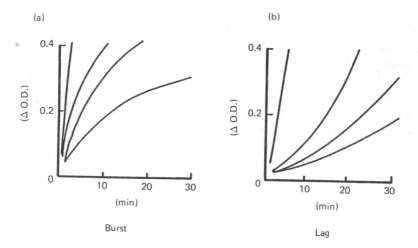

Figure 2 Reaction progress curves for inhibitors exhibiting slow binding. (a) Burst; (b) lag phases. See text for experimental conditions leading to these curves.

EI the collision complex, and EI* the tightened complex. Under saturating conditions, the half-life $(T_{1/2})$ for slow binding occurs on a time scale of seconds to minutes, i.e., on time scales much longer than expected on the basis of substrate turnover (typically in milliseconds), so that the fast binding predicted for transition state analog inhibitors on the basis of Figure 1 (vide infra) is not realized. Note that these half-lives have been determined at high enough concentrations of enzyme and inhibitor to preclude slow rates of bimolecular association which are often observed with high-molecular-weight inhibitors obeying the mechanism in Scheme Va.

Enzymologists and medicinal chemists have speculated over the cause or causes for slow binding of inhibitors to enzymes, but few detailed molecular mechanisms account for the observed kinetic behavior. Slow-binding inhibitors can be classified into two types: those that resemble the structures of transition states or high-energy reaction pathway intermediates, and those that do not resemble these intermediates. The rate of binding of the latter class of inhibitor to the enzyme is unpredictable; fast-weak, slow-weak, or fast-tight bindings are all possible.

The most common explanation for slow-binding inhibition is that a slow change in the conformation of the enzyme occurs after the inhibitor binds which leads to tighter binding between enzyme and inhibitor. A major change in the protein conformation can often be detected by spectroscopic methods (UV, CD, x-ray) and must occur at the slow rate detected kinetically. Although x-ray crystallography can establish the existence of multiple

(a)

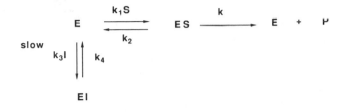

(b)

(c)

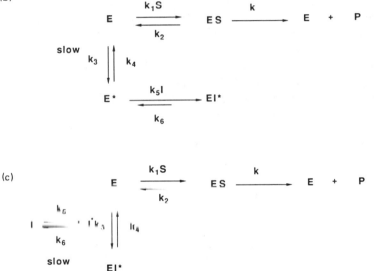

Scheme V

complexes, the method is too slow to ascertain if the structural changes occur on the same time scale as the slow-binding steps. For this purpose, fast, resolved spectroscopy is needed. Slow binding can result from slow interconversions between different enzyme forms (Scheme Vb) or from slow interconversions of inhibitor conformations (Scheme Vc). Generally, this process is associated most often with the latter mechanism. Examples include cis to trans isomerization of amides in the activation of prothrombin precursor (35). However, it is possible that both conformations of an inhibitor could bind to the enzyme, and, if isomerization occurred without dissociation of the complex, slow binding consistent with Scheme VI would result.

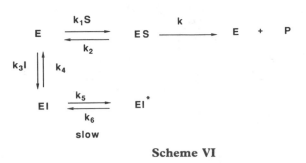

Scheme VI

The rate of binding of transition state analog inhibitors to enzymes deserves more comment. Many slow-binding inhibitors are thought to be reasonably good analogs of transition states (23,24), but if the inhibitor binds to the enzyme by a pathway that closely approximates the binding of substrate and its conversion to TX, then one would expect that the transition-state analog inhibitor would bind faster to the enzyme than substrate binds to the enzyme. This was depicted earlier in the free-energy profile in Figure 1 in which inhibitors that mimic TX cross a lower-energy barrier than substrate had to cross. The corollary of this is that the more potent inhibitors should bind faster than the weaker inhibitors. However, if inhibitors form complexes analogous to TX by completely different pathways, then no correlation between transition-state inhibitors and rate of binding would be expected. But since many transition-state analog inhibitors are very close structural analogs of substrates, it has been difficult to envision why such analogs would bind by a pathway other than that used by substrate. Attempting to rationalize the slow binding by invoking a slow conformational change in the protein only sidesteps the issue; one is then forced to rationalize why the structurally related transition-state analog inhibitor, but not the substrate, requires the slow conformational change.

In preparing this article, we have attempted to identify molecular processes that could be used to explain the slow-binding behavior of transition-state analog inhibitors. In the following discussion, we examine closely four slow-binding inhibitors of enzymes. Two of these have been shown to be reasonably good mimics of reaction pathway intermediates, either of the transition state or of the tetrahedral intermediate. The binding of certain inhibitors to aspartic proteinases and to thermolysin is slower than predicted from Figure 1 owing to an additional factor, the slow (or rare) de-solvation of the active site that must occur before the inhibitor can establish all the interactions with the enzyme needed for tight-binding inhibition. Thus, bound solvent forces the inhibitor into an alternative binding pathway.

Consideration of the kinetic mechanism of other slow-binding inhibitors has suggested additional slow-binding processes that have little to do with the expected catalytic mechanism for the reaction. These examples are described in the following sections.

A. Pepstatin-Derived Inhibitors of Aspartic Proteinases. Substrate (Water) Extrusion as a Cause of Slow Binding

Pepstatin, Iva–Val–Val–Sta–Ala–Sta (1), where Sta is 3S,4S-4-amino-3-hydroxy-6-methyl heptanoic acid (2), is an extremely effective inhibitor of several aspartic proteinases (36,37). Pepstatin has been used to clarify the catalytic mechanism and binding pockets of several aspartic proteinases (31,32), and specific inhibitors of selected aspartic proteinases have been devised by inserting statine for dipeptides in substrate sequences for renin (38,39), penicillopepsin (17), pepsin (40), and chymosin (41).

Pepstatin is a slow, tight-binding inhibitor of pepsin (16a). The slow binding was analyzed in terms of the two-step mechanism (Scheme VI, in which the collision complex is transformed to the tightened complex in a slow process. Structure-activity studies established that the 3S-hydroxyl group in the central statine residue (P_1–$P_{1'}$ in 1) is needed for the slow step. Deletion of the hydroxyl group, or epimerization to the 3R stereochemistry, decreases binding to pepsin about 1000-fold (42). The difference between the initial binding and tightened binding is substantial (> 500- to 1000-fold) for some inhibitors). However, the rate constant for the slow transition is 0.022 sec^{-1}, which is too slow for the formation of a putative II complex, because the analogous formation of a TX complex must proceed with an apparent rate constant equivalent to the enzyme-catalyzed formation of product (see Fig. 1). Fruton has measured with stopped-flow kinetic methods the rates of amide bond cleavage of peptide substrates and determined that the rate constant for the cleavage step exceeds 430 sec^{-1} (43). Additional stopped-flow kinetic studies of pepsin inhibition by the pepstatin analog Ac–Val–Val–Sta–Ala–Sta revealed, in addition to the slow first-order process already described, a second, much faster, first-order step in the binding process (44). Thus, the interaction between pepstatin and pepsin evidently must proceed via the minimal mechanism presented in Eq. (5). Formation of the "intermediate" complex in Eq. (5) is as fast as or faster than the fastest measured steps (sp^2–sp^3) for cleavage of an amide bond, as would be expected for an inhibitor that can bind to an enzyme without requiring sp^2–sp^3 distortion (vide supra).

$$E + I \rightleftharpoons EI \rightleftharpoons EI' \rightleftharpoons EI^* \qquad (5)$$
$$\text{collision} \qquad \text{intermediate} \qquad \text{tightened}$$

Other strong pepsin inhibitors bind to the enzyme much faster than pepstatin does. Ketone analogs **3** and **4** bind quickly even though the carbonyl group is converted from sp^2 to sp^3 (45,47). Ketones **3** and **4** have been shown by ^{13}C NMR to be converted to the tetrahedral gem diol adducts **5** and **6** upon binding to pepsin via enzyme-catalyzed addition of water (shown by ^{18}O-induced shifts of the ^{13}C NMR resonance for the gem diol) (47–49). The addition is too fast to be detected kinetically without resorting to stopped-flow methods, so the upper limit for the half-life for the addition of water is $\ll 20$ sec.

Thus, both the fast first-order process detected in the binding of pepstatin to pepsin and the addition of water to ketone pseudosubstrates in the active site of pepsin proceed much more quickly than the slow transition controlling the onset of inhibition. The fast step would likely involve partial closure of the "flap" region of the enzyme, since x-ray crystal data of the complex between penicillopepsin and Iva–Val–Val–Sta–OEt (**7**) show that, upon inhibitor binding, the "mobile" flap region, comprising protein amino acids 71–83, moves more than 2 Å relative to native enzyme to close the active site about the inhibitor (14). Again, kinetic data for substrates and difference UV and CD kinetic data for inhibitors show that this process occurs faster ($k_{app} > 10$– 15 sec^{-1}) than the slow onset of inhibition of pepsin.

What causes the slow binding? These same crystal structures show that, apart from the mobile "flap" region of the enzyme, the bulk of atoms of the protein backbone in the penicillopepsin–**7** complex remain at their positions in the native enzyme (14). Small reshufflings of side chains are evident, but these can be expected to occur quickly, since they involve small rotations about single bonds. Thus, major conformational changes that might be slow are not apparent, yet the kinetic data establish that some slow process occurs that stabilizes binding several thousandfold.

The slow displacement of a single, tightly bound water molecule from the active site of aspartic proteinases by the critical 3S-hydroxyl group in pepstatin has been offered as a possible mechanism for the slow onset of inhibition of these enzymes by pepstatin analogs (31). This idea was suggested by the realization that the critical 3S-statine hydroxyl group in pepstatin analogs in the penicillopepsin–**7** complex and in the *R. chinensis*–pepstatin complex occupies the same site as what appears to be the substrate water molecule in the native enzymes (see Fig. 3). Thus, inhibitor binding must be accompanied by displacement or extrusion of an enzyme-bound water molecule.

As illustrated schematically in Figure 4, the "intermediate" complex between pepsin and pepstatin would be stabilized by the normal peptide side chain and amide bond interactions plus a weak hydrogen bond to the statine hydroxyl group as it occupies the substrate carbonyl binding site. (Eventu-

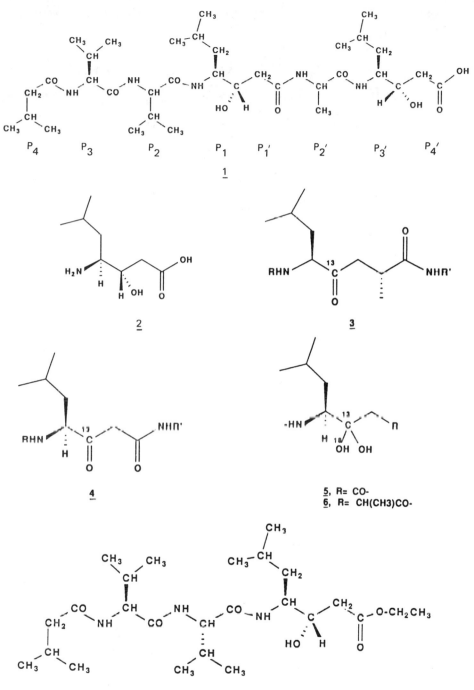

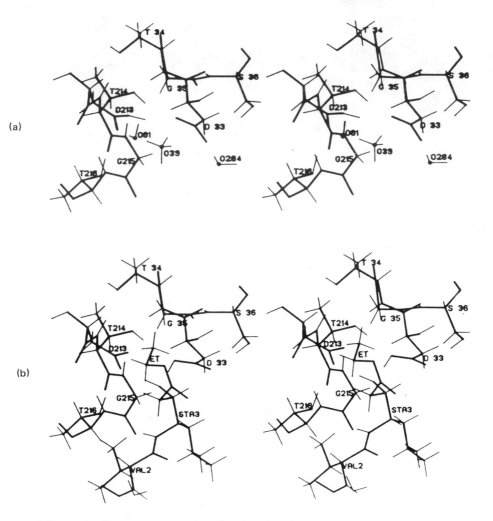

Figure 3 Stereo representation of active site of penicillopepsin. Penicillopepsin with the statine-containing inhibitor **7** bound. Data reproduced with permission (31).

(a) Mechanism of aspartic proteinases

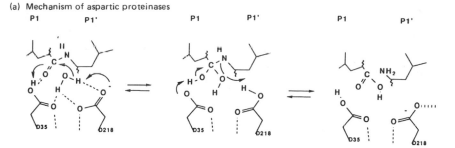

(b) Pepstatin bound in collision complex

(c) Pepstatin bound in tightened complex

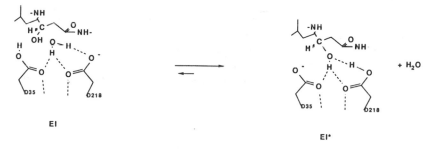

EI

EI*

Figure 4 Schematic representations for water extension by pepstatin. (a) hydrolysis of substrate by pepsin (20). (b) Intermediate complex for pepstatin-pepsin; (c) Tightened complex for pepstatin binding to pepsin.

ally, the 3S-hydroxyl group will occupy the bound water site in the tightened complex, but the carbonyl site is suggested for the "intermediate" complex, since there must be space within the active site to permit substrate carbonyl groups to bind.) The "intermediate" complex is metastable owing to steric interactions between the statine C3 proton and the enzyme-bound water molecule. As the water is displaced by the statine 3S-hydroxyl group via a serendipitous, uncatalyzed process, the "tightened" complex forms. This would be bound more tightly because of removal of the offending steric interactions and, possibly, because of a favorable entropic contribution, that of return of bound water to bulk solvent.

If water extrusion is the slow-binding process, then additional substituents on C3 of statine which retard water loss could slow even further the conversion of the intermediate complex to the tightened complex. Statine derivatives in which the proton on C3 of 3R-Sta analogs has been replaced with a methyl group (3R-MeSta[3]), e.g., **8**, are slower-binding inhibitors than the corresponding statine analogs (50). Thus, onset of inhibition for analog **8**

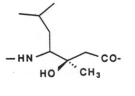

<u>8</u>

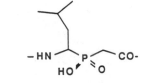

<u>9</u>

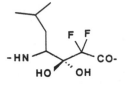

<u>10</u>

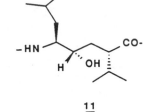

<u>11</u>

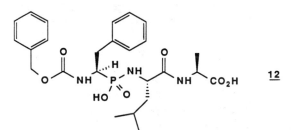

<u>12</u>

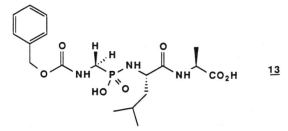

<u>13</u>

is 10 times slower ($T_{1/2} > 300$ sec vs. 31 sec). An even slower binding inhibitor ($T_{1/2} = 155$ min) is the phosphinic acid analog of statine (Sta^P; **9**) (51). The difluorostatone derivatives, e.g., **10**, which are extensively hydrated in solution to the gem diols, are very tight-binding inhibitors of pepsin which would displace the bound water molecule (52). It is probable that the hydroxyethylene isosteres, e.g., **11**, will act by a similar mechanism. Recent crystallographic data show that the hydroxyl group of inhibitor **11** occupies the putative substrate water site (15).

B. Phosphorus-Containing Inhibitors of Thermolysin. Nonsubstrate Water Extrusion as a Cause of Slow Binding

The naturally occurring N-phosphoryl dipeptide phosphoramidon is a slow, tight-binding inhibitor of the metalloprotease thermolysin (53). Bartlett and Marlowe (54) have synthesized a series of phosphonamidate and phosphonate peptide derivatives as potential transition-state analog inhibitors of thermolysin and, in collaboration with Tronrud et al. (55), have characterized the interactions of the inhibitors with thermolysin by x-ray crystallography. These models have served an important role in clarifying enzyme inhibitor interactions and catalytic mechanism. Related studies have suggested that these analogs closely resemble the transition state for the enzyme-catalyzed hydrolysis of substrate. Two recent examples have suggested a new molecular mechanism for slow binding between enzyme and inhibitor (30,56).

Cbz-Phe^P-Leu-Ala (**12**) is a slow, tight-binding inhibitor of thermolysin ($k_{on} = 10^4$ M^{-1} sec^{-1}), whereas the closely related analog Cbz-Gly^P-Leu-Ala (**13**) is less potent but fast-binding ($k_{on} = > 10^6$ M^{-1} sec^{-1}). The crystal structures of both inhibitors complexed with thermolysin have been solved and the structures refined to a resolution of 1.7 Å (56). The differences in protein conformation between native thermolysin and these two inhibitor-enzyme complexes are small. With respect to the S$_{1'}$ and S$_{2'}$ sites, both inhibitors bind essentially identically to thermolysin. However, the configurations of the Cbz–Phe^P and Cbz–Gly^P moieties are very different. In the Cbz–Gly^P complex, a water molecule is interposed between the inhibitor carbamate group and the enzyme in the S$_2$ site (Fig. 5), whereas with the corresponding α-branched analog, Cbz–Phe^P–Leu–Ala, the water molecule has been displaced. In this case, the carbonyl group of the Cbz group has been rotated by about 120° and forms a direct hydrogen bond to the enzyme. Bartlett and Marlowe (30) and Holden et al. (56) postulated that upon binding to the enzyme, the slow-binding inhibitor cannot form the tightened complex until the bound water molecule in the S$_2$ site is absent. When this occurs, a direct hydrogen bond between the Cbz carbonyl group and the Trp

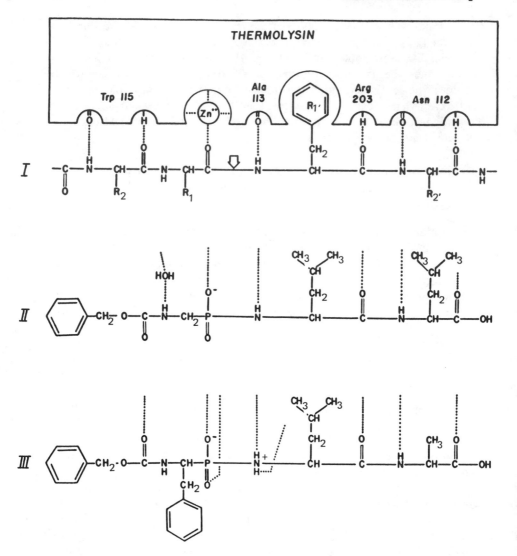

Figure 5 Schematic representations of binding of different thermolysin inhibitors to thermolysin. I. Substrate binding. II. Fast-binding inhibitors with water present. III. Slow-binding inhibitors with water gone. From B. W. Matthews, personal communication (56).

115 NH can form and stabilize the enzyme inhibitor complex. Thus the slow-binding behavior of **12** appears to be caused by the slow displacement of a single, nonsubstrate water molecule (Fig. 5). As Bartlett and Marlowe (30) and Holden et al. (56) point out, the slow process could be caused by the inhibitors' binding to a rare form of the enzyme that lacks this water, or the S_2-bound water could prevent formation of an observable, tightened complex until the bound water slips out. The latter mechanism should give saturation kinetics (Scheme VI), but these were not detected. Thus, which mechanism is operative is not yet known (57).

It is recognized that native enzymes, whether aspartic proteinases or thermolysin, retain a large number of water molecules in the substrate-binding pockets and that these waters are normally displaced either by substrates or inhibitors far too rapidly to account for slow-binding inhibitors. The slowly displaced water molecules described in Sections IIA and IIB differ in that they may be extensively hydrogen-bonded as might be needed for optimal attack of substrate water on peptide substrate or they may be accidentally "trapped" by the relatively large inhibitors, with escape to bulk solvent hindered by the inhibitor structure. In either case the inhibitor covers the active site, thereby preventing what would otherwise be a rapid de-solvation process.

The forgoing discussion was presented to illustrate that extreme care must be taken when attempting to rationalize slow binding between enzyme and inhibitor. If any general lesson can be drawn from the preceding examples, it is that all substrates and products must be considered when transition-state analog inhibitors are "docked" in the enzyme's active site. About 40 examples of slow-binding inhibitors are known (33). Although some of these bind via covalent mechanisms and some via oxidative mechanisms etc., many of the inhibited enzymes catalyze the addition or elimination of water or another small molecule. The supposedly "free" enzyme may still bind these small molecules in solution (certainly the water molecules are bound), and, if these must be displaced from the active site of the enzyme in order for the transition-state analog inhibitor to complete its maximal binding inter-actions, one can anticipate that slow binding will result as these prebound, trapped ligands struggle to escape the active site (57).

C. Alternate Mechanisms for Slow Binding

One can conceive of other mechanisms by which slow binding might be observed. If an inhibitor can bind in two modes, one closely related to substrate, and another structurally different but very tight, then slow-binding kinetics can result. If the inhibitor switches from one mode to the other slowly and without leaving the enzyme active site, then the kinetics will follow the two-step inhibition mechanism (Scheme VI). The inhibition of dihydrofolate reductase by methotrexate might follow this scheme.

The first enzyme inhibitor to be analyzed according to the kinetic equations of Morrison was methotrexate (58), an inhibitor of dihydrofolate reductase (DHFR). Methotrexate (MTX; **14**) binds to DHFR in a two-step process (Scheme VI) in which the initially formed collision complex (EI) is slowly transformed to a tightened complex (EI*). MTX inhibits DHFRs from other sources in the same way, and it has been shown that the slow step in this process increases binding by factors ranging from 150 to 390. Diaminopyrimidines—e.g., trimethoprim (TPM; **15**)—also inhibit DHFR by the two-step mechanism (59). In these cases the initial binding interaction is actually stronger than for MTX, but the net equilibrium favoring the tightened complex is somewhat weaker.

These results clearly show that multiple forms of EI complexes exist when folate antagonists bind to various DHFRs. The kinetic data are consistent with at least one detectable collision complex (EI) and one tightened complex (EI*). X-ray crystal structures for both binary (MTX:DHFR) and tertiary (MTX:DHFR;NADPH) complexes have been reported, and these are presumably for the tightened complex (60). Surprisingly, the crystal structures indicate that the diaminopyrimidine inhibitors bind "backward" relative to binding of substrate in the active site of the enzyme. Thus, the dia-minopyrimidine ring system in the inhibitors has been "rotated" 180° about the C6–C9 bond relative to the folate ring system in the substrates. This orientation is shown in Figure 6. In this case, it is unlikely that the inhibitor binding is mechanistically related to the binding of substrate during catalysis. Thus, the crystal structures suggest that the tightened complex for MTX:DHFR binding is not related in any way to what might be expected for an inhibitor that is a transition-state analog of the substrate. This appears to be a clear case where very tight binding between enzyme and inhibitor and very slow binding of inhibitor to enzyme are not associated with an analog of the transition state.

The DHFR-MTX system is an unusually well-characterized, slow, tight-binding inhibitor system. The catalytic mechanism is known, the inhibition kinetics are done exceptionally well, and excellent x-ray crystal structures are available. In spite of the availability of these data, the molecular events that take place during the slow, first-order transformation of collision to tightened complex have not been established. In molecular terms, this slow process could involve a single, slow transition, such as a major conformation change within the protein, or it could involve the sum of many subtle, small interactions between enzyme and inhibitor. We suggest that a simple explanation could be that the inhibitor is bound like substrate in the collision complex and bound in the observed "backward" mode in the tightened

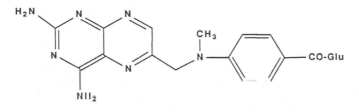

MTX, <u>14</u>

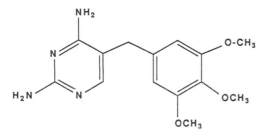

TMP, <u>15</u>

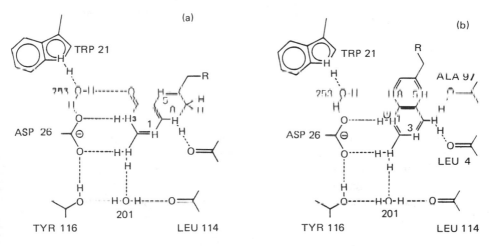

Figure 6 Schematic representation of hydrogen bonding between dihydrofolate reductase and the pteridine portions of (a) 7,8-dihydrofolate (hypothetical) and (b) methotrexate. "R" represents p-aminobenzoyl-L-glutamate. Residues are numbered according to the sequence of the *L. casei* enzyme. The interactions with methotrexate (b) are observed in high-resolution crystallographic studies of *E. coli* and *L. casei* dihydrofolate reductases. Interactions with dihydrofolate (a) are predicted by model-building experiments described in the text. The unlabeled carbonyl oxygen hydrogen bonded to N8 in the proposed enzyme-substrate complex might be Leu-4, Ala-97, or both.

213

complex, rotating from the first to the second at a slow rate. For this latter mechanism to be consistent with the kinetic data, the rotation of the diaminopyrimidine ring system would have to occur while the inhibitor remains on the enzyme, and the rate of rotation would have to occur at a rate consistent with k_5 in Scheme VI. Such slow rotations of aromatic ring systems within proteins have been observed by NMR and are likely due to steric constraints of the surrounding protein structure (2). One would also anticipate that rotations of the aromatic group in the inhibitor would be faster for the smaller aromatic ring in TMP than for MTX, as has been observed.

D. Novel Modes of Binding

The foregoing discussion illustrated the use of enzyme kinetics to characterize multiple enzyme-inhibitor forms where the inhibitor is binding at the expected site on the enzyme. In this section, we describe how synthetic analogs and enzyme kinetic studies were used to uncover an unanticipated binding interaction between inhibitor and enzyme.

Bestatin (**16**) and amastatin (**17**) are two aminopeptidase inhibitors discovered by Umezawa as a result of screening efforts to identify novel inhibitors of therapeutically important enzymes (61). The compounds get their names from the fact that bestatin inhibits aminopeptidase B (APB), the enzyme that cleaves basic residues from the N terminus of peptide chains, whereas amastatin inhibits aminopeptidase A (APA), the enzyme that cleaves acidic amino acids from the N terminus of peptide chains. Each inhibitor also inhibits other aminopeptidases, e.g., leucine aminopeptidase (LAP) and aminopeptidase M (APM) (62), to varying degrees.

Bestatin and amastatin are slow-binding inhibitors of various aminopeptidases (62). The binding of amastatin to APM was studied extensively by enzyme kinetics and synthetic analogs, and it was found that the inhibitor bound in the two-step process (Scheme VI). The structure-activity data for several closely related analogs were consistent with the binding of the hydroxyl stabilizing the collision complex, whereas increasing the length of

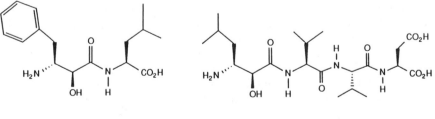

16   17

the peptide chain stabilized the tightened complex. The binding of bestatin to other aminopeptidases follows similar kinetics (63).

The close resemblance of the structures of the N-terminal amino acids in bestatin and amastatin to putative tetrahedral intermediates for amide bond hydrolysis (Fig. 7a) led to proposals that these inhibitors bind to the metallopeptidases in a mechanistically related fashion. Takita et al. (64) suggested that bestatin binds to the active site of aminopeptidases by a mechanism in which the critical 2S-hydroxyl and 3R-amino groups chelated the active-site zinc ion (Fig. 7b). Powers, on the other hand (65), suggested that the critical 2S hydroxyl group was paired with the C-1 carbonyl group during chelation to the active-site zinc ion (Fig. 7c). Both modes of binding placed the aromatic side chain of AHMHA in the P1 position where it would bind to the S_1 enzyme pocket.

If the critical 2S hydroxyl group interacts strongly with the active-site zinc in the tightened complexes, then substitution of the hydroxyl by sulfhydryl should lead to tighter binding inhibitors (66). This strategy has proved successful for the development of inhibitors of the zinc-metallopeptidase angiotensin-converting enzyme (ACE), e.g., Captopril (67), and of enkephalinase, e.g., Thiorphan (68). Consistent with this postulate was the finding that leucine thiol (18) is a very potent inhibitor of LAP (69) and APM (66) that binds to the target enzymes nearly 10,000 times tighter than the corresponding alcohol, leucinol (18b). Subsequently, lysinethiol 19a (70) was shown to inhibit APB (K_i = 0.1 nM) extremely well, binding about 10,000 times more tightly to APB than the alcohol 19b. However, when replacement of hydroxyl by thiol was carried out on bestatin to form thiol bestatin 20, a much weaker inhibitor was produced (66). Structure-activity data for a series of substituted leucine thiols showed that substituents α to the thiol were responsible for the diminished binding (66).

The inhibition of aminopeptidases by amino acid thiol derivatives is clearly consistent with other evidence that these enzymes are zinc metalloproteases. Furthermore, these results indicate that the strategy of using thiol ligands to stabilize the enzyme-inhibitor complex ought to work for aminopeptidases. Assuming that the thiol group in thiol bestatin binds to the enzyme in the same fashion as the hydroxyl group in bestatin, the hydroxyl group in bestatin does not coordinate with the active site zinc in these enzymes.

Detailed kinetics for the inhibition of APB by a reduced amide analog of bestatin 21 have suggested an alternate binding mode for bestatin that does not require the critical 2S hydroxyl group to be near the active-site zinc (71). Double reciprocal plots for the inhibition of APB by 21 were consistent with noncompetitive inhibition against the normal aminopeptidase substrate Arg–ONp. Replots of the slope and intercepts indicated that inhibition of

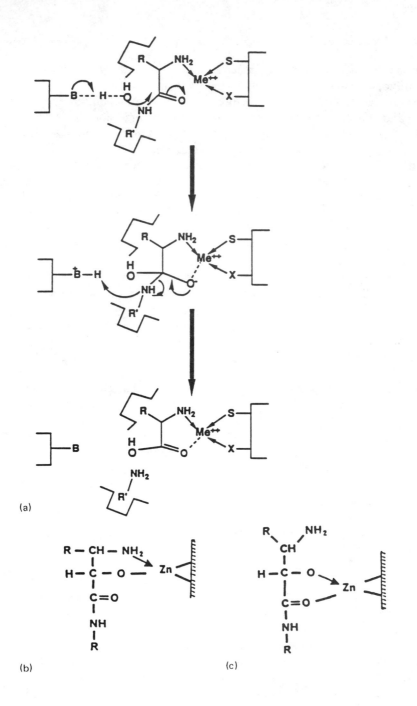

(a)

(b)

(c)

Figure 7 (a) Hydrolysis of substrate by leucine aminopeptidase (LAP). (b) Possible mechanism for inhibition of LAP by bestatin. (c) Alternate possible chelating mechanism for inhibition of LAP by bestatin. Note that N-terminal amino acid binds to S1 in both mechanisms.

APB by **21** followed an unusual inhibitory mechanism called slope-linear, intercept-hyperbolic, noncompetitive inhibition (see Section IV, Fig. 15). A kinetic scheme consistent with these data is shown in Scheme VIIa; Scheme VIIb illustrates the same mechanism in terms of the chemical species involved. The key feature of these schemes is that the inhibitor must be able to bind to the enzyme after an irreversible step in the hydrolytic reaction. This is illustrated as EQI in Scheme VIIa and as the [Arg...RBestatin] complex in VIIb. In order to accommodate the simultaneous binding of the Arg product (which is at S_1) and the reduced bestatin inhibitor, the inhibitor must bind to the $S'_1-S'_2$ enzyme pockets rather than exclusively to the substrate binding sites, $S_1-S'_1$, as required for the proposed mechanisms in Figure 7. This places the aromatic group of the reduced bestatin derivative in the S'_1 binding pocket of the enzyme.

Structure-activity data for a series of ketomethylene inhibitors provide additional evidence for favorable binding of aromatic side chains in the S'_1 pocket of APB (71). Ketomethylene (KM) inhibitors correspond to the replacement of the amide nitrogen in depeptides with a methylene group. Arphamenines (**22a,b**) are naturally occurring ketomethylene inhibitors isolated and characterized by Umezawa and co-workers (72). The structure-activity relationships for a series of these compounds closely correspond with those expected on the basis of the substrate specificity of APB (Table 2). Thus, the best inhibitors contain a basic side chain at the N terminus (22,23), as expected from the fact that APB cleaves Arg and Lys from peptide chains. This implies a favorable interaction between substrate and inhibitor basic side chains and the S_1 binding sites on the enzyme. The structure-activity data also reveal unexpectedly that the binding of a benzyl side chain at S'_1

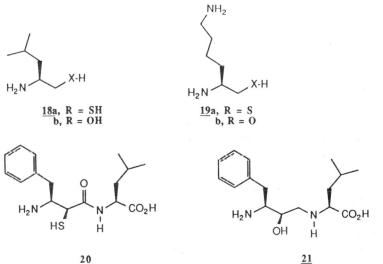

18a, R = SH
 b, R = OH

19a, R = S
 b, R = O

20

21

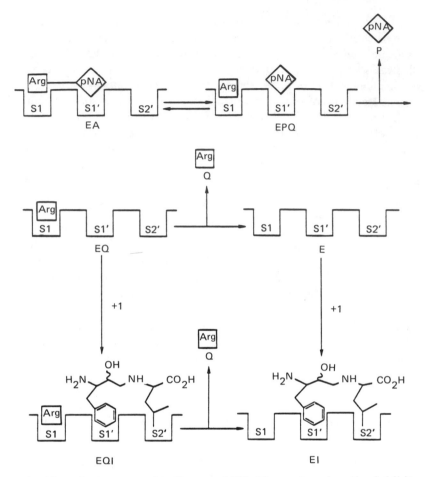

significantly increases binding to APB. Thus, changing the inhibitor side chain from methyl to benzyl increases binding 500- to 760-fold (e.g., **23** vs. **24**; **25** vs. **26** in Table 2).

The structure-activity data for inhibition of APB by bestatin analogs also support the binding of benzyl side chains to the S_1' enzyme site. Changing the second residue side chain from methyl to benzyl in bestatin derivatives (e.g., **16** vs. **27** in Table 2) increases binding 620-fold, an increase quantitatively similar to that found for the N terminus substituted ketomethylene analogs (**24, 26**). In contrast, placing a basic side chain at the N terminus in bestatin does not enhance binding; instead, inhibition is slightly weakened (compare **16** with **28, 29**).

Thus, both structure-activity data for two series of APB inhibitors and the mechanism for inhibition of APB by the reduced bestatin analog **21** are consistent with the binding of aromatic groups to the S_1' site on the enzyme.

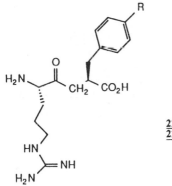
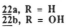

22a, R = H
22b, R = OH

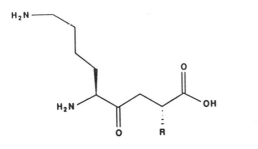

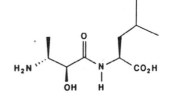

27

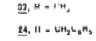

23, R = CH₃

24, R = CH₂C₆H₅

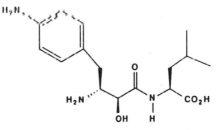

28

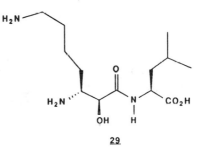

25, R = CH₃

26, R = benzyl

29

Table 2   Structure-Activity Relationships for Bestatin Analogs and Ketomethylene Isostere Inhibitors of Aminopeptidase B

		Bestatin analogs					Ketomethylene substrate analogs			
Cpd #	*	R	R'	IC_{50} (μM)	Relative affinity	Cpd #	R	R'	K_i	Relative affinity
16	(S)	(R)-Benzyl	i-Butyl	0.16		25	(S)-i-Butyl	CH_3	0.13 mM	
		vs.					vs.			65X
28	(S)	(R)-p-NH_2-Benzyl	i-Butyl	0.31	−1.9X	23	(S)-$(CH_2)_4NH_2$	CH_3	2.0 μM	
29	(S)	(S)-Benzyl	i-Butyl	4.0	negl.	26	(S)-i-Butyl	Benzyl	0.17 μM	
	(RS)	(S)-$(CH_2)_4NH_2$	i-Butyl	4.8			vs.			42X
	(S)	(R)-Benzyl	i-Butyl	0.16	−25X	24	(S)-$(CH_2)_4NH_2$	Benzyl	4.0 nM	
		vs.					(R)-i-Butyl	Benzyl	0.77 μM	4.5X
	(S)	(S)-Benzyl	i-Butyl	4.0			vs.			
27	(RS)	(R)-CH_3	i-Butyl	100.	620X		(S)-i-Butyl	Benzyl	0.17 μM	
		vs.				25	(S)-i-Butyl	CH_3	0.13 mM	760X
16	(S)	(R)-Benzyl	i-Butyl	0.16			vs.			
	(S)	(R)-Benzyl	CH_3	1.01	−11X	26	(S)-i-Butyl	Benzyl	0.17 μM	
	(S)	(R)-Benzyl	Benzyl	11.2		23	(S)-$(CH_2)_4NH_2$	CH_3	2.0 μM	500X
						24	(S)-$(CH_2)_4NH_2$	Benzyl	4.0 nM	

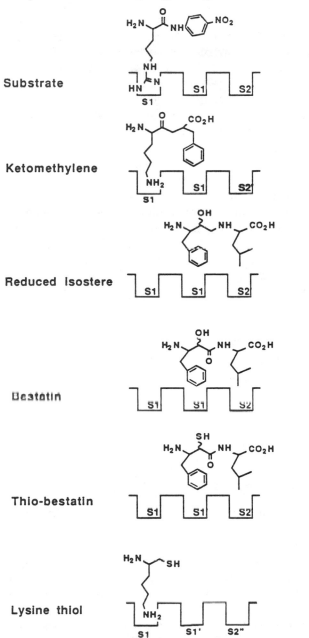

Figure 8 Binding of thiol inhibitors, ketomethylene inhibitors, and bestatin derivatives to aminopeptidase B.

This requires the reduced bestatin to be bound to the $S_1'-S_2'$ enzyme sites as shown in Figure 8 and not at the S_1-S_1' sites, as previously proposed. The fact that the 2-thiol bestatin derivatives are not improved inhibitors relative to bestatin suggests that the 2-hydroxyl group in bestatin does not strongly interact with the zinc ion at the active site. Figure 8 illustrates the different ways each of these inhibitors could bind to APB. The function of the 2S hydroxyl group in bestatin, which is clearly necessary for maximal inhibition of all aminopeptidases (62), remains unknown. The hydroxyl group could displace the second substrate water molecule in a fashion analogous to that suggested for aspartic proteinase (31) and thermolysin inhibitors (56,30), or it might function by a completely new mechanism.

The significance of the bestatin and methotrexate studies with respect to this chapter is to emphasize that tight-binding inhibition and slow-binding inhibition may arise in surprising ways. Just because an inhibitor looks and acts like our preconceptions of a transition-state analog does not mean that it is mimicking the reaction pathway intermediate we suspect. Detailed enzyme kinetic evaluation of natural or synthetic inhibitors of enzymes should be carried out whenever possible in conjunction with molecular modeling efforts to validate the expected mechanism of inhibition.

IV. EFFECTS OF MULTIPLE FORMS ON ENZYME INHIBITION: STRATEGIES OF EXPERIMENTAL DESIGN AND GUIDES FOR EVALUATING KINETIC DATA

The purpose of this section is to focus attention on such practical problems encountered in the study of inhibitors that derive from multiple forms of enzyme and changes between forms.

A. Tight-Binding and Slow-Binding Inhibitors

Enzyme inhibition has traditionally been considered in terms of complexes with free enzyme (giving competitive inhibition as in the mechanism of Scheme Va) or with free enzyme plus the enzyme-substrate complex (giving noncompetitive inhibition as in Scheme VIII). During the last decade, additional forms of enzyme-inhibitor complexes had to be proposed and considered in order to understand the kinetics of tight-binding and slow-binding inhibitors (73).

In the mechanism of Scheme VI, kinetics consistent with tight-binding behavior arise from a lower value for k_6 than k_5; kinetics for slow-binding behavior arise from k_5 itself having a low value relative to catalysis. The mechanism applies to many tight-binding inhibitors, and the two forms of

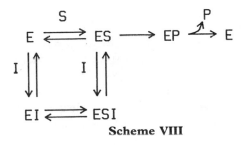

Scheme VIII

enzyme that figure into the inhibition are the collision complex and the tightened complex. The inhibition constant is not a simple dissociation constant but includes the equilibrium constant for the isomerization between the collision and tightened complex, as shown in Eq. (6).

$$K_i = \frac{k_4 k_6}{k_3 (k_5 + k_6)} \tag{6}$$

In addition, because of the slow onset of inhibition, there is a change in the distribution of enzyme forms during the time that would normally be considered the steady-state region of a kinetic assay. As illustrated in Figure 9, instead of the usual linear initial velocity during the first 10% of reaction

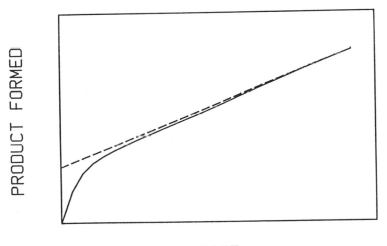

Figure 9 Progress curve for an enzymatic assay in the presence of a slow-binding inhibitor.

(assuming the reaction is started with the addition of enzyme), one observes a more rapid reaction near time zero which then relaxes to the slower, true steady-state velocity, which expresses the full measure of inhibition.

In the mechanism of Scheme Va, kinetics consistent with tight-binding behavior arise from a low value for k_4; kinetics for slow-binding behavior arise from low values for both k_3 and k_4. The mechanism does not invoke a need for additional forms of enzyme over those found in simple competitive inhibition, but one nevertheless still has to contend with a change in form during assays of inhibited enzyme. Regardless of mechanism, when assaying inhibited enzymes, it is necessary that both the sensitivity of one's assay and the length of time over which data are collected be sufficient to detect a possible transition between forms. Obviously, a single-point, fixed-time assay (e.g., a radioactivity assay) cannot detect the curvature shown in Figure 9; instead, a continuous monitor of the time course of a reaction is preferred (e.g., a spectrophotometric assay). But if a fixed-time assay cannot be avoided, then it is necessary to collect many data points, extending from very early to very late in the assay, in order to identify correctly the level of inhibition of the enzyme in the steady state (e.g., the dashed line in Fig. 9). To determine the slope of the dashed line accurately, computer fitting is usually essential, because the progress curve approaches the dashed line asymptotically and will fall away eventually owing to substrate depletion [see Eqs. (1)–(6), Appendix 1]. [For a general discussion of other practical problems of obtaining steady-state velocities from enzymatic assays, see Allison and Purich (74), and for a discussion of the kinetics of tight-binding inhibitors, see Williams and Morrison (58).]

B. Multiple Forms of Free Enzyme

These may be either stable forms of different polypeptides (i.e., isozymes) or slowly interconverting forms of the same peptide. Multiple forms of both kinds have been heavily documented in the literature, and both can confound the results of in vitro screening and analysis of potential drugs. For example, human liver alcohol dehydrogenase was once thought of as a single enzyme, whereas extensive studies during the past 15 years have shown that it is highly polymorphic, consisting of several dozen dimeric isozymes, assembled from five subunits. Moreover, the isozymes differ in substrate specificity and susceptibility to inhibition by 4-methylpyrazole. Class I isozymes prefer long-chain alcohols and display inhibition constants as low as 0.13 μM, whereas the class II isozyme prefers aromatic alcohols and has an inhibition constant of 2000 μM (75). It follows that the use of an artificial substrate, because of its ease of assay, or an uncommon substrate, because of its low cost, must be accompanied by a demonstration of the relationship of its isozymic susceptibility to that of the specific substrate whose metabolism one wishes to inhibit. One simple test that is applicable to the artificial substrate (if it is the only reactant detected in the assay) is to examine the kinetics of apparent inhibition by the natural substrate and compare its pseudo inhibition constant with its Michaelis-Menten constant, determined in a separate assay which measures turnovers of the natural substrate; these should agree if the artificial and natural substrates are both acted on by the same enzyme or isozymes.

A particularly difficult problem can arise with slowly interconverting but catalytically different forms of the same enzyme, because substrates and inhibitors may shift the equilibria between forms in vitro, and which forms are functional in vivo is usually unknown. For example, Williams and Northrop (76) observed an inhibition constant of 0.37 μM for competitive inhibition of 3N-aminoglycoside acetyltransferase I by neomycin B when tobramycin was the varied substrate, but also obtained a much larger value of 30 μM when sisomicin was the varied substrate. Because an enzyme binds a competitive inhibitor only during the absence of the varied substrate, the enzyme should not "remember" the substrate when binding the inhibitor. These data therefore show that tobramycin and sisomicin bind to different forms of enzyme. A failure to separate these two forms on a neomycin affinity column argued against the presence of different isozymes, and a lag present in assays of tobramycin but not of sisomicin supported slowly interconverting enzyme conformers. More recently, Marti (77) has observed similar differences in inhibition constants for paromomycin versus 12 aminoglycoside substrates; four sets of inhibition constants have been determined, suggesting four conformers of enzyme. If one wishes to consider a paromomycin-like derivative as a possible drug for combating antibiotic resistance mediated by this particular enzyme, it then becomes necessary to be specific regarding which aminoglycoside antibiotic one wishes to protect.

C. Analysis of Enzyme Kinetic Data

The traditional method of analyzing the velocities of enzymatic reactions as a dependent function of concentrations of substrate is by graphical analysis, setting reciprocal velocities against reciprocal concentrations, as first formulated by Lineweaver and Burk (78) and illustrated in Figure 10A. The Michaelis-Menten constant was obtained by extrapolation to the horizontal axis and taking the negative reciprocal of the value at the point of intersection. In order to get an equal spacing of data points as shown and thus obtain a more balanced contribution from each assay performed, equally spaced dilutions of a stock solution—e.g., 1/20, 5/20, 9/20, 13/20, etc.—are prepared, and equal amounts of each are used in the separate assays.

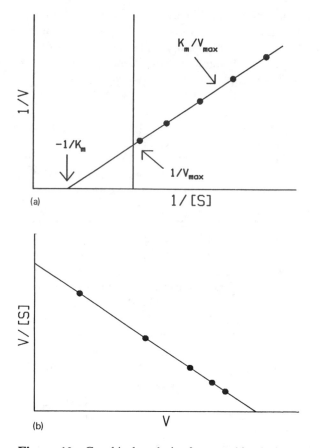

Figure 10   Graphical analysis of enzyme kinetic data. (a) Double-reciprocal plot. (b) Eadie-Hofstee plot.

Considerable objection from statisticians such as Dowd and Riggs (79) have been raised against the use of the double-reciprocal plot, and alternatives such as the Eadie-Hofstee plot, shown in Figure 10b, have been championed. Also, not all enzymes obey the Michaelis-Menten equations under all conditions, and the Eadie-Hofstee plot is more sensitive to deviations from linearity. Nevertheless, the double-recriprocal plot remains the favored means for illustrating data, for the simple reason that it is the only linear formulation of the Michaelis-Menten equation that separates the dependent and independent variables on the two graphical axes. Also, the fundamental kinetic constants are easily noted in the slopes and intercepts of the plot. The statistical objections are serious, however, and fitting normal data to the Michaelis-Menten equation by nonlinear regression has therefore replaced graphical analysis as a means of extracting unbiased kinetic constants [see Appendix 1, Eq. (4)]. In practice, regression usually precedes graphics, in order to provide the correct coordinates for the line. The program written by Duggleby (80) for small computers and reproduced in Appendix 1 has proved to be especially useful for kinetic applications.

D. Competitive Inhibition

Inhibitory analogs of substrates are expected to bind in the active site of an enzyme and completely displace the substrate. Both mechanisms of Schemes Va and VI will give rise to the normal kinetic pattern for competitive inhibition—but only if true steady-state velocities are analyzed (vide infra) and only if the enzyme concentration is significantly below the lowest concentration of inhibitor (vide supra). Structural similarity alone, however, is not sufficient to presume competitive binding, because partial or unusual bindings of analogs can occur; hence, the competitiveness of the inhibitor must be documented. To do so, one determines the initial velocity of the enzyme at various concentrations of substrate and inhibitor and constructs a double-reciprocal plot as shown in Figure 11.

The diagnostic portion of the plot is the intersection of the lines on the vertical intercept. For this reason, it is desirable to choose high concentrations of substrate (i.e., the solid circles) rather than low concentrations (i.e., the open circles) in order to focus on the vertical intercept and avoid a long extrapolation from less precise data. To establish the commonality of the intersection point, *each line* should be fitted to the hyperbolic form of the

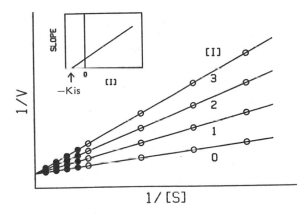

Figure 11 Competitive inhibition pattern.

Michaelis-Menten equation by nonlinear regression. If competitive inhibition is present, it will be identified by a set of apparent values of V_{max}, one for each line, of similar values whose standard errors overlap.

To extract the inhibition constant, all of the velocities should be fitted to the general rate equation for competitive inhibition:

$$V = \frac{V[S]}{K_m(1 + [I]/K_{is}) + [S]} \tag{7}$$

where v is the observed steady-state velocity, V is the maximal velocity, $[S]$ is the concentration of substrate, K_m is the Michaelis-Menten constant, $[I]$ is the concentration of inhibitor, and K_{is} is the inhibition constant. Alternatively, in the days of graphical analysis of enzyme kinetic data, one plotted the slopes of the individual lines from the double-reciprocal plot against the concentrations of inhibitor and obtained the inhibition constant by extrapolating a straight line through the data points to the horizontal axis (see inset to Fig. 11). Computer fitting is preferred, however, because it avoids bias due to improper weighting; moreover, it can provide standard errors for each parameter. These should be included in publications of results to give the reader a proper measure of the precision of the inhibition constant. Nevertheless, it is still useful to make replots of slopes and intercepts from the results of individual line fits in order to detect partial inhibition or other specialized patterns (vide supra).

E.   Classical Noncompetitive Inhibition

Noncompetitive inhibition of unireactant enzymes is usually depected as binding of inhibitor and substrate to different sites on the enzyme surface, allowing the formation of an enzyme-substrate-inhibitor complex. Thus, the inhibitor binds to two forms of enzyme, both free and complexed with the substrate. In the classical or textbook mode, the inhibitor is assumed to bind equally well to both forms, and lines in double-reciprocal plots of inhibited velocities cross on the horizontal axis, as shown in Figure 12. However, this is usually found not to be the case in the laboratory when, inhibition lines are examined individually and the results are properly compared. As a result, data from a kinetic pattern should not be examined only as a set of lines expected to intersect solely on the horizontal axis—or on the vertical axis, for that matter. Rather, as described above, each line should again be fitted to the Michaelis-Menten equation; if classical noncompetitive inhibition is present, it will be identified by a set of apparent values of K_m of similar value whose standard errors overlap. When the errors do not overlap, the noncompetitive data reveal the presence of either binding antagonism or binding synergism between substrate and inhibitor. For example, Figure 13 illustrates a noncompetitive inhibitor that synergizes the binding of substrate.

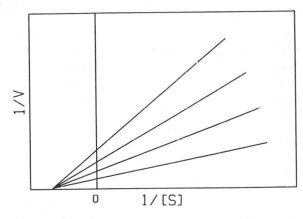

Figure 12   Classical noncompetitive inhibition pattern.

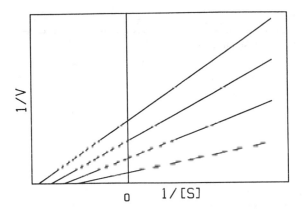

Figure 13   Nonclassical noncompetitive inhibition pattern.

Fitting each inhibitory line to the Michaelis-Menten equation yields apparent values of K_m which decrease with increasing concentrations of inhibitor. Moreover, fitting the entire data set to the general rate equation for noncompetitive inhibition:

$$V = \frac{V[S]}{K_m(1 + [I]/K_{is}) + [S](1 + [I]/K_{ii})} \tag{8}$$

will give different values for K_{is} and K_{ii}. K_{is} expresses the effect of the inhibitor on the slopes of the lines in the kinetic pattern and is a true dissociation constant for the release of inhibitor from the enzyme-inhibitor complex; K_{ii} expresses the effect on intercepts and is a true dissociation constant for the release of inhibitor from the enzyme-substrate-inhibitor complex. The difference between values of K_{is} and K_{ii} (or between slope and intercept effects) reveals the presence and degree of binding synergism ($K_{is} > K_{ii}$) or antagonism ($K_{is} < K_{ii}$). If the difference is significant, it can have relevance to expected levels of inhibition in vivo. With binding synergism, the level of inhibition increases as the concentration of substrate increases, which potentiates the blocking effect.

F. Nonclassical Noncompetitive Inhibition

Few enzymes are unireactant, and in bireactant or higher systems, noncompetitive inhibition frequently arises by inhibitors combining with forms of enzyme-cosubstrate complexes or with other forms of enzyme which lie downstream from the binding of substrates. To illustrate, consider the multiple binding of an inhibitor to an enzyme obeying a bireactant-ordered mechanism.

Given an inhibitor that is an analog of the second substrate, its binding to free enzyme may be very slight or nonexistent. Therefore the concentration of the first substrate—the one *not* resembling the inhibitor—is an important consideration in kinetic analyses, because it may control the distribution of enzyme between susceptible and unsusceptible forms of enzyme (e.g., EA and E, respectively, in Scheme IX). For example, inhibitory analogs of folic acid bind as much as 50,000-fold more tightly to the NADPH enzyme form of dihydrofolate reductase than to free enzyme (59). It is thus very important that the physiological concentration of the nonvaried or cosubstrate is known and reproduced in assays of the inhibited enzyme.

The sole combination of inhibitor with EA to form EAI in Scheme IX is competitive with the binding of B, so a slope effect is expressed in kinetic patterns where the concentration of B is varied. But if the inhibitor is also an analog of the first product, which is likely, it may also bind to EQ to form EQI. This secondary binding is uncompetitive to the binding of B, so an intercept effect is expressed. The combination of both effects resulting from the binding of inhibitor to two different forms of enzyme during one turnover generates a noncompetitive inhibition pattern in which the slope and intercept effects are independent of each other. This kinetic pattern is

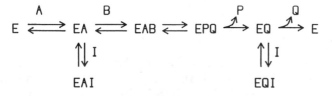

Scheme IX

indistinguishable from that which one would obtain for a classical noncompetitive inhibitor, where the slope and intercept effects are related; yet the binding of the inhibitor is essentially competitive versus the second substrate in this nonclassical case.

Moreover, while K_{is} is again a true dissociation constant (for the release of I from EAI, if measured at saturating concentrations of A), K_{ii} is not. The latter inhibition constant is dependent not only on the dissociation constant for EQI but also on the amount of total enzyme present as EQ during steady-state turnover at saturating levels of both substrates A and B. Given equal true dissociation constants for EAI and EQI, when the catalytic segment is rate-limiting, very little EQ will be present, K_{ii} will be much higher than K_{is}, and the kinetic pattern will approach that of simple competitive inhibition.

On the other hand, if the release of the second product, Q, is the rate-limiting segment, then virtually all of the enzyme will be present as EQ, K_{ii} will equal K_{is}, and the kinetic pattern will approach the classical noncompetitive pattern with intersection on the horizontal axis. Factors such as pH, temperature, and concentrations of other reactants or activators which change the distribution of the forms of enzyme, either toward or away from EQ, will change the sensitivity of this enzyme to inhibition, even though the true dissociation constants remain unchanged. For example, glutamate dehydrogenase follows an ordered mechanism similar to Scheme IX, in which uncompetitive substrate inhibition by α-ketoglutarate arises from the formation of an enzyme-NADP-ketoglutarate complex (i.e., EQI). Rife and Cleland (84) observed that the inhibition was enhanced (i.e., the apparent K_{ii} was lowered) by the addition of stock NADP+ to the assay cuvettes, which shifted the distribution of free enzyme forms toward EQ during reaction turnovers. Physiologically, one would expect NADP+ to be present at a significant level at all times. Thus, the addition of some product to the kinetic assays provides a more realistic measure of the susceptibility of this enzyme to substrate inhibition than would be obtained from standard measurements of initial velocities.

G. Parabolic Inhibition

Changes in slopes and intercepts need not be linear functions of the concentration of inhibitor. If more than a single combination of inhibitor with enzyme can occur, or if the combination with one form enhances a second combination later in the reaction, then the inhibitor appears self-activating. This behavior is expressed as a parabolic curve when the changes in slopes or intercepts are replotted as a function of the concentration of inhibitor, as illustrated in Figure 14.

Parabolic inhibition is uncommon [product inhibition of liver alcohol dehydrogenase by ethanol is an example, however (82)], probably owing

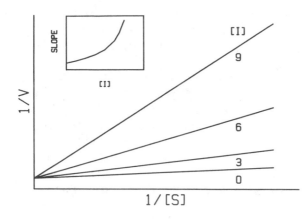

Figure 14 Parabolic competitive inhibition pattern.

more to a lack of complete kinetic studies than to a low incidence. Because it is more likely to occur with small inhibitors of large substrates (which allows for multiple bindings to the active site), one should be on the lookout for parabolic inhibition when investigating enzymes acting on polymeric substrates (e.g., proteins, carbohydrates, and nucleic acids) and inhibited by monomeric or dimeric inhibitors. The practical significance of parabolic inhibition is that one obtains much more inhibition at high concentrations of inhibitor than one would predict based on an inhibition constant determined at low or moderate concentrations.

H. Hyperbolic Inhibition

More common origins of nonlinear inhibition, however, are combinations of inhibitor with enzyme that fail to completely block further progress toward an enzymatic turnover and give as a result only partial inhibition. This second type of nonlinear inhibition is expressed as a hyperbolic curve when the changes in slopes or intercepts are replotted as a function of the concentration of inhibitor. For example, Gates and Northrop (83) have shown that aminoglycoside nucleotidyltransferase also catalyzes an ordered reaction as shown in Scheme IX, in which A is Mg:ATP, B is aminoglycoside, P is pyrophosphate, and Q is AMP-aminoglycoside. The enzyme is inhibited by neomycin, which combines with both EA and EQ, but unlike the mechanism in Scheme IX, the EQI complex is not dead-ended; rather, Q can escape from it, albeit at a slower rate than from EQ, and this second pathway of product release produces partial inhibition, expressed as a hyperbilic effect on the intercepts of the noncompetitive inhibition pattern, illustrated in Figure 15.

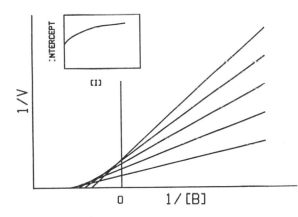

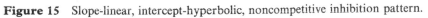

Figure 15 Slope-linear, intercept-hyperbolic, noncompetitive inhibition pattern.

Partial inhibition is important to document because it can severely limit the effectiveness of even the most tightly bound of inhibitors. (See Section III for the hyperbolic inhibition of aminopeptidases by inhibitor **21**.)

I. Artifactual Noncompetitive Inhibition

Morrison (34) noted that tight-binding competitive inhibitors generate what appear to be noncompetitive inhibition patterns if the concentrations of inhibitor are comparable to the concentration of active sites of an enzyme, as illustrated in Figure 16. The reason for this is the nonlinearity of the inhibited lines of the pattern. At very high concentrations of substrate, the lines curve downward and converge at a common intersection point on the vertical axis, as they should in a competitive inhibition pattern. But at low concentrations of substrate, the lines approach linear asymptotes which do not intersect on the vertical axis. These asymptotes reflect a progressive decrease in the amount of unbound inhibitor as the concentration of substrate decreases. With weaker inhibitors, the amount of bound inhibitor is insignificant compared to total inhibitor, and therefore the amount of unbound inhibitor is constant for a given line. Like others before it, this pattern can be detected by replotting slopes and intercepts; if artifactual noncompetitive inhibition is present, the slope replot will show upward curvature much like parabolic replots. It may also be possible to identify this pattern by the downward curvature of the primary plots, but because this occurs only at very high concentrations of substrate, this curvature is often excluded from the experimental data. When present, artifactual noncompetitive inhibition may be analyzed by the graphical method of Henderson (85) or by computer fitting directly to Morrison's equation [see Eqs. (14–17), Appendix 1].

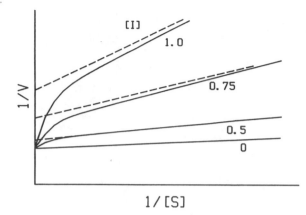

Figure 16 Competitive inhibition pattern by a tight-binding inhibitor. [After Morrison (34).]

J. Multiple Inhibition

A powerful but underused kinetic method for probing the binding sites of inhibitors is the multiple inhibition approach of Yonetani and Theorell (89,90). In their design, the substrate is held constant at a level below its K_m while two competitive inhibitors are varied against each other. The data are plotted as reciprocal velocities versus the concentration of one inhibitor, at fixed concentrations of the other, as shown in Figure 17. If the two competitive inhibitors are also competitive against each other, then the pattern consists of a set of parallel lines, governed by an equation of the form [cf. Eq. (7)]:

$$v = \frac{V[S]}{K_m(1 + [I]/K_I + [J]/K_J) + [S]} \tag{9}$$

where J is the second inhibitor.

If, on the other hand, the two inhibitors are not competitive with each other but occupy subsites of the enzyme active center, then the lines are intersecting, governed by a more complex equation:

$$v = \frac{V[S]}{K_m(1 + [I]/K_I + [J]/K_J + [I][J]/\alpha K_I K_J) + [S]} \tag{10}$$

in which α is an interaction constant. When α is greater than 1, the inhibitors are antagonistic [e.g., when $\alpha = \infty$, inhibitors are totally antagonistic, and

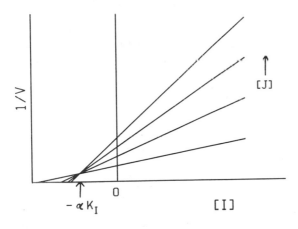

Figure 17 Yonetani-Theorell plot of multiple inhibition for two synergistic competitive inhibitors.

Eq. (10) reduces to Eq. (9)]; when α is less than 1, the inhibitors are synergistic. Yonetani (90) notes than "ion-dipole, interionic, interdipole, hydrophobic, and hydrophilic interactions, as well as simple steric hinderence and protein-conformational changes, may be involved" in the antagonism or synergism. As a practical note, the design of experiments to examine the value of α should include relatively high concentrations of both inhibitors, because these concentrations are multiplied together in the α term of Eq. (10); hence high concentrations of both enhance the expression of the α term.

In addition, Northrop and co-workers (76,77,91,92) have extended the method to inhibitors that are not competitive with substrate and that do not resemble each other as a means to identify the form of enzyme to which an inhibitor binds and to demonstrate changes in the steady-state distribution of enzyme. For example, in the ordered reaction mechanism illustrated in Scheme IX, part of the inhibition arises from the combination of I with EQ to form EQI. If the amount of enzyme present as EQ during steady-state turnovers were small, this origin of inhibition might be unimportant. But if Q were added as a product inhibitor and it raised the steady-state level of EQ, then the sensitivity to inhibition by I would be increased, and the inhibitors would be said to be synergistic. Similar experimental designs of multiple inhibition can be devised that might document changes in the distribution of enzyme forms by many known inhibitors, which to date have not been subjected to multiple inhibition kinetics with a second inhibitor.

V. SUMMARY

The foregoing kinetic discussion can be summarized below as a strategy for obtaining useful data and analyzing appropriate patterns to characterize enzyme inhibitors.

1. Investigate the kinetics of inhibition as a function of the substrate or substrates of interest in vivo. If an artificial substrate is to be used for ease of assay, establish its kinetic equivalency to the natural substrate.
2. Use a sensitive assay, continuous if possible, or collect multiple fixed-time data points if not, to ensure that the true steady-state velocity is the reaction rate being detected.
3. If a burst or lag is present in the assay, analyze the transient by nonlinear regression to obtain the true steady-state velocity.
4. Collect rate data at concentrations of inhibitor and varied substrate that will be diagnostic for the expected pattern of inhibition—e.g., high concentrations of both if the pattern is competitive.
5. Select a sufficient number and range of concentrations of inhibitor to establish linearity of both slope and intercept functions. Investigate a larger number and wider range, if nonlinearity is detected, to document hyperbolic or parabolic functions.
6. Be sure that the concentrations of inhibitor are in excess of the concentration of active sites when using standard patterns and rate equations for data analysis.
7. Illustrate kinetic data on double-reciprocal plots, but locate each line separately by fitting normal velocity data to the Michaelis-Menten equation using nonlinear regression.
8. Identify the pattern of inhibition by examining changes in the slopes and intercepts of the double-reciprocal plot independently of each other.
9. Extract the inhibition constant(s) by a fit of *all* velocity data to the appropriate rate equation.
10. Final kinetic constants for enzyme inhibition should be based on data collected under as close to physiological conditions as possible.
11. Address enzyme kinetics in terms of V and V/K_m. Do not take references to Michaelis-Menten constants and rate-limiting steps too seriously.

ACKNOWLEDGMENTS

This work was supported in part by a grant to D.B.N. from IBM, Inc., through Project Trochos of the University of Wisconsin, Madison. Additional support from NIH (DK 20100) is gratefully acknowledged. We thank Professor Paul Bartlett for helpful discussion and criticism and Professor Brian Matthews for communicating data prior to its publication.

APPENDIX 1

A method of statistical analysis of enzyme kinetic data using nonlinear least-squares analysis was developed by Wilkinson (86) and popularized by the FORTRAN computer programs of Cleland (7). Recently, Duggleby (80) has translated Cleland's FORTRAN matrix solution subroutine into BASIC and inserted it into a more efficient and general program for use on personal computers. It is reprinted in IBM BASIC with permission from *Computers in Biology and Medicine*, Vol. 14, by R. G. Duggleby, *Regression Analysis of Nonlinear Arrhenius Plots: An Emperical Model and a Computer Program*, 1984 Pergamon Press, Ltd. Before running the program, the equation to be fitted must be inserted. Some sample equations consistent with this chapter are the following. [For a recent discussion of the need, theory, and practical problems of statistical analysis of enzyme kinetic data, see Cleland (7).]

```
5100 G1=B(2)*X(1)
```
(1)
```
5110 G2=ABS(G1)
```
(2)
```
5130 IF G2<75 THEN 5160
```
(3)
```
5140 G1=.9*G1
```
(4)
```
5150 GOTO 5100
```
(5)
```
5160 G=B(4)+B(2)*X(1)-(B(2)-B(1))*(1-EXP(-G1))/B(3)
```
(6)
```
5100 G=B(1)*X(1)/(B(2)+X(1))
```
(7)
```
5100 G=B(1)*X(1)/(B(2)*(1+X(2)/B(3))+X(1))
```
(8)
```
5100 G=B(1)*X(1)/(B(2)*(1+X(2)/B(3))+X(1)*(1+X(2)/B(4)))
```
(9)
```
5100 G=B(1)*X(1)/(B(2)+X(1)*(1+X(2)/B(3)))
```
(10)
```
5100 G=B(1)*X(1)/(B(2)*(1+X(2)/B(3))^2+X(1))
```
(11)
```
5100 G=B(1)*X(1)/(B(2)*(1+X(2)/B(3))/(1+X(2)/B(4)))+X(1))
```
(12)
```
5100 G=B(1)*X(1)/(B(2)*(1+X(2)/B(3))+X(1)*(1+X(2)/B(4))/(1+X(2)/B(5)))
```
(13)
```
5100 G1=(B(2)+X(1))*B(3)/B(2)
```
(14)
```
5110 G2=G1+X(2)-X(3)
```
(15)
```
5120 G3=(G2^2+4*X(3)*G2)^.5
```
(16)
```
5130 G=B(1)*X(1)*(G3-G2)/(2*(B(2)+X(1)))
```
(17)
```
5100 G=B(1)/(1+X(1)/B(2)+X(2)/B(3)+X(1)*X(2)/(B(2)*B(3)*B(4)))
```
(18)

Equations (1) through (6), inserted together, describe the progress curve for an enzymatic assay in the presence of a slow transition from an initial reaction velocity, $B(1)$, to a steady-state velocity, $B(2)$, governed by the first-order rate constant, $B(3)$, and offset from zero by $B(4)$. It may be used to fit either bursts or lags [see Eq. (24) or Ref. 58].

Equation (7) is the Michaelis-Menten equation where here, and in the remaining equations, parameters $B(1)$ and $B(2)$ are V and K_m, respectively. Equation (8) represents competitive inhibition where $B(3)$ is K_{is} and $X(2)$ here and below is the concentration of inhibitor. Equation (9) represents noncompetitive inhibition where $B(3)$ is K_{is} and $B(4)$ is K_{ii}. Equation (10) represents uncompetitive inhibition where $B(3)$ is K_{ii}. Equation (11) represents parabolic competitive inhibition where $B(3)$ is K_{is}, $B(4)$ is K_{id}. Equation (12) represents hyperbolic competitive inhibition where $B(3)$ is K_{is}, $B(4)$ is K_{id}. Equation (13) is slope-linear, intercept-hyperbolic partial noncompetitive inhibition where $B(3)$ is K_{is}, $B(4)$ is K_{ii}, and $B(5)$ is K_{id}. Equations (14) through (17), inserted together, represent Morrison's equation for a tight-binding competitive inhibitor where $B(3)$ is K_{is}, $X(3)$ is the concentration of enzyme (or active sites).

Equation (18) describes multiple inhibition where $B(1)$ is the uninhibited velocity at a substrate concentration less than K_m, $X(1)$ is the concentration of inhibitor I, $B(2)$ is K_I, $X(2)$ is the concentration of inhibitor J, $B(3)$ is K_J, and $B(4)$ is α, the interaction constant.

```
1000 REM
1010 REM    NONLINEAR REGRESSION PROGRAM FOR UP TO 5 PARAMETER EQUATIONS
1020 REM
1030 REM    WRITTEN BY R.G.DUGGLEBY, DEPT. OF BIOCHEMISTRY, UNIVERSITY
1040 REM    OF QUEENSLAND, ST.LUCIA, AUSTRALIA
1050 REM-----------------------------------------------------------------
1060 REM    THE FOLLOWING ARRAYS ARE USED:
1070 REM            X1          INDEPENDENT VARIABLES
1080 REM            Y           DEPENDENT VARIABLE
1090 REM            W           WEIGHTING FACTORS
1100 REM            X           CURRENT VALUES OF THE INDEPENDENT VARIABLES
1110 REM            B           THE PARAMETERS
1120 REM            B0          RECENT PARAMETER VALUES, MASKS AND BOUNDS
1130 REM            P           PARTIAL DERIVATIVES. ALSO USED IN CALCULATING THE
1140 REM                        CORRECTION VECTOR, STD ERRORS, AND IN SOLVING S
1150 REM            S           THE ARRAY OF CROSS-PRODUCTS WHICH IS SOLVED
1160 REM            T           COPY OF S, USED FOR SUBITERATIONS
1170 REM            S1          VECTOR USED FOR SOLVING ARRAY S
1180 REM-----------------------------------------------------------------
1190 DIM X(3),X1(3,50),Y(50),W(50),B(5),B0(4,5),P(6),S(6,7),T(6,7),S1(6)
1200 REM-----------------------------------------------------------------
1210 REM    THE FOLLOWING VARIABLES ARE USED:
1220 REM            I,J,K,L     LOOP INDICES
1230 REM            M           NUMBER OF PARAMETERS
1240 REM            M3          NUMBER OF ACTIVE PARAMETERS
1250 REM            M1,M2       M3+1 AND M3+2, RESPECTIVELY
1260 REM            V1          THE NUMBER OF INDEPENDENT VARIABLES
1270 REM            N1          NUMBER OF DATA POINTS
1280 REM            S0,T0       SUMS OF SQUARES CALCULATED IN REGRESSION
1290 REM            G           THEORETICAL VALUE OF Y
1300 REM            C           CONVERGENCE TEST QUANTITY. ALSO, THE
```

```
1310 REM                     VALUE OF G USED IN CALCULATING P
1320 REM           V         RESIDUAL VARIANCE.  ALSO USED FOR THE
1330 REM                     STD. DEV. OF DATA POINTS (IF SPECIFIED)
1340 REM           I1,I2     ITERATION COUNTERS
1350 REM           R1,R2     MARQUARDT'S LAMBDA AND NU
1360 REM
1370 REM    THE STRING Q$ IS USED TO DETERMINE WEIGHTING
1380 REM    AND THE RESPONSE TO ASSORTED OTHER QUESTIONS
1390 REM--------------------------------------------------------------------
1500 REM    THE SECTION BEGINNING ON LINE 7000 IS A BASIC TRANSLATION OF THE
1510 REM    FORTRAN MATRIX SOLUTION SUBROUTINE POPULARISED BY CLELAND, ADVANCES
1520 REM    IN ENZYMOLOGY,1967. IT HAS BEEN CHANGED TO USE MARQUARDT'S METHOD BY
1530 REM    MULTIPLYING THE DIAGONAL ELEMENTS OF S (THE MATRIX WHICH IS SOLVED)
1540 REM    BY A CONSTANT FACTOR, 1+R1.  AFTER SOLUTION, ELEMENT P,1 CONTAINS
1550 REM    THE CORRECTION FOR THE P'TH PARAMETER, WHILE THE REMAINDER OF S IS
1560 REM    PROPORTIONAL TO THE VARIANCE-COVARIANCE MATRIX.  TO OBTAIN THE
1570 REM    LATTER, MULTIPLY BY THE RESIDUAL VARIANCE.
1580 REM--------------------------------------------------------------------
2000 PRINT "HOW MANY PARAMETERS & INDEPENDENT VARIABLES ", : INPUT M,V1
2010 PRINT "HOW MANY DATA POINTS ", : INPUT N1
2020 PRINT  : PRINT "SPECIFY WEIGHTS ...." : PRINT "  CONSTANT STD DEV     (C)"
2030 PRINT "  PROPORTIONAL STD DEV (P)" : PRINT "  BETWEEN THE ABOVE      (B)"
2040 PRINT "  STD DEV SUPPLIED      (S)" : INPUT Q$2045 GOTO 9000
2050 PRINT  : PRINT "INPUT INDEPENDENT VARIABLE(S), DEPENDENT VARIABLE";
2060 IF Q$="S" OR Q$="s" THEN PRINT " AND STD DEV";
2070 REM---INPUT THE DATA-------------------------------------------------
2080 PRINT  : FOR I=1 TO N1 : PRINT I, : IF Q$="S" OR Q$="s" THEN 2160
2090 ON V1 GOTO 2100,2110,2120
2100 INPUT X1(1,I),Y(I) : GOTO 2130
2110 INPUT X1(1,I),X1(2,I),Y(I) : GOTO 2130
2120 INPUT X1(1,I),X1(2,I),X1(3,I),Y(I)
2130 W(I)=1 : IF Q$="C" OR Q$="c" THEN 2210
2140 W(I)=1/Y(I) : IF Q$="B" OR Q$="b" THEN 2210
2150 W(I)=W(I)^2 : GOTO 2210
2160 ON V1 GOTO 2170,2180,2190
2170 INPUT X1(1,I),Y(I),V : GOTO 2200
2180 INPUT X1(1,I),X1(2,I),Y(I),V : GOTO 2200
2190 INPUT X1(1,I),X1(2,I),X1(3,I),Y(I),V
2200 W(I)=1/V^2
2210 NEXT I
2500 PRINT  : PRINT "ENTER ESTIMATES OF THE PARAMETERS, MASKS AND BOUNDS"
2510 M3=0 : FOR I=1 TO M : PRINT I,
2520 LINE INPUT B0$ : GOSUB 8000 : IF B0(2,I)=0 THEN M3=M3+1
2530 NEXT I
2540 M1=M3+1 : M2=M1+1
2550 REM---CALCULATE THE INITIAL SUM OF SQUARES---------------------------
2560 GOSUB 6010 : PRINT  : PRINT "INITIAL SUM OF SQUARES = ",S0 : PRINT
2570 IF M3<>0 THEN 3010
2580 PRINT "ALL PARAMETERS MASKED. SIMULATION ONLY" : GOTO 4180
3000 REM---BEGIN NONLINEAR ITERATIONS-----------------------------------
3010 I1=0 : R1=.1 : R2=10
3020 T0=S0
3030 I1=I1+1 : IF I1<11 THEN 3100
3040 REM---TOO MANY ITERATIONS------------------------------------------
3050 PRINT "INTERRUPTED AFTER 10 ITERATIONS"
3060 PRINT "ACCEPT (A), CONT. (C), NEW EST. (N) OR QUIT (Q) ", : INPUT Q$
3065 IF Q$="A" OR Q$="a" THEN I1=-1 : GOTO 3470
3070 IF Q$="Q" OR Q$="q" THEN 4210
3080 IF Q$="N" OR Q$="n" THEN 2500
3090 GOTO 2560
```

```
3100 I2=1
3110 FOR I=1 TO M1 : FOR J=1 TO M2 : T(I,J)=0 : NEXT J : NEXT I
3120 REM---LOOP OVER THE DATA TO CALCULATE THE ARRAY TO BE SOLVED--------------
3130 FOR I=1 TO N1
3140 FOR K=1 TO V1 : X(K)=X1(K,I) : NEXT K
3150 REM---CALCULATE THE PARTIAL DERIVATIVES----------------------------------
3160 K=0 : FOR J=1 TO M : IF B0(2,J)<>0 THEN 3190
3170 K=K+1 : B(J)=1.02*B(J) : GOSUB 5100 : C=G
3180 B(J)=B(J)*.98/1.02 : GOSUB 5100 : B(J)=B(J)/.98 : P(K)=(C-G)/(.04*B(J))
3190 NEXT J
3200 REM---CALCULATE THE RESIDUAL AND FORM THE VARIOUS SUMS------------------
3210 GOSUB 5100 : P(M1)=Y(I)-G : FOR J=1 TO M3 : FOR K=1 TO M1
3220 T(J,K)=T(J,K)+W(I)*P(J)*P(K) : NEXT K : NEXT J
3230 NEXT I
3240 REM---CORRECT THE PARAMETERS, CALCULATE SSQ AND CHECK FOR CONVERGENCE-----
3250 FOR I=1 TO M1 : FOR J=1 TO M2 : S(I,J)=T(I,J) : NEXT J : NEXT I3255 IF I1=0
THEN GOSUB 7010 : GOSUB 6010 : GOTO 4010
3260 GOSUB 7010 : PRINT : PRINT "ITERATION ",I1," SUBITERATION ",I2
3270 PRINT "PARAMETERS ...." : L=1 : C=0 : I=0
3280 FOR J=1 TO M : IF B0(2,J)<>0 THEN 3310
3290 I=I+1 : P(I)=S(I,1) : C=C+ABS(P(I)/B(J)) : B0(1,J)=B(J)
3300 B(J)=B(J)+P(I) : IF SGN(B(J)-B0(3,J))*(B0(4,J)-B(J))<0 THEN L=-1
3310 PRINT B(J), : NEXT J
3320 PRINT : GOSUB 6010 : PRINT "CURRENT SUM OF SQUARES = ";S0," LAMBDA = ",R1
3330 IF R2=0 THEN 4010
3340 IF R1*L<0 THEN 3390
3350 IF R1*S0<=R1*T0*1.00001 THEN 3450
3360 REM---CORRECTIONS ARE TOO BIG--PARAMETERS VIOLATE LIMITS; OR--------------
3370 REM---THE SSQ HAS INCREASED.    MULTIPLY R1 BY R2, REMOVE THE--------------
3380 REM---CORRECTIONS TO THE PARAMETERS AND REPEAT THE ITERATION--------------
3390 R1=R1*R2 : FOR I=1 TO M : IF B0(2,I)<>0 THEN 3410
3400 B(I)=B0(1,I)
3410 NEXT I                     .
3420 I2=I2+1 : IF I2>10 THEN 3050
3430 GOTO 3250
3440 REM---SSQ HAS NOT INCREASED.  DIVIDE R1 BY R2 FOR THE NEXT ITERATION------
3450 R1=R1/R2 : IF R1>.0002 THEN 3020
3460 IF C>(M3*.003)^2 THEN 3020
3470 R1=0 : R2=0 : GOTO 3020
4000 REM---RUN HAS CONVERGED.  CALCULATE FINAL RESULTS------------------------
4010 V=S0/(N1-M3) : I=0 : FOR J=1 TO M : P(J)=0 : IF B0(2,J)<>0 THEN 4030
4020 I=I+1 : P(J)=SQR(V*S(I,I+1))
4030 NEXT J
4040 PRINT : PRINT "FINAL VALUES ...." : PRINT
4050 FOR I=1 TO M : PRINT B(I)," +/- ",P(I) : NEXT I
4060 PRINT : PRINT "PRINT COVARIANCES AND CORRELATIONS (Y/N) ", : INPUT Q$
4070 IF Q$="N" OR Q$="n" THEN 4160
4080 FOR I1=1 TO 2 : PRINT : K=0 : FOR J=1 TO M : IF B0(2,J)=0 THEN K=K+1
4090 L=0 : FOR I=1 TO J : IF B0(2,I)<>0 THEN 4140
4100 IF B0(2,J)<>0 THEN 4140
4110 L=L+1 : IF I1=2 THEN 4130
4120 PRINT V*S(K,L+1), : GOTO 4150
4130 PRINT S(K,L+1)/SQR(S(K,K+1)*S(L,L+1)), : GOTO 4150
4140 PRINT 0,
4150 NEXT I : PRINT : NEXT J : NEXT I1
4160 PRINT : PRINT "PRINT RESIDUAL TABLE (Y/N) ", : INPUT Q$
4170 IF Q$="N" OR Q$="n" THEN 4210
4180 PRINT : PRINT "Y(EXPTL)","Y(FITTED)","DIFFERENCE" : PRINT
4190 FOR I=1 TO N1 : FOR K=1 TO V1 : X(K)=X1(K,I) : NEXT K
4200 GOSUB 5100 : PRINT Y(I),G,Y(I)-G : NEXT I
4210 PRINT : PRINT "END OF PROGRAM" : GOTO 7200
5000 REM-----------------------------------------------------------------------
```

```
5010 REM    INSERT FITTED FUNCTION HERE IN THE FORM:
5020 REM         G=F(B(1),B(2)....;X(1),X(2)....)
5030 REM------------------------------------------------------------------
5100 PRINT "Insert your equation in line 5100 ":BEEP:BEEP:GOTO 7200
5200 RETURN
6000 REM---CALCULATE THE CURRENT SUM OF SQUARES-----------------------------
6010 SO=0 : FOR I=1 TO N1
6020 FOR K=1 TO V1 : X(K)=X1(K,I) : NEXT K6030 GOSUB 5100 : SO=SO+W(I)*(Y(I)-G)^2
6040 NEXT I
6050 RETURN
7000 REM---SOLVE THE MATRIX S TO OBTAIN CORRECTIONS-------------------------
7010 FOR K=1 TO M3 : S1(K)=SQR(S(K,K)) : IF S1(K)<=0 THEN S1(K)=1
7020 S(K,K)=(1+R1)*S1(K)*S1(K) : S1(K)=1/S1(K) : NEXT K
7030 S1(M1)=1 : FOR J=1 TO M1 : FOR K=1 TO M3
7040 S(K,J)=S(K,J)*S1(K)*S1(J) : NEXT K : NEXT J
7050 P(M1)=-1 : S(1,M2)=1 : FOR L=1 TO M3
7060 FOR K=1 TO M3 : P(K)=S(K,1) : NEXT K
7070 FOR J=1 TO M1 : FOR K=1 TO M3
7080 S(K,J)=S(K+1,J+1)-P(K+1)*S(1,J+1)/P(1) : NEXT K
7090 NEXT J : NEXT L
7100 FOR K=1 TO M3 : S(K,1)=S(K,1)*S1(K) : FOR J=2 TO M1
7110 S(K,J)=S(K,J)*S1(K)*S1(J-1) : NEXT J : NEXT K
7120 RETURN
7200 END
8000 BO$=BO$+",,,," : PC=INSTR(1,BO$,",") : IF PC<2 THEN 8020
8010 B(I)=VAL(LEFT$(BO$,PC-1))
8020 BO$=MID$(BO$,PC+1) : BO(2,I)=0 : BO(3,I)=-1E+20 : BO(4,I)=1E+20
8030 FOR J=2 TO 4 : PC=INSTR(1,BO$,",") : IF PC<2 THEN 8050
8040 BO(J,I)=VAL(LEFT$(BO$,PC-1))
8050 BO$=MID$(BO$,PC+1) : NEXT J : RETURN
9000 PRINT : PRINT "DATA FILENAME (OR NULL FOR TERMINAL) "; : INPUT F$
9010 IF F$="" THEN 2050 ELSE OPEN F$ FOR INPUT AS #1
9020 FOR I=1 TO N1 : IF Q$="S" OR Q$="s" THEN 9100
9030 ON V1 GOTO 9040,9050,9060
9040 INPUT #1,X1(1,I),Y(I) : GOTO 9070
9050 INPUT #1,X1(1,I),X1(2,I),Y(I) : GOTO 9070
9060 INPUT #1,X1(1,I),X1(2,I),X1(3,I),Y(I)
9070 W(I)=1 : IF Q$="C" OR Q$="c" THEN 9150
9080 W(I)=1/Y(I) : IF Q$="B" OR Q$="b" THEN 9150
9090 W(I)=W(I)^2 : GOTO 9150
9100 ON V1 GOTO 9110,9120,9130
9110 INPUT #1,X1(1,I),Y(I),V : GOTO 9140
9120 INPUT #1,X1(1,I),X1(2,I),Y(I),V : GOTO 9140
9130 INPUT #1,X1(1,I),X1(2,I),X1(3,I),Y(I),V
9140 W(I)=1/V^2
9150 NEXT I
9160 CLOSE#1 : GOTO 2500
```

Once entered into a computer, the equations may be saved as separate files and merged to an already loaded regression program to avoid future typographical errors. Alternatively, to reduce keystrokes, allow for refitting with alternative weighting, and to provide a hard copy printout, the following code was written. This example, when merged to the NONLINEAR REGRESSION PROGRAM, provides a dedicated version for fitting kinetic data to competitive inhibition. It is easily changed to generate dedicated versions for fitting data to the other equations.

```
100   REM---------DEDICATED VERSION OF DUGGLEBY'S REGRESSION PROGRAM----------
110   REM   TO CREATE NEW VERSION, CHANGE STATEMENTS 120-160, 5100
120   T$="FIT TO COMPETITIVE INHIBITION"   : REM   TITLE
130   E$="v = V[S]/{Km(1+[I]/Ki)+[S]}"     : REM   ALGEBRAIC EQUATION
140   M=3                                  : REM   NUMBER OF PARAMETERS
150   V1=2                                 : REM   NUMBER OF INDEPENDENT VARIABLES
160   B1$="V " : B2$="Km" : B3$="Ki"       : REM   NAMES OF PARAMETERS
170   KEY OFF:CLS
180   PRINT T$: PRINT
190   PRINT E$: PRINT
1600  PRINT: GOTO 2010
2045  IF Q2$="Y" OR Q2$="y" THEN 2560 ELSE GOTO 9000
4210  PRINT: PRINT "REPEAT WITH NEW WEIGHTING",: INPUT Q2$
4220  IF Q2$="Y" OR Q2$="y" THEN 2020
4230  PRINT: PRINT "PRINT HARD COPY",: INPUT Q1$
4240  IF Q1$="Y" OR Q1$="y" THEN 4250 ELSE 4270
4250  PRINT : PRINT "ENTER IDENTIFYING COMMENTS (NO COMMAS):"
4260  PRINT : INPUT C$ : GOTO 10000
4270  PRINT : PRINT "END OF PROGRAM" : GOTO 7200
5100  G=B(1)*X(1)/(B(2)*(1+X(2)/B(3))+ X(1))
10000 REM----------ROUTINE TO PRINT HARD COPY OF RESULTS-----------------
10010 LPRINT T$
10020 LPRINT E$
10030 LPRINT
10040 LPRINT C$ : LPRINT
10050 LPRINT B1$;" =" ;B(1);" +/- ";P(1)
10060 LPRINT B2$;" = ";B(2);" +/- ";P(2): IF M=2 THEN 10100
10070 LPRINT B3$;" = ";B(3);" +/- ";P(3): IF M=3 THEN 10100
10080 LPRINT B4$;" = ";B(4);" +/- ";P(4): IF M=4 THEN 10100
10090 LPRINT B5$;" = ";B(5);" +/- ";P(5)
10100 LPRINT : LPRINT "  X","Y(EXPTL)","Y(FITTED)","DIFFERENCE"
10110 FOR I=1 TO N1 : FOR K=1 TO V1 : X(K)=X1(K,I) : NEXT K
10120 GOSUB 5100 : LPRINT X1(1,I),Y(I),G,Y(I)-G : NEXT I
10130 LPRINT: LPRINT "DATAFILE = ",F$
10140 LPRINT "ITERATIONS =",I1
10150 LPRINT "R. G. DUGGLEBY'S NON-LINEAR REGRESSION ROUTINE"
10160 LPRINT "REFERENCE;  COMPUT. BIOL. MED. 14, 447-455 (1984)"
10170 GOTO 4210
```

APPENDIX 2

The rate equations for Scheme III can be derived most easily by employing the net rate concepts of Cleland (1975). Starting with the final, irreversible step, the net rate constants (indicated by primes) are:

$$k_9' = k_9 \tag{1}$$

$$k_7' = \frac{k_7 k_9'}{k_8 + k_9'} \tag{2}$$

$$k_5' = \frac{k_5 k_7'}{k_6 + k_7'} \tag{3}$$

$$k_3' = \frac{k_3 k_5'}{k_4 + k_5'} \tag{4}$$

$$K'_1 = \frac{[S]k_1 k'_3}{k_2 + k'_3} \tag{5}$$

By substituting each equation into the successive one, a complete expression for the right-hand side of each equation can be obtained free of primes. The maximal velocity is the reciprocal of the sum of reciprocals of the net rate constants not including a substrate concentration term, or;

$$V = \frac{1}{1/k'_3 + 1/k'_5 + 1/k'_7 + 1/k'_9} \tag{6}$$

By substituting individual rate constants for net rate constants and rearranging,

$$V = \frac{k_3 k_5 k_7 k_9}{k_4 k_6 k_8 + k_4 k_6 k_9 + k_4 k_7 k_9 + k_5 k_6 k_9 + k_3 k_6 k_8} +$$
$$k_3 k_6 k_9 + k_3 k_7 k_9 + k_3 k_5 k_8 + k_3 k_5 k_9 + k_3 k_5 k_7 \tag{7}$$

The expression for V/K_m is $K'_1/[S]$ or

$$\frac{V}{K_m} = \frac{k_1 k_3 k_5 k_7 k_9}{k_2 k_4 k_6 k_8 + k_2 k_4 k_6 k_9 + k_2 k_4 k_7 k_9 + k_2 k_5 k_7 k_9 + k_3 k_5 k_7 k_9} \tag{8}$$

Their ratio is

$$K_m = \frac{k_2 k_4 k_6 k_8 + k_2 k_4 k_6 k_9 + k_2 k_4 k_7 k_9 + k_2 k_5 k_7 k_9 + k_3 k_5 k_7 k_9}{k_1(k_4 k_6 k_8 + k_4 k_6 k_9 + k_4 k_7 k_9 + k_5 k_6 k_9 + k_3 k_6 k_8)} +$$
$$k_3 k_6 k_9 + k_3 k_7 k_9 + k_3 k_5 k_8 + k_3 k_5 k_9 + k_3 k_5 k_7) \tag{9}$$

If k_9 is small relative to all other rate constants, then all denominator terms containing k_9 are removed, leaving

$$V = \frac{k_3 k_5 k_7 k_9}{k_4 k_6 k_8 + k_3 k_6 k_8 + k_3 k_5 k_8 + k_3 k_5 k_7} \tag{10}$$

$$\frac{V}{K_m} = \frac{k_1 k_3 k_5 k_7 k_9}{k_2 k_4 k_6 k_8} \tag{11}$$

$$K_m = \frac{k_2 k_4 k_6 k_8}{k_1(k_4 k_6 k_8 + k_3 k_6 k_8 + k_3 k_5 k_8 + k_3 k_5 k_7)} \tag{12}$$

The rate equations for Scheme II can be derived by setting $k_6 = 0$ in Eqs. (7)–(9). Canceling $k_7 k_9$ terms yields

$$V = \frac{k_3 k_5 k_7 k_9}{k_4 k_5 k_9 + k_5 k_7 k_9 + k_3 k_7 k_9 + k_3 k_5 k_8 + k_3 k_5 k_9 + k_3 k_5 k_7} \tag{13}$$

$$\frac{V}{K_m} = \frac{k_1 k_3 k_5}{k_2 k_4 + k_2 k_5 + k_3 k_5} \tag{14}$$

$$K_m = \frac{k_7 k_9 (k_2 k_4 + k_2 k_5 + k_3 k_5)}{k_1 (k_4 k_7 k_9 + k_5 k_7 k_9 + k_3 k_7 k_9 + k_3 k_5 k_8 + k_3 k_5 k_9 + k_3 k_5 k_7)} \tag{15}$$

Under conditions where k_5 is small relative to other rate constants, the denominator terms containing k_5 are removed. Canceling $k_7 k_9$ leaves

$$V = \frac{k_3 k_5}{k_3 + k_4} = \frac{k_5}{1 + k_4/k_3} \tag{16}$$

$$\frac{V}{K_m} = \frac{k_1 k_3 k_5}{k_2 k_4} = \frac{k_5}{(k_2/k_1)(k_4/k_3)} \tag{17}$$

$$K_m = \frac{k_2 k_4}{k_1 k_3 + k_1 k_4} = \frac{k_2 (k_4/k_3)}{k_1 (1 + k_4/k_3)} \tag{18}$$

REFERENCES

1. Ringe, D., and G. A. Petsko, Mapping Protein Dynamics by X-Ray Diffraction. *Prog. Biophys. Mol. Biol. 45*(3): 197–235 (1985).
2. Jardetzky, O., NMR studies of macromolecular dynamics. *Am. Chem. Res. 14*:291–298 (1981).
3. Karplus, M., and J. A. McCammon, Dynamics of proteins: Elements and function. *Am. Rev. Biochem. 52*:263–300 (1983).
4. Michaelis, L., and M. L. Menten, Die kinetic der invertinwirkung. *Biochem. Z. 49*:333–369 (1913).
5. Briggs, G. E., and J. B. S. Haldane, A note on the kinetics of enzyme action. *Biochem. J. 19*:338–339 (1925).
6. Northrop, D. B., Determining the absolute magnitude of hydrogen isotope effects. In *Isotope Effects in Enzyme-Catalyzed Reactions*. University Park Press, Baltimore, pp. 122–152 (1977).
7a. Cleland, W. W., Steady state kinetics. In *The Enzymes*, 3rd Ed., Vol. 2. Academic Press, New York, pp. 1–65 (1970).
7b. Cleland, W. W., Statistical analysis of enzyme kinetic data. *Methods Enzymol. 63*:103–138 (1979).
8a. Northrop, D. B., Minimal kinetic mechanism and general equation for deuterium isotope effects on enzymic reactions: Uncertainty in detecting a rate-limiting step. *Biochemistry 20*:4056–4061 (1981).
9. Ray, W. J. Jr., Rate-limiting step: A quantitative definition. Application to steady-state enzymic reactions. *Biochemistry 22*:4625–4637 (1983).
10. Johnston, H. S., *Theory of Complex Reactions*, Chap. 16, Roland Press, New York (1966).
11. Boyd, R. K., Some common oversimplifications in teaching chemical kinetics. *J. Chem. Educ. 55*:84–89 (1978).

12. Radika, K., and D. B. Northrop, The kinetic mechanism of kanamycin acetyltransferase derived from the use of alternative antibiotics and coenzymes. *J. Biol. Chem. 259*:12543–12546 (footnote 3) (1984).

13. Nageswara Rao, B. D., and M. Cohen, ^{31}P NMR studies of enzyme-bound substrates of rabbit muscle pyruvate kinase. *J. Biol. Chem. 254*:2689–2696 (1979).

14. James, M. N. G., A. Sielicki, F. Salituro, D. H. Rich, and T. Hofmann, Conformational flexibility in the active sites of aspartyl proteinases revealed by a pepstain fragment binding to penicillopepsin. *Proc. Natl. Acad. Sci. USA 79*:6137–6141 (1982).

15. Foundling, S. I., J. Cooper, F. E. Watson, A. Cleasby, L. H. Pearl, B. L. Sibanda, A. Hemmings, S. P. Wood, T. L. Blundell, M. J. Vallner, C. G. Norey, J. Kay, J. Boger, B. M. Dunn, B. J. Leckie, D. M. Jones, B. Atrash, A. Hallett, and M. Szelke, High resolution x-ray analyses of renin inhibitor-aspartic proteinase complexes. *Nature 327*:349–352 (1987).

16a. Rich, D. H., and E. T. O. Sun, Mechanism of inhibition of pepsin by pepstatin. Effect of inhibitor structure on dissociation constant and time-dependent inhibition. *Biochem. Pharmacol. 29*:2205–2212 (1980).

16b. Rich, D. H., E. T. O. Sun, and E. Ulm, Synthesis of analogues of the carboxyl protease inhibitor pepstatin. Effect of structure on inhibition of pepsin and renin. *J. Med. Chem. 23*:27–33 (1980).

17. Salituro, F. G., N. Agarwal, T. Hofmann, and D. H. Rich, Inhibition of aspartic proteinases by peptides containing lysine and ornithine side-chain analogues of statine. *J. Med. Chem. 30*:286–293 (1987).

18a. Hammes, G., and P. Schimmel, Rapid reactions and transient states. In *The Enzymes*, 3rd Ed., Vol. 2, P. Boyer, ed. Academic Press, New York, p. 67 (1970).

18b. Cleland, W. W., The statistical analysis of enzyme kinetic data. *Adv. Enzymol. 29*:1–29 (1967).

19. Bott, R., E. Subramanian, and D. R. Davies, Three dimensional structure of the complex of the *Rhizopus chinensis* carboxyl proteinase and pepstatin at 2.5-Å resolution. *Biochemistry 21*:6956–6962 (1982).

20. Sugana, K., E. A. Padlan, C. W. Smith, W. D. Carlson, and D. R. Davies, Binding of a reduced peptide inhibitor to the aspartic proteinase from *Rhizopus chinensis*: Implications for a mechanism of action. *Proc. Natl. Acad. Sci. USA 84*: 7009–7013 (1987).

21a. Jencks, W. P., Binding energy, specificity and enzymatic catalysis: The circle effect. *Adv. Enzymol. 43*:219–490 (1975).

21b. Crosby, J., R. Stone, and G. E. Lienhard, Mechanisms of thiamine-catalyzed reactions. Decarboxylation of 2-(1-carboxy-1-hydroxyethyl)-3,4-dimethyl-thiazolium chloride. *J. Am. Chem. Soc. 92*:2891 (1970).

22. Pauling, L., Molecular architecture and biological reactions. *Chem. Eng. News 24*:1375 (1946).

23. Wolfenden, R., Analog approaches to the structure of the transition state in enzyme reactions. *Acc. Chem. Res. 5*:10–18 (1972).

24. Leinhard, G. E., Enzymatic catalysis and transition-state theory. *Science 180*:149 (1973).

25. Dewar, M. J. S., and D. M. Storch, Alternative view of enzyme reactions. *Proc. Natl. Acad. Sci. USA 82*:2225–2229 (1985).

26. Hammond, G., A correlation of reaction rates. *J. Am. Chem. Soc. 77*:334 (1955). (This adjustment is made on the basis that as TX is stabilized, the transition state will more closely approach substrate and therefore be at a lower energy state.)

27. Westerik, J. O., and R. Wolfenden, Aldehydes as inhibitors of papain. *J. Biol. Chem. 247*:8195–8197 (1972).

28. Thompson, R. C., Use of peptide aldehydes of generate transition-state analogs of elastase. *Biochemistry 12*:47–51 (1973).

29. Bartlett, P. A., and C. K. Marlowe, Phosphonamidates as transition-state analogue inhibitors of thermolysin. *Biochemistry 22*:4618–46524 (1983).

30. Bartlett, P. A., and C. K. Marlowe, Transition state analogs and slow-binding inhibition: Kinetic studies of phosphorus-containing inhibitors of thermolysin. *Biochemistry 26*:8553–8561 (1987).

31. Rich, D. H., Pepstatin-derived inhibitors of aspartic proteinases, a close look at an apparent transition-state analogue inhibitor. *J. Med. Chem. 28*:263–273 (1985).

32. Holladay, M. W., F. G. Salituro, and D. H. Rich, Synthetic and enzyme inhibition studies of pepstatin analogues containing hydroxyethylene and ketomethylene dipeptide isosteres. *J. Med. Chem. 30*:374–383 (1987).

33. Morrison, J. F., and C. T. Walsh, The behavior and significance of slow-binding enzyme inhibitors. *Adv. Enzymol. 61*:201–301 (1988).

34. Morrison, J. F., Kinetics of the reversible inhibition of enzyme-catalyzed reactions by tight-binding inhibitors. *Biochim. Biophys. Acta 185*:269–286 (1969).

35a. Marsh, H. C., P. Robertson Jr., M. E. Scott, K. A. Koehler, and R. G. Hiskey, Magnesium and calcium ion binding to bovine prothrombin fragment 1. *J. Biol. Chem. 254*:10268–10275 (1979).

35b. Galardy, R. E., and M. Leakopoulou-Kyriakides, The rate of s-cis/s-trans isomerization in angiotensin II is at least 70-fold greater than in His–Pro and is not rate limiting in receptor binding. *Int. J. Peptide Protein Res. 20*:144–148 (1982) and references therein.

36. Umezawa, H., Low molecular weight enzyme inhibitors of microbial origin. *Annu. Rev. Microbiol. 36*:75–99 (1982).

37. Rich, D. H., Inhibitors of aspartic proteinases. In *Proteinase Inhibitors*, A. J. Barrett and G. Salveson, eds. Elsevier, New York, pp. 179–217 (1986).

38. Boger, J., N. S. Lohr, E. H. Ulm, M. Poe, E. H. Blaine, G. M. Fanelli, T.-Y. Lin, L. S. Payne, T. W. Schorn, B. I. Lamont, T. C. Vassil, I. I. Stabilito, D. F. Veber, D. H. Rich, and A. S. Boparai, Novel renin inhibitors containing the amino acid statine. *Nature 303*:81–84 (1983).

39. Boger, J., Inhibition of cathepsin D by synthetic oligopeptides. In *Aspartic Proteinases and Their Inhibitors*, V. Kostka, ed. Walter de Gruyter, Berlin, pp. 401–420 (1985).

40. Maibaum, J., and D. H. Rich, Inhibition of porcine pepsin by two substrate analogues containing statine. The effect of histidine at the P_2 subsite on the inhibition of aspartic proteinases. *J. Med. Chem. 31*:625–629 (1988).

41. Hallett, A., D. M. Jones, B. Atrash, M. Szelke, B. J. Leckie, S. Beattie, B. M. Dunn, M. J. Valler, C. E. Rolph, J. Kay, S. I. Foundling, S. P. Wood, L. H. Pearl, F. E. Watson, and T. L. Blundell, Inhibition of aspartic proteinases by transition-

state substrate analogues. In *Aspartic Proteinases and Their Inhibitors*, V. Kostka, ed. Walter de Gruyter, Berlin, pp. 467–478 (1985).

42. Rich, D. H., E. Sun, and J. Singh, Synthesis of dideoxy-pepstatin. Mechanism of inhibition of porcine pepsin. *Biochem. Biophys. Res. Commun. 74*:762–767 (1977).

43. Fruton, J. S., The mechanism of the catalytic action of pepsin and related acid proteinases. *Adv. Enzymol. 44*:1–36 (1976).

44. Kitagishi, K., H. Nakatani, and K. Hiromi, Static and kinetic studies on the binding between pepsin and streptomyces pepsin inhibitor with a fluorescent probe. *J. Biochem. 87*:573–579 (1980).

45. Rich, D. H., A. S. Boparai, and M. S. Bernatowicz, Synthesis of a 3-oxo-4(S)-amino acid analog of pepstatin. A new inhibitor of carboxyl (acid) proteinase. *Biochem. Biophys. Res. Commun. 104*:1127–1133 (1982).

46. Rich, D. H., and M. S. Bernatowicz, Oxidation of statine-containing peptides to ketone analogues via novel peptide sulfonium ylides. *J. Org. Chem. 38*:1999–2001 (1983).

47. Rich, D. H., M. S. Bernatowicz, and P. G. Schmidt, Direct carbon-13 NMR evidence for a tetrahedral intermediate in the binding of a pepstatin analog to porcine pepsin. *J. Am. Chem. Soc. 104*:3535–3536 (1982).

48. Schmidt, P. G., M. W. Holladay, F. G. Salituro, and D. H. Rich, Identification of oxygen nucleophiles in tetrahedral intermediates: ^{2}H and ^{18}O induced isotope shifts in ^{13}C NMR spectra of pepsin-bound peptide ketone pseudosubstrates. *Biochem. Biophys. Res. Commun. 129*:597–602 (1985).

49. Holladay, M. W., F. G. Salituro, P. G. Schmidt, and D. H. Rich, Pepsin-catalysed addition of water to a ketomethylene peptide isostere: Observation of the tetrahedral species by ^{13}C-nuclear-magnetic-resonance spectroscopy. *Biochem. Soc. Trans. 13*:1046–1048 (1985).

50. Kawai, M., A. S. Boparai, M. S. Bernatowicz, and D. H. Rich, Synthesis of novel 3 methylstatine analogues. Assignment of absolute configuration. *J. Org. Chem. 48*:1876–1879 (1983).

51. Bartlett, P. A., and W. B. Kezer, Phosphinic acid dipeptide analogue: Potent slow-binding inhibitors of aspartic peptidases. *J. Am. Chem. Soc. 106*:4282–4283 (1984).

52. Gelb, M. H., J. P. Svaren, and R. H. Ables, Fluoroketone inhibitors of hydrolytic enzymes. *Biochemistry 24*:1813–1817 (1985).

53. Kam, C.-M., N. Nishino, and J. C. Powers, Inhibition of thermolysin and carboxypeptidase A by phosphoramidate. *Biochemistry 18*:3032–3038 (1979).

54. Bartlett, P. A., and C. K. Marlowe, Evaluation of intrinsic binding energy from a hydrogen bonding group in an enzyme inhibitor. *Science 235*:569–571 (1987) and references therein.

55. Tronrud, D. E., H. M. Holden, and B. W. Matthews, Structures of two thermolysin-inhibitor complexes that differ by a single hydrogen bond. *Science 235*:571–574 (1987) and references therein.

56. Holden, H. M., D. E. Tronrud, A. F. Monzingo, L. H. Weaver, and B. W. Matthews, Slow- and fast-binding inhibitors of thermolysin display different modes of binding: A crystallographic analysis of extended phosphonamidate transition state analogues. *Biochemistry 26*:8542–8553 (1987).

57. It again bears pointing out that trapped water molecules will impose an additional barrier to inhibitor binding. Thus, the rapid binding of transition-state analog inhibitors, predicted in Figure 1, will not occur, since the inhibitor must find an alternative pathway to the tightened complex. This model also suggests that the collision complex dissociation constants could be much greater than K_D for substrate because of an additional steric interaction between the additional inhibitor atoms (a proton or oxygen) and solvent water that is not present with substrate. This could made it difficult to observe saturation kinetics.

58. Williams, J. W., and J. F. Morrison, The kinetics of reversible tight-binding inhibition. *Methods Enzymol. 63*:437–467 (1979).

59. Stone, S. R., and J. F. Morrison, Mechanism of inhibition of dihydrofolate reductases from bacterial and vertebrate sources by various classes of folate analogues. *Biochim. Biophys. Acta 869*: 275–285 (1986).

60. Bolin, J. T., D. J. Filman, D. A. Matthews, R. C. Hamlin, and J. Kraut, Crystal structures of *Escherichia coli* and *Lactobacillus casei* dihydrofolate reductase refined at 1.7 Å resolution. *J. Biol. Chem. 257*:13650–13662 (1982).

61. Umezawa, H., Small molecular microbial products enhancing immune response. *Antibiotic Chemother. (Basel) 24*:9–18 (1979).

62. Rich, D. H., S. Harbeson, and B. J. Moon, Inhibition of aminopeptidases by amastatin and bestatin derivatives. Effect of inhibitor structure on slow-binding processes. *J. Med. Chem. 27*:417–422 (1984).

63. Wilkes, S. H., and J. M. Prescott, The slow tight binding of bestatin and amastatin to aminopeptidases. *J. Biol. Chem. 24*:13154–13162 (1985).

64. Nishizawa, R., T. Saino, T. Takita, H. Suda, T. Aoyagi, and H. Umezawa, Synthesis and structure-activity relationships of bestatin analogues, inhibitors of aminopeptidase B. *J. Med. Chem. 20*:510–515 (1977).

65. Nishino, N., and J. C. Powers, Design of potent reversible inhibitors for thermolysin peptides containing zinc coordinating ligands and their use in affinity chromatography. *Biochemistry 18*:4340–4347 (1979).

66. Ocain, T. D., and D. H. Rich, L-lysinethiol: A subnanomolar inhibitor of aminopeptidase B. *Biochem. Biophys. Res. Commun. 145*:1038–1042 (1987).

67. Ondetti, M. A., and D. W. Cushman, Inhibition of the renin-angiotensin system. A new approach to the therapy of hypertension. *J. Med. Chem. 24*:355–361 (1981).

68. Fournié-Zaluski, M. C., P. Chaillet, R. Bouboutou, A. Couland, P. Chérot, G. Waksman, J. Costentin, and B. P. Roques, Analgesic effects of kelatorphan, a new highly potent inhibitor of multiple enkephalin degrading enzymes. *Eur. J. Pharmacol. 102*:525–528 (1984).

69. Chan, W. W.-C., L-Leucinthiol—a potent inhibitor of leucine aminopeptidase. *Biochem. Biophys. Res. Commun. 116*:297–302 (1983).

70. Ocain, T. D., and D. H. Rich, L-Lysinethiol: A subnanomolar inhibitor of aminopeptides B. *Biochem. Biophys. Res. Commun. 145*: 1038–1042 (1987).

71. Harbeson, S. L., and D. H. Rich, Inhibition of Arginine Aminopeptidase by Bestatin and Arphamenine Analogues. Evidence for a New Mode of Binding to aminopeptidases. *Biochemistry 27*:7301–7310 (1988).

72. Umezawa, H., T. Nakamura, S. Fukatsu, T. Aoyagi, and J. Tatsuta, Synthesis of arphamenine A and epi-arphamenine A. *Antibiotics 36*:1787–1788 (1983).

73. Knight, G. C., The characterization of enzyme inhibition. In *Proteinase Inhibitors*, A. J. Barrett and G. Salvesen, eds. Elsevier, New York, pp. 38–42 (1986).

74. Allison, R. D., and D. L. Purich, Practical considerations in the design of initial velocity enzyme rate assays. *Methods Enzymol. 63*:2–22 (1979).

75. Bosron, W. F., and T.-K. Li, Catalytic properties of human liver alcohol dehydrogenase isoenzymes. *Enzyme 37*:19–28 (1987).

76. Williams, J. W., and D. B. Northrop, Kinetic mechanisms of gentamicin acetyltransferase I. Antibiotic-dependent shift from rapid to nonrapid equilibrium random mechanisms. *J. Biol. Chem. 253*:5902–5907 (1978).

77. Marti, K. M. B., Kinetic characterization of aminoglycoside acetyltransferase-3-I. Ph.D. dissertation. University of Wisconsin, Madison, 1987.

78. Lineweaver, H., and D. Burk, The determination of enzyme dissociation constants. *J. Am. Chem. Soc. 56*:58–66 (1934).

79. Dowd, J. E., and D. S. Riggs, A comparison of estimates of Michaelis-Menten kinetic constants from various linear transformations. *J. Biol. Chem. 240*:868–869 (1964).

80. Duggleby, R. G., Regression analysis of nonlinear Arrhenius plots: An empirical model and a computer program. *Comput. Biol. Med. 14*:447–455 (1984).

81. Wilkinson, G. N., Statistical estimations in enzyme kinetics. *Biochem. J. 80*:324–332 (1961).

82. Wratten, C. C., and W. W. Cleland, Product inhibition studies of yeast and liver alcohol dihydrogenases. *Biochemistry 2*:935–941 (1963).

83. Gates, C. A., and D. B. Northrop, Alternative substrate and inhibition kinetics of aminoglycoside nucleotidyltransferase 2″-I in support of a Theorell-Chance kinetic mechanism. *Biochemistry 27*:3826–3833 (1988).

84. Rife, J. E., and W. W. Cleland, Determination of the chemical mechanism of glutamate dehydrogenase from pH studies. *Biochemistry 19*:2321–2328 (1980).

85. Henderson, P. J. F., Statistical analysis of enzyme kinetic data. *Biochem. J. 127*:321–333 (1972).

86. Cleland, W. W., Partition analysis and the concept of net rate constants as tools in enzyme kinetics. *Biochemistry 14*:3220–3224 (1975).

87. Hermes, J. D., C. A. Roeske, M. H. O'Leary, and W. W. Cleland, Use of multiple isotope effects to determine enzyme mechanisms and intrinsic isotope effects. Malic enzyme and glucose-6-phosphate dehydrogenase. *Biochemistry 21*:5106–5114 (1982).

88. For example, of five NAD(P)-dependent oxidative decarboxylases, four catalyze hydride transfer separate from decarboxylation. See Hermes, J. D., P. A. Tipton, M. A. Fisher, M. H. O'Leary, J. F. Morrison, and W. W. Cleland, Mechanisms of enzymatic and acid-catalyzed decarboxylation of prephenate. *Biochemistry 23*:6263–6275 (1984).

89. Yonetani, T., and H. Theorell, Studies on liver alcohol dehydrogenase complexes. III. Multiple inhibition kinetics in the presence of two competitive inhibitors. *Arch. Biochem. Biophys. 106*:243–251 (1964).

90. Yonetani, T., The Yonetani-Theorell graphical method for examining overlapping subsites of enzyme active centers. *Methods Enzymol.* 7:500–509 (1982).

91. Northrop, D. B., and W. W. Cleland, The kinetics of pig heart triphosphopyridine nucleotide-isocitrate dehydrogenase. *J. Biol. Chem.* 249:2928–2931 (1974).

92. Gates, C. A., and D. B. Northrop, Determination of the rate-limiting segment of aminoglycoside nucleotidyltransferase 2″-I by pH- and viscosity-dependent kinetics. *Biochemistry* 27:3834–3842 (1988).

Applications

7

Computer-Aided Design and Evaluation of Angiotensin-Converting Enzyme Inhibitors

David G. Hangauer
Merck Sharp & Dohme Research Laboratories, Rahway, New Jersey

I. INTRODUCTION

Angiotensin-converting enzyme (ACE) is a member of the renin-angiotensin-aldosterone system, which plays an important role in the control of blood pressure. ACE is the enzyme responsible for cleavage of the C-terminal dipeptide unit His-Leu from the decapeptide angiotensin I to produce the potent vasoconstrictor angiotensin II. The vasodilating peptide bradykinin is also destroyed by ACE. Aldosterone, which is a sodium-retaining steroid, is released from the adrenals in response to angiotensin II. The combined effect of these activities is to raise blood pressure by increasing fluid volume and vascular resistance (1,2). Inhibition of ACE has proved to be a very effective approach to the control of hypertension. A number of reviews have been published that outline the development of ACE inhibitors (3–8). It is the purpose of this chapter to give an overview of the role rational design has played in the development and understanding of ACE inhibitors with particular emphasis on the use of computers as an aid in this process.

II. DESIGN OF CAPTOPRIL WITH THE AID OF A CONCEPTUAL MODEL FOR ANGIOTENSIN-CONVERTING ENZYME

The earliest work on the design of ACE inhibitors was carried out at the Squibb laboratories by Cushman, Ondetti, and co-workers and led to the discovery of the first ACE inhibitor to be approved for use in treating human hypertension. This drug carries the generic name captopril. Although this early work did not utilize computers, it exemplifies the potential advantages of rational drug design from a working (and evolving) model for the target enzyme, a process that can be aided by computer modeling. The discussion in this section will be limited to work relating to the use of a conceptual model for ACE as a guide in the discovery of captopril. The reader is referred to previous reviews (5–8) for a more complete account.

In 1974 the Squibb group began an effort directed toward the design of low-molecular-weight ACE inhibitors that might be expected to have oral activity. This work drew partly on the previous results obtained with peptide inhibitors derived from snake venom. These peptide inhibitors contained from five to 13 amino acid residues. One of the peptides, a nonapeptide called teprotide (SQ 20,881), was used as a pharmacological tool to demonstrate the effectiveness of ACE inhibition in humans for blood pressure control. Since teprotide was not orally active, it had to be administered intravenously.

Structure-activity studies were carried out to elucidate the sequence specificity for inhibition with peptide inhibitors. The structure-activity data generated on the pentapeptide inhibitor BPP_{5a} (<Glu–Lys–Trp–Ala–Pro) was of particular value. It was found that the C-terminal sequence was responsible for most of the activity of these peptides, and Ala–Pro was particularly good as the C-terminal dipeptide. The Ala–Pro dipeptide itself had significant activity against ACE ($IC_{50} = 2.3 \times 10^{-4}$ M). It was expected that di- or tripeptide-based inhibitors would have a better chance of being orally active. Consequently, it became desirable to find a structural modification of the C-terminal small-peptide inhibitors that would raise the potency dramatically (i.e., about 4 or 5 orders of magnitude) while resulting in a compound with the required properties for good oral bioavailability.

To address this challenge, the Squibb group constructed the conceptual working model for the ACE active site shown in Figure 1 by using the crystallographically characterized active site of carboxypeptidase A as a guide (9). It was recognized that both enzymes are zinc peptidases and probably have similar mechanisms for catalyzing the cleavage of peptide bonds. Carboxypeptidase A cleaves the C-terminal amino acid from a typical substrate, whereas ACE cleaves the C-terminal dipeptide from most of its substrates. It was assumed that both enzymes utilize the zinc atom in the active site to activate the scissile peptide bond toward cleavage. It was postulated that a positively charged residue, possibly an Arg, forms a salt bridge with the C-terminal carboxyl group of the substrate in the active site of ACE, much the same as was proposed for Arg-145 of carboxypeptidase A.

In developing the model, the distance from this positive charge to the zinc atom was increased from the length of one amino acid unit in carboxypeptidase A to that of a dipeptide unit in ACE to accommodate the difference in positioning of the labile peptide bond for their respective

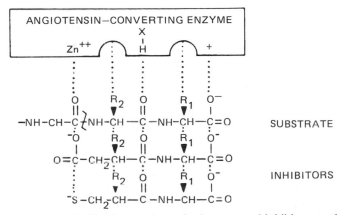

Figure 1 Binding interactions of substrates and inhibitors to the initial conceptual model for ACE as proposed by Cushman et al. (9). Reproduced with permission.

substrates. The Squibb group also assumed that ACE may form a hydrogen bond to the C-terminal peptide carbonyl group of the substrate. Finally, the affinity of ACE for the side chains (R_1 and R_2) of the terminal dipeptide unit was expected to result from two binding sites as depicted in Figure 1 with no direct analogy to carboxypeptidase A. Information regarding the specificity of ACE for the R_1 and R_2 side chains was obtained initially from structure-activity data on the peptide inhibitors mentioned above as well as substrates.

The Squibb group reasoned that if the peptide cleavage mechanisms of carboxypeptidase A and ACE were indeed similar, then inhibitor designs that are effective on carboxypeptidase A might also be effective on ACE. Byers and Wolfenden (10,11) had reported that D-benzylsuccinic acid is a potent competitive inhibitor ($K_i = 4.5 \times 10^{-7}$ M) of carboxypeptidase A and proposed that this compound was a biproduct analog—i.e., one that combines certain binding interactions of both products with the enzyme in one molecule. The Squibb group assumed that the D-benzylsuccinic acid carboxyl group, which mimics the product carboxyl group, binds to the zinc atom. It was postulated that a carboxyl group might be able to bind to the ACE active-site zinc in a similar way and could be incorporated into a dipeptide ACE inhibitor by substituting a carboxylalkyl group for the dipeptide amino group as shown in Figure 1. According to this model, substituted succinyl amino acids would have the right number of main-chain atoms to interact with the zinc and form the other binding interactions shown. Since Ala-Pro was a good dipeptide sequence to use as a starting point, methylsuccinyl-Pro inhibitor [1] was prepared and found to have an $IC_{50} = 22 \times 10^{-6}$ M (Table 1) for the diastereomer with stereochemistry corresponding to that in Ala–Pro (the other diastereomer was much less active). Variations in chain length for the carboxyalkyl groups were also investigated, and it was found that an additional methylene, resulting in glutaryl-Pro analogs, resulted in more potent inhibitors. The methylglutaryl-Pro inhibitor [2] (Table 1), with stereochemistry corresponding to that of Ala–Pro, showed a fivefold improvement in the IC_{50}. The additional methylene present in the glutaryl derivatives presumably results in a more favorable positioning of the carboxyl group as a zinc ligand.

In the conceptual model used by the Squibb group for ACE, it was postulated that the glutaryl and succinyl carboxyl groups were binding to the active-site zinc atom. Therefore, it was further postulated that if this carboxyl was replaced with a group having a higher affinity for zinc, then a more potent inhibitor should result. Indeed, the substitution of a sulfhydryl group for this carboxyl (Fig. 1) in methylsuccinyl-Pro [1] resulted in captopril [3] (Table 1) which showed a 1000-fold improvement in in vitro activity and good oral bioavailability. The optimal chain length was found to be that corresponding to the sulfhydryl for carboxyl substitution in the succinyl-Pro

Table 1 Comparison of Carboxyalkanoyl-
and   Mercaptoalkanoyl-Proline   ACE
Inhibitors

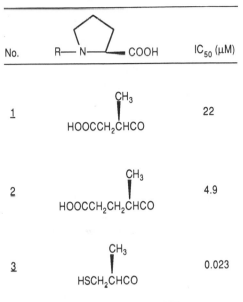

No.	R—N—⟨ ⟩—COOH	IC$_{50}$ (µM)
1	CH$_3$ | HOOCCH$_2$CHCO	22
2	CH$_3$ | HOOCCH$_2$CH$_2$CHCO	4.9
3	CH$_3$ | HSCH$_2$CHCO	0.023

Source: Data from Cushman et al. (9).

series rather than the glutaryl-Pro series. The difference in optimal chain
lengths for the inhibitors providing a carboxyl zinc ligand as compared to
those providing a sulfhydryl zinc ligand presumably reflects a different
preferred geometry for binding near the zinc. Subsequently, the crystal
structure of the complex between thermolysin (another closely related zinc
peptidase) and an inhibitor that utilizes a sulfhydryl group for binding to the
active site zinc was solved (12). The crystal structure verified the Squibb
hypothesis that the sulfhydryl group would displace the zinc-coordinated
water molecule in zinc proteases from the native enzyme, resulting in a new
tetrahedral zinc complex.

The Squibb group continued to refine their conceptual model for ACE as
more structure-activity data became available, evolving to the model shown
in Figure 2 (6). The X—H group in the region of the S$_1$, subsite was proposed
to be a Tyr and provide the proton required for the departing nitrogen of the
scissile peptide group based on analogy to the mechanistic proposals for
carboxypeptidase A at the time (the carboxypeptidase A mechanism was later
revised, and the Tyr was no longer proposed as the proton source for the

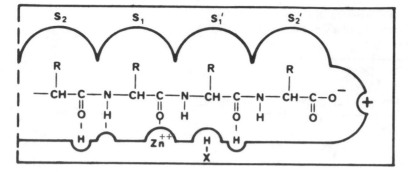

Figure 2 Revised conceptual model for ACE as proposed by Petrillo and Ondetti (6). Reproduced with permission.

departing nitrogen (13,14)). A hydrogen bond donor and acceptor were added for interacting with the peptide linkage to the P_2 residue, and pockets for the P_1 and P_2 side chains were added to extend the model further down the active site. The proposed (6) binding modes for a variety of inhibitors to this conceptual model are shown in Figure 3.

The success of the Squibb work in developing ACE inhibitors from the initial peptide leads appears to stem from their use of a conceptual model for ACE as a general guide in conjunction with the more classical medicinal chemistry approach of exploring structural modifications in a largely empirical fashion. The ACE model was considered a "working model" and consequently was adjusted to accommodate structure-activity data as it became available. In this way the model can continually evolve toward a more accurate representation of the target enzyme. A model generated and continually adjusted in this way might be considered a convenient conceptual framework within which a large amount of inhibitor and substrate structure-activity data, along with structural and mechanistic data for related enzymes, can be distilled down to their essence. Models of this type can now be made more detailed and more three-dimensional with the use of computer graphics, particularily if the sequence of the target enzyme is known and high homology exists with a related enzyme for which a crystal structure is available.

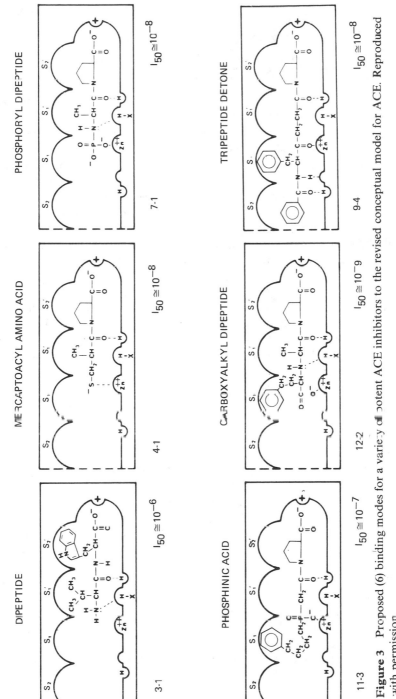

Figure 3 Proposed (6) binding modes for a variety of potent ACE inhibitors to the revised conceptual model for ACE. Reproduced with permission.

III. MOLECULAR MECHANICS-AIDED DESIGN OF CONFORMATIONALLY RESTRICTED CAPTOPRIL ANALOGS

The discovery of captopril by Squibb provided a good inhibitor design for initial testing of the effects of conformational restrictions on in vitro activity. Freely rotating bonds in inhibitors, which lose much of their rotational freedom when the inhibitor binds to the enzyme, can reduce the inhibitor activity by as much as an order of magnitude because of an inhibitor entropy loss of up to 1.5 kcal/mol (15). Consequently, if one or more bonds in the inhibitor can be fixed into the conformation preferred by the enzyme, without introducing repulsive interactions into the inhibitor:enzyme complex, then substantial increases in activity are possible.

The first conformationally restricted captopril analogs reported contained five- and six-membered ring lactams which tethered the alanine methyl group to the peptide nitrogen of a terminal glycine or substituted glycine. Two examples are inhibitors [4] and [5] in Table 2. These compounds were first described by Klutchko and co-workers (16). They concluded that these lactams are considerably less active than captopril largely owing to the absence of proline at the C terminus. Later Squibb researchers also reported the six-membered ring lactam [5] (17). It was noted that the amide bond is fixed in the trans orientation in inhibitor [5]. They concluded that this *trans*-amide geometry is preferred by ACE based on a comparison of IC_{50} data with analogous acyclic inhibitors and cis/trans populations of acyclic inhibitors vs. activity. Neither of these research groups reported larger ring lactams or discussed the effect of ring size on the psi angle of the alanine fragment (Fig. 4).

Thorsett and co-workers (18) had begun investigating similar lactam inhibitors shortly after captopril was announced. The methyl group of the alanine residue in captopril was known to contribute significantly to the high activity of this inhibitor. Thorsett et al. postulated that this activity enhancement was due to a combination of an effect on the conformation of the dipeptide region of the inhibitor as well as a possible interaction of the methyl group with a binding pocket on ACE. They assumed that the conformation of captopril in the captopril:ACE complex would be a member of the family of low-energy conformers. Since Ala–Pro is the C-terminal dipeptide in many of the more potent peptide inhibitors and is largely incorporated into the captopril structure, they began by studying the conformation of Ala–Pro.

The molecular mechanics feature of the Merck Molecular Modeling System (19) was used to identify families of low-energy conformations for Ala–Pro. Thorsett and co-workers found the trans conformation of the peptide

Table 2 Conformationally Restricted Captopril Analogs: Mercaptomethyl Lactams

No	Compound[a]	IC$_{50}$(μM)
4	HS— (five-membered lactam ring), N—CO$_2$H, =O	3.7 [b]
5	HS— (six-membered lactam ring), N—CO$_2$H, =O	3.4, 1.0 [b], 10 [c]
6	HS— (seven-membered lactam ring), N—CO$_2$H, =O	0.17
7	HS— (eight-membered lactam ring), N—CH(CH$_3$)—CO$_2$H, =O	0.053 [d]
8	HS— (five-membered lactam ring), N—CH(CH$_3$)—CO$_2$H, =O	4.9 [d]
9	HS— (six-membered lactam ring), N—CH(CH$_3$)—CO$_2$H, =O	0.5 [d]
3	HS-CH$_2$CH(CH$_3$)-C(=O)-N (proline ring) CO$_2$H	0.023

[a]All lactams tested as racemic mixtures.
[b]Ref. 16.
[c]Ref. 17.
[d]Most active racemate.
Source: Reproduced with permission from Ref. 18.

bond to be of lower energy than the cis, in agreement with earlier studies, and the range of psi angles that corresponds to the low-energy conformers was identified. They noted that the trans conformation of the peptide bond and the psi angle can be fixed by introducing a carbon chain that connects the Ala methyl group to the proline C 5 methylene as in structure [10] of Figure 4

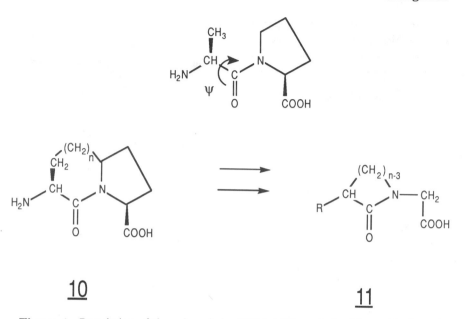

Figure 4 Restriction of the psi angle in ACE inhibitors derived from Ala–Pro via lactam formation (18).

To facilitate the synthesis, these lactams were simplified to the monocyclic inhibitors [11] after substituting the mercaptomethylene group for the dipeptide nitrogen (i.e., R = CH$_2$SH). Low-energy conformations for inhibitors [11] were then identified via molecular mechanics calculations focusing particularly on the psi angle. It was found that only the large-ring lactams— i.e., the seven- to nine-membered ring lactams—had low-energy conformations with psi angles corresponding to the low-energy psi angles for Ala–Pro. Based on these calculations and their initial assumptions, Thorsett and co-workers predicted that the most active lactam inhibitors would have ring sizes greater than 6. Indeed, subsequent synthesis and testing of these inhibitors verified their prediction. The IC$_{50}$ data for the inhibitors given in Table 2 shows that the five- and six-membered lactams have equivalent activity, whereas the seven-membered lactam [6] has an activity 20 times better than the smaller-ring lactams.

   Thorsett and co-workers then began to build pieces of the proline ring back into these lactam inhibitors as illustrated by inhibitors [7], [8], and [9]. A comparison of [5] and [9] indicated that the addition of pieces of the proline ring might improve the activity, although in this comparison the improvement was only about threefold (assuming [5] is a 1/1 mixture of

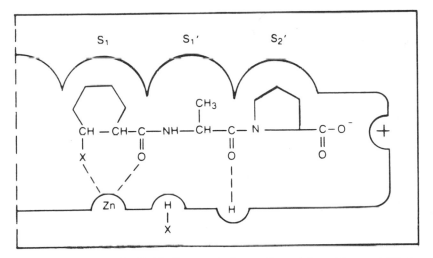

Figure 5 Proposed (20) binding mode for cyclic acyldipeptides to ACE. Reproduced with permission.

diastereomers and one of the diastereomers is relatively inactive). When the lactam ring size was increased to 8 and a methyl group was added to the carboxymethyl side chain (inhibitor [7]), the activity was improved to the extent of reaching essentially equal potency with captopril [3] (Table 2). This added methyl group constitutes another piece of the missing proline ring and was thought to contribute to the high activity by enhancing hydrophobic binding to ACE and also producing a favorable rotational restriction of the carboxymethyl side chain.

The Squibb group has used their conceptual model for ACE as an aid in the design of ACE inhibitors with a conformational restriction adjacent to the zinc-binding ligand (20). Acyl groups were designed for extending Ala-Pro-based inhibitors into the S_1 subsite while providing a carboxyl or a mercapto group in a suitable constrained orientation for binding to the active-site zinc. The proposed binding mode for these inhibitors is illustrated in Figure 5, where X = SH or CO_2H. The structure-activity data obtained for this series of inhibitors demonstrated the importance of the zinc ligand and the stereochemistry, as shown in Table 3. The most active inhibitor obtained in this series [14] has an in vitro potency nearly 10 times better than captopril [3] (Table 2). This study also included acyl groups containing carbocyclic rings larger and smaller than the cyclohexane ring as well as cis substitution of the zinc ligand and the amide group on the ring. An optimal dihedral angle range of 30–60° between the bonds to the zinc ligand and the

Table 3   Relationship of the Zinc Ligand and Its Stereochemistry to In Vitro Potency in Cyclic Acyl-Dipeptides

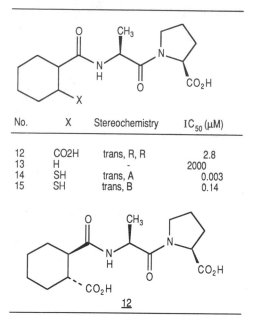

No.	X	Stereochemistry	IC_{50} (µM)
12	CO2H	trans, R, R	2.8
13	H	-	2000
14	SH	trans, A	0.003
15	SH	trans, B	0.14

12

Source: Reproduced with permission from Ref. 20.

amide group was identified from an analysis of these analogs. These data are valuable for refining a three-dimensional model for ACE in the region of the S_1 subsite.

IV.   MOLECULAR MECHANICS-AIDED DESIGN OF CONFORMATIONALLY RESTRICTED ENALAPRILAT ANALOGS

The announcement of captopril by Squibb encouraged Patchett and co-workers at Merck to focus their efforts on finding an orally active ACE inhibitor that does not utilize a sulfhydryl group for binding to the active site zinc. The Merck researchers hypothesized that the sulfhydryl group present in captopril was related to some of the side effects observed in humans during initial clinical trials with this drug. In 1978 enalaprilat [16] (Fig. 6) was discovered by the Merck group and later found to be orally active as its prodrug monoethylester, enalapril (21). Enalapril was the second ACE

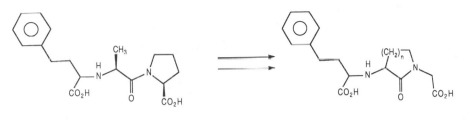

Figure 6 Restriction of the psi angle in enalaprilat analogs via lactam formation (24).

inhibitor to be marketed as an antihypertensive drug. The design of enalaprilat, like that of captopril, can be traced back to Byers and Wolfendens' collected product inhibitor design and has been described in several reviews (3,4,22).

Thorsett and co-workers decided to shift their attention toward, applying the lactam conformational restriction concept to the enalaprilat design (23,24). Enalaprilat contains the dipeptide unit Ala–Pro, similar to captopril, so the transfer of the lactam design to enalaprilat was thought to be a logical next step. However, the presence of a phenethyl side chain for binding in the S_1 subsite may affect the conformation of the Ala–Pro region of the inhibitor and lead to a change in the optimal lactam ring size. As before, the Ala methyl group was tethered to the C-5 carbon atom of proline, and the C-3 and C-4 carbon atoms of the proline ring were excluded to facilitate the synthesis. This conceptual process is illustrated in Figure 6. The IC_{50} data for the resulting inhibitors [17;a–e] (Table 4) show that the optimum activity is reached at the eight-membered ring inhibitor [17;d], analogous to the captopril-based lactams, and suggesting that the phenethyl side chain did not alter the preferred Ala–Pro conformation.

A detailed investigation of the conformations of the lactam rings present in inhibitors [17; a–e] was carried out with molecular mechanics calculations to better define the relationship of the activity to the psi angle (24). The simplified lactams [18; a–e] (Fig. 7) were chosen for these calculations in order to focus on the effect of ring size on the psi angle. The starting geometries for the five- and six-membered lactams [18; a] and [18; b] were generated by inputting approximate known low-energy conformations for these ring systems into the minimization program. The starting geometries for the seven- to nine-membered lactams [18; c–e] were not as intuitively obvious, and therefore the RINGMAKER/BAKMOD computational

Table 4 Comparison of ACE Inhibitory Activities and Minimum Energy ψ Angles for Lactam Inhibitors 17; a-e] and Enalaprilat [16]

Compound	No.	Ring size	IC$_{50}$ (isomer A)[a]	IC$_{50}$ (isomer B)[a]	Model[b]	ψ_{calcd}	ψ_{x-ray}
17; a	1	5	1.2×10^{-5}	1.9×10^{-5}	18; a	-132 (132)[c]	
17; b	2	6	4.3×10^{-7}	1.7×10^{-6}	18; b	-138 (138)[c]	
17; c	3	7	7.0×10^{-7}[d]	1.9×10^{-8}	18; c	166	166[e]
17; d	4	8	1.7×10^{-6}	4.8×10^{-9}	18; d	145	159[f]
17; dSS	4	8		2.0×10^{-9}			
17; dRR	4	8		9.2×10^{-8}			
17; e	5	9	1.3×10^{-6}	8.1×10^{-9}	18; e	135	
16				1.2×10^{-9}[g]		140	143

[a]IC$_{50}$ concentrations are molar. Isomer A is the first diester isomer to elute from silica gel and B is the second. All compounds tested as racemic mixtures unless otherwise noted.
[b]Model lactam used to obtain ψ_{calcd} from Table 5.
[c]Values in parentheses are for lactams having R configuration at C-3.
[d]Approximately 5% isomer B present by HPLC.
[e]From crystal structure of 17; c.
[f]From crystal structure of a related compound.
[g]Value from S,S,S enantiomer.
Source: Data from Ref. 24.

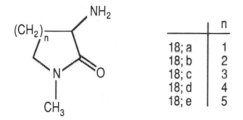

	n
18; a	1
18; b	2
18; c	3
18; d	4
18; e	5

Figure 7 Model lactams for molecular mechanics calculations (24).

programs of Still and Galynker (25) were used to generate conformations for subsequent minimization.

The complexity of the larger-ring lactams is exemplified by the identification of 407 rough starting conformations for the cis isomer of the nine-membered lactam [18; e] using the RINGMAKER program. After refining the conformations by energy minimization, sorting by relative strain energy, and applying a program to remove redundant conformations, a total of 19 conformations within 4 kcal of the minimum-energy conformer remained. The same procedure was applied to the seven- and eight-membered lactams [18; c,d], resulting in six and four unique conformations, respectively. The relative energies, population distribution (calculated from a Boltzmann distribution function), and psi angles are listed in Table 5 for the five- to nine-membered lactams [18; a–e].

The computed global minimum energy conformations for the seven to nine-membered [18; c–e] lactams were in good agreement with the x-ray-determined conformations for similar lactams. The computed conformations for the five- and six-membered lactams [18; a,b] were similar to the known conformations for cyclopentene and cyclohexene, respectively. The agreement of computed conformations to experimentally determined conformations for similar compounds remarkably extended to a comparison of the conformational population distributions. The reported interpretations of NMR, infrared, and circular dichrosim data for lactams similar to those subjected to the molecular mechanics calculations in this study showed striking correspondence in their conformational population distributions.

The psi angles for the lactam inhibitors [17; a–e] were derived by analogy with the computed psi angles for the model lactams [18; a–e] and are listed in Table 4 along with the IC_{50} data. The computed and x-ray-derived psi angles for enalaprilat [16] and the available x-ray-derived psi angles for the lactam inhibitors are also listed in Table 4. If one assumes that the high binding affinity of enalaprilat and the large-ring lactams to ACE is partially due to the bound conformation's being close to the global minimum-energy

Table 5 Relative Energies, ψ Values, and Relative Populations[a] for Low-Energy Conformations of Five- to Seven-Membered N-Methyl-3-Amino Lactams 18; a–e Derived from MM2 Calculations

	E^b	ψ	$\%^c$		E^b	ψ	$\%^c$
18; a ($n = 1$)				18; e ($n = 5$)			
a	0.0	−132	52.0	a	0.0	135	42.5
b	0.04	−106	48.0	b	0.6	−64	15.4
				c	0.8	143	11.0
18; b ($n = 2$)				d	0.9	116	9.3
a	0.0	−138	88.4	e	1.1	129	6.6
b	1.2	−111	11.6	f	1.5	−45	4.0
				g	1.5	116	3.4
18; c ($n = 3$)				h	1.6	131	2.9
a	0.0	166	75.0	i	1.8	−60	2.2
b	0.7	−72	23.0	j	2.1	135	1.2
c	2.3	−98	1.5	k	2.4	169	0.7
d	3.3	−109	0.3	l	3.0	124	0.3
e	3.9	−149	0.1	m	3.4	146	0.1
f	3.9	−155	0.1	n	3.4[d]	145	0.1
				o	3.7	169	0.08
18; d ($n = 4$)				p	3.8[d]	139	0.07
a	0.0	145	69.4	q	3.9[d]	120	0.06
b	0.5	144	29.8	r	4.0[d]	130	0.05
c	2.7	−48	0.7	s	4.0	−80	0.05
d	3.9	−89	0.1				

[a]Relative populations were calculated from the discrete Boltzmann distribution function: $P_i = 1/\exp[(E_i - E_j)/KT]$ as the mole ratio.
[b]Relative energies, kcal/mol.
[c]Population distribution.
[d]Trans isomers.
Source: Reproduced with permission from Ref. 24.

conformation, then the data indicate that ACE will accept inhibitors with psi angles between about 130° and 170°.

Interpretation of the results for the psi angle vs. IC_{50} with the small-ring lactams [17; a,b] is more complex. The psi angles for the five- and six-membered lactams with S stereochemistry at the carbon atom corresponding to the C-alpha of Ala in enalaprilat are about 50–60° out of the acceptable range of 130–170°, which may explain the large drop in activity for these inhibitors. The psi angles for the five- and six-membered lactams [17; a,b] with R stereochemistry at the same carbon atom are in the acceptable range.

However, the R stereochemistry corresponds to that of a D-Ala in an enalaprilat inhibitor. Published data on the D-Ala analog of enalaprilat (3) shows that inversion of the stereochemistry at this position reduces the activity by nearly 3 orders of magnitude. If one holds the psi angle of bound enalaprilat in the acceptable range and then inverts the stereochemistry at the Ala to R, the methyl side chain is moved considerably, so that a repulsive interaction with a different region of the active site might occur and/or a favorable hydrophobic interaction with the active site might be lost. In addition, inversion of the Ala side chain to the R configuration could affect the conformation of the phenylbutyric side chain. Consequently, the five- and six-membered lactams with R configuration might have an acceptable psi angle, but a repulsive interaction, alteration in positioning of the phenyl-butyric side chain, and/or loss of a hydrophobic interaction might have occurred, analogous to a D-Ala substitution in enalaprilat, rationalizing the drop in activity.

Thorsett and co-workers continued to elaborate the enalaprilat-based lactam inhibitors (26). Methyl groups were added to the seven- and eight-membered lactam inhibitors to mimic the C-3 and C-4 carbons of proline in enalaprilat. The x-ray-derived psi angles and the computed psi angles for these lactams were again near the 130–170° range. The IC_{50}'s were improved to the point of being equal with the activity of enalaprilat. Ultimately the entire proline ring was fused onto both the seven- and eight-membered lactams to give inhibitors [19] and [20] (Table 6). The IC_{50}'s and psi angles for these inhibitors and enalaprilat are listed in Table 6. Interestingly, the completion of the proline ring provided no further improvement in activity over the previous methyl-substituted analogs. Since further restricting the active conformation of the inhibitor would be expected to increase the activity, this result suggests that these bicyclic inhibitors may not be in precisely the optimum conformation or that a necessary degree of conformational mobility has been lost.

Wyvratt and co-workers (3,27) prepared analog [21] (Table 6) of the bicyclic seven-membered lactam [19] wherein the C-4 carbon atom of the proline ring has been replaced with a sulfur atom. The psi angle determined by x-ray was again near the acceptable 130–170° range. The substitution of sulfur for carbon improved the activity by fivefold over the corresponding bicyclic seven-membered lactam [19]. Thorsett suggests (26) that the increased flexibility of the thiazolidine ring in [21] over the corresponding proline ring in [19] may account for the improvement in activity. This suggestion is based on the finding of Bull and co-workers (28) that the mechanism of ACE inhibition by enalaprilat is a two-step process involving an initial loose complex followed by conversion to a tightly bound complex.

Inversion of the stereochemistry at the carbon atom of inhibitor [21]

Table 6 Bicyclic Enalaprilat Analogs Containing
Proline or Thiaproline

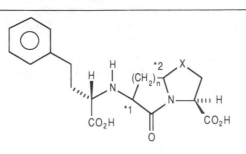

Compd	X	n	*1	*2	IC$_{50}$(nM)	ψx-ray
19	CH$_2$	3	IIIIIH	IIIIIH	2.9	174
20	CH$_2$	4	IIIIIH	IIIIIH	3.4	–
21	S	3	IIIIIH	IIIIIH	0.6	168
22	S	3	IIIIIH	——H	4.0	199[b]
23	S	3	——H	IIIIIH	1,700	168
16	(enalaprilat)		IIIIIH	–	1.2	143

[a]Calculated (3).

Source: Data from Refs. 26 and 27.

mimicking the C-alpha of Ala so that the stereochemistry corresponding to a
D-Ala is present gives inhibitor [23] (Table 6). This compound has a
computed psi angle of 156° and an x-ray-derived psi angle of 168° (3). Even
though these angles are within the 130–170° window suggested by the earlier
lactam work, the inhibitor is relatively inactive. Wyvratt and Patchett (3)
suggest that the low activity may be due to the R stereochemistry's causing an
unfavorable interaction with the active site analogous to the reduced activity
of inhibitors with a D-Ala at this position. This result corroborates the results
for the five- and six-membered monocyclic lactams discussed above which
also have stereochemistry corresponding to D-Ala along with an "acceptable" psi angle. The additional possible rationalizations mentioned
above for the reduced activity of these monocyclic lactams could also be
applied to inhibitor [23].

Interestingly, bicyclic lactam isomer [22] (Table 6) is only slightly less
active than isomer [21], even though the psi angle for [22] is calculated to be
outside of the "acceptable" window of 130–170° (3). Wyvratt and Patchett

(3) suggest that particularly effective hydrophobic interactions may be compensating for the unfavorable psi angle. These results highlight the importance of considering, inasmuch as possible, additional interactions (attractive as well as repulsive) with the active site which might result from the introduction of a conformational restriction into an inhibitor.

V. COMPUTER-AIDED DESIGN OF CILAZAPRIL

A group at Roche has also designed conformationally restricted bicyclic analogs of captopril [3] (29,30) and later enalapril at [16] (31,32) with the aid of computer studies. As described below, these studies ultimately led to the design of cilazapril, which is undergoing clinical testing in man as an antihypertensive agent.

Initially the binding of captopril to ACE was conceptually reduced to three essential binding interactions. The proline carboxyl group was assumed to interact with a positively charged active-site residue. The amide linkage was assumed to be trans, and the carbonyl group of the amide was postulated to function as a hydrogen bond acceptor with an NH group from ACE. The ACE donor NH was assumed to form an optimum angle of 150–180° with the amide carbonyl bond and be positioned with the hydrogen atom about 1.8 Å from from the carbonyl oxygen. The conformations of the two C–C bonds emanating from the amide carbonyl toward the SH were studied by molecular mechanics, and all high-energy conformations for these bonds were eliminated from consideration as possible bound conformations. Finally, the C–S bond was assumed to be in the less sterically crowded anti conformation when the sulfur coordinates with the active-site zinc.

All of these assumptions and results were combined to produce a range of possible binding conformations for captopril to the three essential binding sites in ACE. These possible binding modes are presented as a composite diagram in Figure 8, where the mesh indicates the range of possible positions for the zinc atom (corresponding to the feasible positions for the inhibitor sulfur atom to which the zinc is coordinated) and the loops indicate the range of possible positions for the other two enzyme groups. The x-ray and major solution conformation (determined by NMR) of captopril are similar and fit within the conformational space accommodated by this plot.

The Roche group used this postulated range of possible binding modes to design the conformationally restricted analogs of captopril shown in Table 7 along with their in vitro activities. They concentrated on restricting the conformation of the Ala-Pro mimicking region of captopril as the Merck group has done. Three bicyclic structural frameworks were chosen based on their ability to explore the conformational space accommodated by the plot in Figure 8 and synthetic accessibility. The conformation of each series

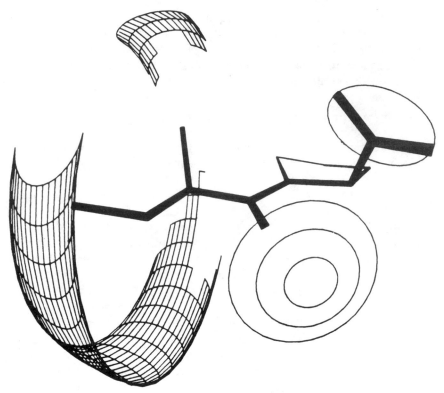

Figure 8 Initial proposed binding conformations for captopril to the postulated active site for ACE. Reproduced with permission from Ref. 29.

was studied by NMR and, when possible, x-ray. The octahydro-6,9-dioxopyridazo[1,2-a]pyridazine-based inhibitor [30] was found to be the most active.

The possible bound positions of the sulfur atoms in captopril and inhibitor [30] were then compared. First the bicyclic framework of [30] was superimposed via computer graphics upon the analogous parts of the proline and amide carbonyl of captopril, then the conformationally feasible positions for the sulfur in inhibitor [30] were traced assuming complete rotation around the previous C–C bond. Since the conformation of the next C–C bond (from the carbon mimicking C-alpha in alanine to the amide carbonyl) is greatly restricted in inhibitor [30], the range of feasible positions for the sulfur atom (common to both inhibitor [30] and captopril) is reduced to the mesh area shown in Figure 9 along with the proposed bound conformation for inhibitor [30].

Table 7 Bicyclic Captopril Analogs

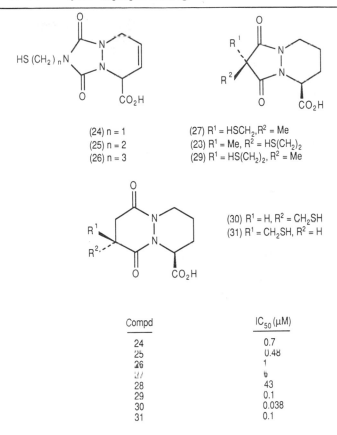

(24) n = 1
(25) n = 2
(26) n = 3

(27) R^1 = HSCH$_2$, R^2 = Me
(28) R^1 = Me, R^2 = HS(CH$_2$)$_2$
(29) R^1 = HS(CH$_2$)$_2$, R^2 = Me

(30) R^1 = H, R^2 = CH$_2$SH
(31) R^1 = CH$_2$SH, R^2 = H

Compd	IC$_{50}$ (μM)
24	0.7
25	0.48
26	1
27	6
28	43
29	0.1
30	0.038
31	0.1

Source: Data from Ref. 30.

The in vitro activity of inhibitor [30] is only fivefold less than that of captopril, so it was assumed that the sulfur atom must be positioned to coordinate reasonably well with the active-site zinc in ACE. When the same procedure was applied to the less active, conformationally restricted inhibitors, different common feasible positions for the sulfur atoms were obtained. The reduction in activity was assumed to arise in part from a reduced interaction with the zinc. Therefore the conformations common to inhibitor [30] and captopril should be useful for locating the probable positions of the active-site zinc relative to the active-site hydrogen bond promoter and salt bridge. To do this it was assumed that the Zn–S–C–C torsion angle would

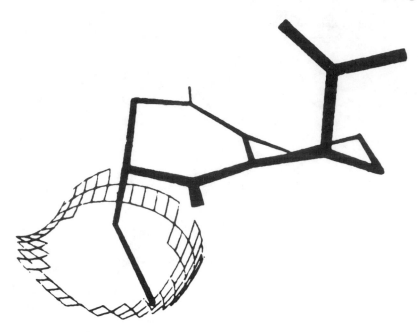

Figure 9 The common possible positions (indicated by mesh area) for the sulfur atoms in captopril and inhibitor [30] when bound to ACE (30). Reproduced with permission.

be anti when inhibitor [30] is complexed to ACE, and a standard geometry was assumed for the $Zn-S-CH_2$ coordination (the same assumptions were applied to captopril when deriving Fig. 8). When these assumptions and the common feasible positions for the sulfur atoms in captopril and inhibitor [30] were considered, the possible positions for the active-site zinc were reduced from the mesh area shown in Figure 8 to the smaller mesh area shown in Figure 10.

If the conformation of the 6,6-bicyclic inhibitor [30] is precisely the same as the bound conformation of captopril, and the binding interactions with the ACE active site are equivalent, one would expect [30] to be more active than captopril owing to a lower entropy loss upon binding. The Roche group compared the psi angle energy profile for Ala in Ala−Pro to the corresponding angle in [30] available from their previous conformational studies. Analogous to the Merck finding with six-membered lactams, the Roche group observed that the psi angle in [30] corresponds to a high-energy psi angle in Ala−Pro (see Gilbert and Thomas (33) for a detailed discussion of NMR conformational studies on this ring system). The high energy of this

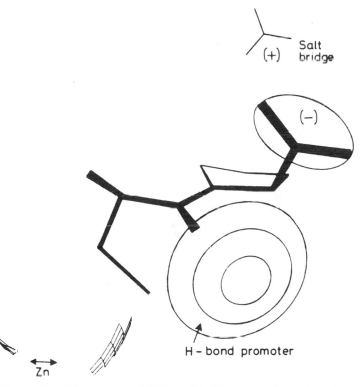

Figure 10 Final proposed (30) possible binding conformations for captopril to the postulated active site for ACE after considering the effect of conformational restrictions on activity. Reproduced with permission.

conformation was due to a close interaction between the alanine side chain methyl group and C-4 of proline. The smaller 5,6-bicyclic inhibitors (e.g., [29]) were even less active and also have a psi angle corresponding to a similar high-energy psi angle in Ala–Pro. The reduced activity for these inhibitors (relative to captopril) was postulated to be due partly to the nonoptimal psi angle.

The Roche group then chose to examine the larger 7,6- and 8,6-bicyclic inhibitor frameworks which, based on molecular graphics simulations, offered better prospects of having a psi angle corresponding to the postulated bound conformation of captopril and cnalaprilat (31,32). It was assumed that the Ala–Pro regions of both captopril and enalapril bind to ACE in the same conformation, and therefore the bicyclic Ala–Pro mimicking framework could be transferred from one series to the other. The 6,6-bicyclic and larger ring inhibitors were then investigated with inhibitors utilizing the enalaprilat design. The psi angles for a representative series of these compounds were derived either from NMR, from crystal structures on model compounds, or by calculation, and are listed in Table 8 along with the activities (see also Thomas and Whitcombe (34) for a detailed discussion of NMR studies on the 7,6-bicyclic ring systems). The data indicated that a psi angle of about 165° is required for optimal activity against ACE. This angle is within the window of 130–170° proposed by the Merck group for the psi angle based on their monocyclic and bicyclic lactams. The most active inhibitor [34] utilizes a 7,6-bicyclic ring system, has a psi angle of 164°, and is slightly more active than enalaprilat (IC_{50} = 1.6 nM vs. 3.3 nM, respectively, against rabbit lung ACE under their assay conditions).

The Roche group combined their results with the information provided by Monzingo and Matthews (35) on the crystal structure of an enalaprilat analog bound to the active site of thermolysin to deduce the binding mode shown in Figure 11 for inhibitor [34] to ACE. The monoethyl ester of inhibitor [34] (cilazapril), analogous to enalapril, is orally active and provides another ACE inhibitor for the treatment of hypertension.

Table 8   Variation of ACE IC_{50} with Ring Size and ψ Angle

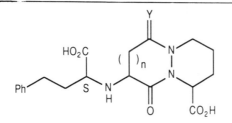

Compd.	n	ψ^a	IC_{50} (nM)	Compd.	n	ψ	IC_{50} (nM)
		Y = H$_2$				Y = O	
32	0	254.9	8000	36	0	237.6	
33	1	245.6	28	37	1	196.6	20
34	2	163.9	1.6	38	2	165.3	4
35	3	142.1 [b]	4.5	39	3	146.4 [b]	15

[a] ψ values obtained from crystal structures of model bicyclic compounds.
[b] Values calculated by MNDO.
Source: Reproduced with permission from Ref. 32.

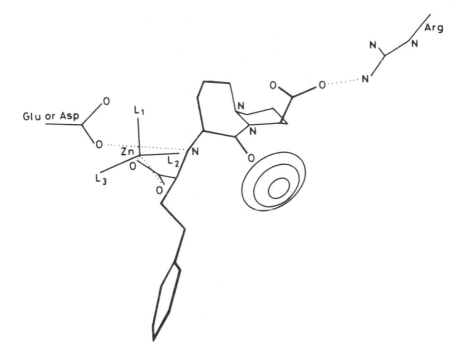

Figure 11   Proposed binding mode for inhibitor [34] to the postulated active site for ACE (32). Reproduced with permission.

VI.   MAPPING THE ANGIOTENSIN-CONVERTING ENZYME ACTIVE SITE FROM A CONFORMATIONAL ANALYSIS OF DIVERSE INHIBITORS

Andrews and co-workers have carried out a conformational analysis of eight structurally diverse ACE inhibitors and concluded that there is a common conformation throughout the series (36). The ACE inhibitors used in this study are listed in Table 9 along with their in vitro activities. Classical potential energy calculations, holding the bond angles and bond lengths at fixed standard values and varying the dihedral angles by 10° increments, were used to identify the low-energy conformations of each of these inhibitors. The phi_1 vs. psi_1 conformational energy map for inhibitors [40], [41], and [3] (captopril) were compared. A common minimum at about $psi_1 = 165°$ was noted. Consequently, Andrews and co-workers concluded that a psi angle of

Table 9 Structures, Activities, and Conformational Variables of ACE Inhibitors Studied

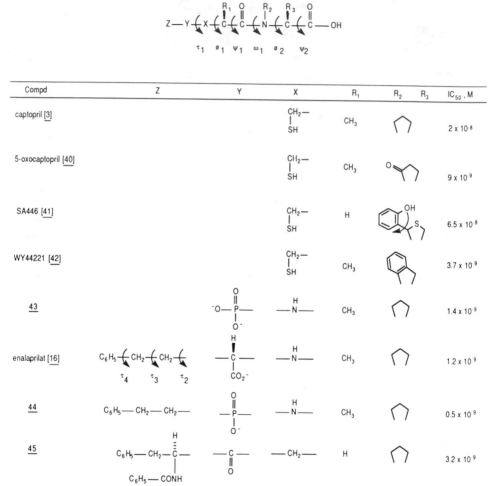

Compd	Z	Y	X	R_1	R_2	R_3	IC_{50}, M
captopril [3]			$\begin{array}{c}CH_2- \\ | \\ SH\end{array}$	CH_3			2×10^{-8}
5-oxocaptopril [40]			$\begin{array}{c}CH_2- \\ | \\ SH\end{array}$	CH_3			9×10^{-9}
SA446 [41]			$\begin{array}{c}CH_2- \\ | \\ SH\end{array}$	H			6.5×10^{-8}
WY44221 [42]			$\begin{array}{c}CH_2- \\ | \\ SH\end{array}$	CH_3			3.7×10^{-9}
43		$\begin{array}{c}O \\ || \\ ^-O-P- \\ | \\ O^-\end{array}$	$\begin{array}{c}H \\ -N-\end{array}$	CH_3			1.4×10^{-9}
enalaprilat [16]	$C_6H_5-(CH_2-(CH_2-()\\ \quad \tau_4 \quad \tau_3 \quad \tau_2$	$\begin{array}{c}H \\ -C- \\ | \\ CO_2^-\end{array}$	$\begin{array}{c}H \\ -N-\end{array}$	CH_3			1.2×10^{-9}
44	$C_6H_5-CH_2-CH_2-$	$\begin{array}{c}O \\ || \\ -P- \\ | \\ O^-\end{array}$	$\begin{array}{c}H \\ -N-\end{array}$	CH_3			0.5×10^{-9}
45	$\begin{array}{c}H \\ C_6H_5-CH_2-\overset{\vdots}{C}- \\ | \\ C_6H_5-CONH\end{array}$	$\begin{array}{c}-C- \\ || \\ O\end{array}$	$-CH_2-$	H			3.2×10^{-9}

Source: Reproduced with permission from Ref. 36.

about 165° is required for binding to ACE, in agreement with the conclusions of the Merck and Roche groups.

The phi_1–psi_1 maps were also used, along with the result on one of the Roche conformationally restricted captopril analogs [24] (Table 7), to conclude that a phi_1 angle of 300° is part of the bound conformation for captopril. The position of the zinc atom in ACE was further defined by carrying out a conformational analysis of phi_1 and tau_1 angles for inhibitors [43], [44], [45], and [16], holding the psi_1 angle at 165°. Only a few accessible orientations for the zinc-binding groups were identified. The position of the S_1 binding site for the phenyl group in inhibitors [44], [45], and [16] was deduced by studying the conformation of the phenethyl side chain and assuming that only the common low-energy conformations available to all three inhibitors are likely to include the active conformation. The active site of ACE was then "mapped" by deriving the position of the enzyme groups thought to interact with the inhibitors from the deduced bound conformations of the inhibitors. A stereo representation of the deduced bound conformations for inhibitors [3], [43], [16], and [45] is shown in Figure 12 along with the active-site zinc (the inhibitor groups binding near the S_1 subsite have been removed for clarity).

All of these inhibitors were analyzed assuming monodentate coordination to the zinc. Later studies with a thermolysin inhibitor (35) containing the enalaprilat inhibitor core have shown that the carboxyl group binds in a bidentate fashion. Recent x-ray studies with thermolysin inhibitors utilizing the phosphonamidate and phosphoramidate inhibitor designs (37,38) have also shown bidentate coordination to the zinc. It has also been suggested that the ketone based inhibitors such as [45] bind as the hydrate (39,40). If this information had been available to Andrews and co-workers at the time of their study, a somewhat different positioning of the ACE active-site zinc

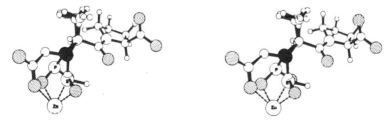

Figure 12 Stereoscopic view of the deduced bound conformations for inhibitors [3], [43], [16], and [45] along with the ACE active-site zinc (the inhibitor regions binding near the S_1 subsite have been removed for clarity) (36). Reproduced with permission.

might have resulted. This underscores the value of having as much experimental information as possible when carrying out a study of this type.

Subsequent to Andrews and co-workers' publication, a paper was published by Ciabatti and co-workers (41) describing a series of conformationally restricted captopril analogs wherein the position of the zinc-binding sulfhydryl group was fixed relative to the alanine-mimicking fragment. The most active compounds reported utilized a four- or five-membered ring to restrict the conformation. The in vitro activities for these compounds, along with some of the less active diastereomers, are listed in Table 10. The most active diastereomers in these series have a trans-substituted ring and are only a factor of 2 less active than captopril. This trans orientation positions the sulfhydryl group close to the position proposed by Andrews and co-workers as shown in Figure 12. Since these conformationally restricted analogs are not more active than captopril, the relative position of the sulfhydryl group may not be ideal, and/or the ring has introduced unfavorable interactions with ACE. Nevertheless, it seems likely that the zinc atom is located in the general vicinity of the position (relative to captopril) proposed by Andrews and co-workers.

Table 10   ACE Inhibitory Activity of Captopril Analogs with a Conformational Restriction Adjacent to the Sulfhydryl Groups

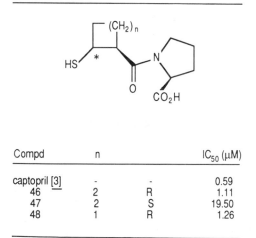

Compd	n		IC_{50} (μM)
captopril [3]	-	-	0.59
46	2	R	1.11
47	2	S	19.50
48	1	R	1.26

Source: Data from Ref. 41.

VII. THERMOLYSIN AS A MODEL FOR ANGIOTENSIN-CONVERTING ENZYME

Thermolysin is a well-studied zinc endopeptidase. A variety of inhibitor, substrate, and crystallographic data have been reported. The crystal and solution conformations appear to correspond closely, based on available experimental comparisons (42). The crystalline enzyme can hydrolyze peptides (43,55), and the conformation changes very little upon binding a reversible inhibitor in the active site (44). The Merck group found that the enalaprilat inhibitor design could be utilized to prepare potent inhibitors of thermolysin (45) but was relatively ineffective against carboxypeptidase A (3). It was for these reasons, and the fact that the crystal structure of the complex between thermolysin and an inhibitor utilizing the enalaprilat design had been solved (35), that Hangauer and co-workers decided to use thermolysin as a model for ACE.

A. MECHANISM OF THERMOLYSIN-CATALYZED PEPTIDE CLEAVAGE AND COMPARISON TO THE BINDING MODE OF AN ENALAPRILAT ANALOG

Hangauer and co-workers, in collaboration with Matthews and co-workers at the University of Oregon, utilized computer graphics, the crystal structure of native thermolysin (46), and various thermolysin: inhibitor complexes to explore plausible mechanisms for peptide cleavage by thermolysin (47,48). A detailed proposed mechanism emerged from this work that both extended and modified previously suggested mechanisms. The main features of this new mechanism have been supported by subsequent crystal structures of transition state and substrate analogs bound to thermolysin (37,38,55,56). The essential elements of this mechanism have also been incorporated into the proposed mechanism for carboxypeptidase A (14,35).

The computer graphics-aided thermolysin mechanism study was stimulated by the x-ray structure of the complex between the enalaprilat analog inhibitor [49] (Table 11) and thermolysin solved by Monzingo and Matthews (35). The crystal structure revealed a bidentate coordination of the carboxyl group to the zinc and extensive hydrogen bonding with the active site in the region where the scissile peptide linkage of a substrate would be expected to bind, as shown in Figure 13.

Since the enalaprilat inhibitor design gives inhibitors of high potency against both ACE and thermolysin, it was of interest to compare the binding mode of the thermolysin/ACE inhibitor [49] to the proposed mechanism for thermolysin-catalyzed peptide cleavage that resulted from the computer graphics study. Coordinates for various points along the reaction pathway

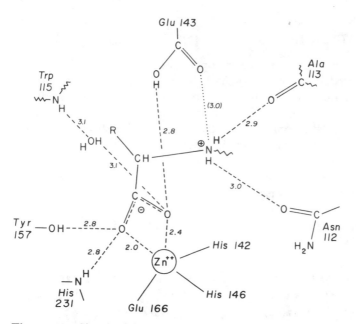

Figure 13   Sketch of the apparent interactions between inhibitor [49] and thermolysin as determined by x-ray (35). Interatomic distances are given in angstroms, and hydrogen bonds are indicated by dotted lines. Reproduced with permission.

with the model peptide substrate Cbz–Phe–Phe–Leu–Trp were compared to the x-ray coordinates for the bound inhibitor. It was concluded that the inhibitor binding mode is most analogous to the transition state for breakdown of the tetrahedral intermediate (47).

This conclusion is consistent with the concept that transition state analog inhibitors bind tenaciously because the enzyme has been constructed to reduce the transition-state energy by maximizing its binding interactions with the substrate at the transition state (49). Therefore, when a compound is presented to the enzyme which, in one of its low-energy states, mimics the high-energy transition state of the substrate, maximum utilization of the binding energy available with the enzyme is possible.

B.   Computer Graphics-Aided Design of New Thermolysin/Angiotensin-Converting Enzyme Inhibitors

Hangauer and co-workers used the crystal structure of the thermolysin:inhibitor [49] complex along with computer graphics and the information they had generated on the mechanism of peptide cleavage to design new inhibitors of both thermolysin and ACE (50). The crystal structure of the thermolysin:inhibitor [49] complex showed the phenethyl side chain binding in the S_1 subsite similar to the model peptide substrate Cbz–Phe–Phe–Leu–Trp when the tetrahedral intermediate was formed (47). Enalaprilat has an analogous phenethyl side chain which was thought to bind in the S_1 subsite of ACE. Previous attempts to append a substituent to enalaprilat that can bind in the S_2 subsite and increase the in vitro potency against ACE were unsuccessful (51). Consequently, a major focus of the computer graphics-aided design work was to explore various substituents that can be appended to the phenethyl side chain and bind in the S_2 subsite of thermolysin and/or ACE resulting in increased in vitro potency. The ability to span the S_2–$S_{2'}$ subsites of various zinc endopeptidases with the enalaprilat inhibitor design was thought to be important for expanding the scope of applications for this class of inhibitors.

A selection of the inhibitors designed with the aid of the thermolysin:inhibitor [49] crystal structure and computer graphics is given in Table 11 along with a few additional inhibitors required to interpret the in vitro activities listed.

A comparison of the structures for inhibitor [50] and the tetrahedral intermediate for the model peptide substrate Cbz–Phe–Phe–Leu–Trp is given in Figure 14. Inhibitor [50] was designed to mimic the transition state for breakdown of the tetrahedral intermediate of a substrate with the sequence Cbz–Phe–Gly–Leu–Trp wherein the Gly–Leu bond is the scissile linkage. The model substrate used in the mechanism study has a Phe at the P_1 position rather than the Gly present in the peptide mimicked by inhibitor [50]. A benzyl side chain for binding in the S_1 subsite was not included in inhibitor [50] and its analogs mainly for synthetic reasons. A comparison of the activities against thermolysin for inhibitors [51] and [52] (Table 11) shows that removing the benzyl group that binds in the S_1 subsite can reduce the activity by a factor of 47. Similarly, removal of the same benzyl group from ACE inhibitors has been shown to reduce the activity by a factor of 24 (3). Consequently, any binding achieved in the S_2 subsite with inhibitor [50] and its analogs would have to more than compensate for the loss in activity that results from removal of the benzyl group.

When the tetrahedral intermediate complex for the model substrate was superimposed on the x-ray coordinates for bound inhibitor [49], it was noted that the zinc-coordinating carboxyl introduces an "extra" C–C bond between the zinc ligands and the main chain of the inhibitor relative to the tetrahedral intermediate. This "extra" bond causes a displacement of the adjacent inhibitor main chain away from the zinc and toward the $S_{2'}$ end of the active site (47). This displacement makes the Cbz–Phe of an analogous extended inhibitor unable to reach the S_1 subsite unless a methylene is inserted into the

Table 11 Thermolysin/ACE Inhibitors Designed with the Aid of the Thermolysin Crystal Structure and Computer Graphics

Compd	K_i (nM, Thermolysin)	IC_{50} (nM, ACE)
49	34	10 ($K_i = 1.03$)
50	11	— ($K_i = 0.78$)
51	600	36
52	28,000	—
53	220	—

Table 11   Continued

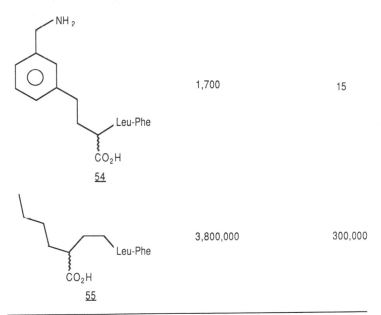

1,700	15
3,800,000	300,000

Source: Data from Ref. 50.

main chain just before the nitrogen which is acylated with the Cbz–Phe. Inhibitor [50] resulted from inserting this methylene into the main chain and removing the benzyl group which could bind in the S_1 subsite.

A stereo view of inhibitor [50] in the active site of thermolysin, as it was originally modeled, is shown in Figure 15. In this modeled complex, the Cbz–Phe is able to make two hydrogen bonds with Trp-115 (Cbz–Phe N–H to Trp-115 C=O 3.0 Å and Cbz–Phe C=O to Trp-115 N–H 2.6 Å (heteroatom distances)), and the Cbz–Phe side chain is buried in the bottom of the active-site cleft analogous to the proposed position of the P_2 Cbz–Phe in the tetrahedral intermediate complex for the model substrate (47). As with the model substrate, the Cbz–Phe side chain is too close to the Asp-150 side chain carboxyl group (closest heteroatom distance 2.1 Å), requiring that the Asp-150 side chain swing out of the way. The Leu–Trp region and the zinc-binding carboxyl group of the inhibitor are positioned identically to the same groups in inhibitor [49] as determined by x-ray.

The modeled inhibitor [50] was found to be a potent inhibitor of both thermolysin and ACE, as shown by the K_i's listed in Table 11. When this inhibitor design was analyzed in a series using Phe for binding in the $S_{2'}$ subsite (i.e., inhibitor [53]), it was found to be 127 times more active against

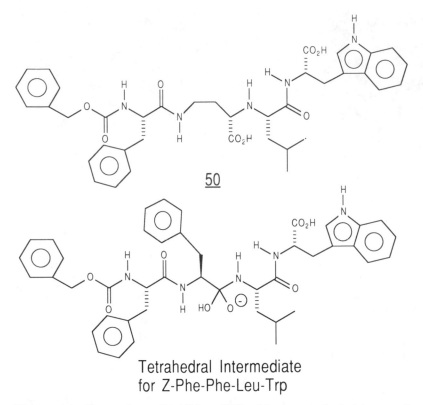

Tetrahedral Intermediate
for Z-Phe-Phe-Leu-Trp

Figure 14 Comparison of inhibitor [50] with the tetrahedral intermediate for hydrolysis of Cbz–Phe–Phe–Leu–Trp (50). Reproduced with permission.

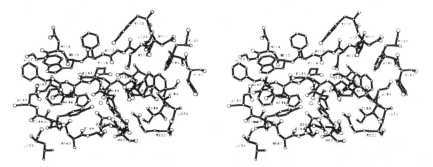

Figure 15 Stereo representation of inhibitor [50] in the active site of thermolysin as originally modeled (50). Reproduced with permission.

thermolysin than inhibitor [52], which also lacks a benzyl group for binding in the S_1 subsite. The modeled inhibitor [50], as a 1/1 mixture of diastereomers, is threefold more active against thermolysin than the most active diastereomer of inhibitor [49], which contains a benzyl group for binding in the S_1 subsite. This improvement in activity is also apparent in the series using Phe for the $S_{2'}$ subsite (i.e., [53] vs. [51]). Against ACE the modeled inhibitor [50] is perhaps slightly more active than inhibitor [49] and considerably more active than inhibitors that lack a substituent for binding in the S_1 subsite (3).

The increase in activity for inhibitor [50] against thermolysin and ACE over inhibitors that lack substituents for binding in the S_1 and S_2 subsites suggested that the modeled inhibitor might have in fact extended into the S_2 subsite as intended. Additional inhibitors of this type were then prepared which substituted Cbz–Ala and Cbz–Gly for Cbz–Phe in the inhibitor series using Phe for binding in the $S_{2'}$ subsite. The K_i's for these inhibitors were compared to the k_{cat}/K_m's and K_m's for a series of analogous substrates as shown in Table 12. No correlation was found between the K_i's and either the k_{cat}/K_m's or the K_m's.

As discussed in the chapter by Rich and Northrop earlier in this book, a correlation between transition state analog K_i's and the k_{cat}/K_m's can be expected only under certain conditions. In fact, Bartlett and Marlow have observed a good correlation for phosphonamidate thermolysin inhibitors when the amino acid fragment that binds in the $P_{2'}$ subsite was varied (57) but

Table 12   Comparison of Thermolysin Inhibition Data for Analogs of [50] to the Kinetic Data for Corresponding Thermolysin Substrates

Inhibitors		Substrates	
		(Morihara & Tsuzuki (1970)	
		Eur. J. Biochem. 15, 374)	
X—N(H)—⟨ ⟩(CO₂H)⟨ ⟩Leu—Phe		X-Gly-Leu-Ala	
X	K_i (nM)	Km (mM)	kcat/Km (sec^{-1} mM^{-1})
Z-Gly	405	12	30
Z-Ala	860	9	606
Z-Phe	220	1	491

not when the amino acid fragment that binds in the P_1 subsite was varied (58). The breakdown in the correlation when the amino acid fragment that binds in the P_1 subsite was varied appears to be due to a change in the rate-limiting step for substrate hydrolysis from the chemical transformation to the diffusion limited for substrate binding. This explanation for a poor correlation appears not to be applicable in the case of the thermolysin inhibitors designed with the aid of computer graphics (50). Consequently, it was concluded (for this and additional reasons) that the variable region of these inhibitors is probably binding differently from both the tetrahedral intermediates and the Michaelis complexes for the analogous substrates.

Alternate binding modes for inhibitor [50] in the active site of thermolysin were explored via computer graphics. The Leu–Trp and zinc-binding carboxyl group were held in the position found for the same groups in the inhibitor [49]:thermolysin complex. Working from the region of the inhibitor held constant toward the Cbz–Phe group, the three staggered conformations about the first C–C bond were generated. For each of these conformations, three staggered conformations about the second C–C bond were generated. The same process was carried out for the next C–C bond, giving a total of 27 rough starting conformations for subsequent fine adjustments and evaluation as plausible bound conformations. The number of possible conformations increases still further when the low-energy conformations for the Cbz–Phe are included. Many of the generated conformations appeared reasonable (after fine adjustments were made) as potential bound conformations based on a visual inspection of their interactions with the active site. Since the number of conformations grows rapidly as one continues this process further and as incremental dihedral angle variations within torsion wells are added, the manual search for additional bound conformations was not exhaustive. A computer-driven generation and subsequent free-energy evaluation of alternate binding modes would clearly be desirable for this kind of study but was beyond the state of the art at the time. Nevertheless, a bound conformation was proposed that involves placement of the Cbz–Phe in the S_1 region of the thermolysin active site and provides a plausible rationalization of the structure-activity data for the analogs. Coordinates for this modeled complex were sent to the laboratories of Matthews and co-workers along with a sample of the inhibitor for an x-ray analysis of the complex with thermolysin. Unfortunately, inhibitor [50] was apparently too large to penetrate the thermolysin crystals, and a crystal structure of the parent inhibitor (i.e., missing the Cbz–Phe) was obtained instead (50).

A number of additional substituents for extending into the S_1 and S_2 subsites were also designed with the aid of computer graphics and the inhibitor [49]:thermolysin crystal structure (50). These substituents were designed to take advantage of various possible binding interactions in the S_1

and S_2 subsites such as salt bridge formation and displacement of a tightly bound water molecule with an inhibitor hydroxyl group. In general the activity of these inhibitors against both thermolysin and ACE showed similar structure-activity relationships with some exceptions. When an aminomethyl group was attached to the phenyl ring of the phenethyl side chain (which binds in the S_1 subsite of both enzymes), resulting in inhibitor [54], the activity against ACE increased twofold, whereas the activity against thermolysin decreased threefold relative to the unsubstituted inhibitor [51]. This result, along with additional results on cationic side chains which bind in the S_1 subsites of both enzymes, suggested that ACE has an Asp or Glu at the edge of the S_1 subsite that can form a salt bridge with the cation, whereas thermolysin has only hydrogen-bonding residues.

The enalaprilat inhibitor design contains a carboxyl and an amino group similar to the cleavage products from a peptide substrate. It is therefore tempting to consider this inhibitor design to be a collected product design. The fact that the nitrogen atom is directly bonded to the carbon atom bearing the carboxyl group means that the amino and carboxy fragments are closer together in space than the bound cleavage products can be without interpenetrating Van der Waals radii. This resulted in the zinc-binding carboxyl group's being positioned on the zinc in closer correspondence to the tetrahedral intermediate oxygens than the cleavage product carboxyl group in the computer graphics study (47). This observation was in part responsible for the classification of the enalaprilat design as an analog of the transition state for breakdown of the tetrahedral intermediate (47).

More experimental information was desired to clarify the relationship of the enalaprilat design to the peptide cleavage mechanism. Consequently, an attempt was made to use computer graphics as an aid in designing an analog that could bind in closer analogy to the cleavage products. Inhibitor [55] (Table 11) was envisioned to contain the carboxy and amino groups found in the cleavage products and in the enalaprilat design. However, the amino and carboxy fragments are not directly bonded to each other (an ethylene bridge is used to connect the two), so the amino and carboxy fragments cannot approach each other closer than Van der Waals contact distance. Also the spacer allowed a more analogous positioning of the carboxyl group and the basic nitrogen in the active site relative to the corresponding groups in the modeled peptide cleavage products from the mechanism study. The butyl side chain was chosen for binding in the S_1 subsite, because alkyl groups of this type were shown to provide equal potency against ACE compared to the phenethyl group, and the increased flexibility of the butyl side chain would allow more possible conformations for binding in the S_1 subsite. As shown in Table 11, the activity of this inhibitor was reduced by 4 orders of magnitude against both thermolysin and ACE relative to the corresponding enalaprilat analog inhibitor [51]. This drop in activity seems too drastic to be completely due to adding two rotatable bonds to the inhibitor. Therefore this result provides some additional support for the classification of the enalaprilat design as an analog of the transition state for breakdown of the tetrahedral intermediate rather than a collected product analog.

Halgren and co-workers (52) made a preliminary attempt to calculate the rank order of the activities of the designed inhibitors against thermolysin. Molecular mechanics calculations were used to calculate and minimize the conformational energy of the inhibitors in the active site while maximizing the attractive interaction between the inhibitor and the enzyme. The initial results indicated that most of the designed inhibitors (including the enalaprilat analog with an ethylene spacer [55]) should be much more potent than inhibitor [51]. When specific waters of hydration were included in the calculations, the magnitude of the predicted improvement in activity decreased, but the rank order of the activities was still not in agreement with experiment. In these calculations the enzyme was held fixed, and entropy and extensive solvation were not considered. Since a prediction of the relative free energy of binding for the various inhibitors is required for an accurate prediction in the general case, this problem remains a formidable one for the present state of the art.

The computer graphics studies were quite useful for eliminating from consideration potential thermolysin inhibitors which have a low probability of being active. Potential inhibitors were eliminated if they would require major changes in the conformation of the protein to fit in the active site or if repulsive groups became adjacent upon docking. In addition, the process of docking various possible inhibitors in the active site of thermolysin via computer graphics was helpful for generating new inhibitor design ideas.

Overall thermolysin proved to be a reasonable qualitative model for ACE in the S_2–S_1 subsites and in the region of the active site where the zinc and catalytic side chains are located. New ACE inhibitors, most of which had good activity, resulted from the use of thermolysin as a model for ACE. A number of these inhibitors would probably not have been explored if thermolysin had not been used as a model. As one would expect, some differences were found between the thermolysin and ACE structure-activity data for the inhibitors designed in this study. These variations provide clues to the differences in the active-site structures of the two enzymes.

VIII. CONCLUSIONS

In this chapter an attempt has been made to review the role rational design has played in the development and understanding of ACE inhibitors, particularly when aided by computer studies. It appears that the first ACE inhibitors to become successful antihypertensive agents, captopril and enalapril, were designed largely from combining a conceptual and working model for ACE (derived primarily from crystal structures of related enzymes) with the more classical approach of analyzing biological data obtained with compounds derived from a lead structure. Computer graphics, theoretical calculations, and x-ray crystal structures of related enzymes were not as available or refined as they are today. If these aids had been as sophisticated and available as they are now, they might well have played a more significant role in the development of the first ACE inhibitors. This is not meant to suggest that the problem of rational design, even in a situation were a large amount of experimental data such as that provided by refined enzyme crystal structures, has now been solved. The free energy of binding an inhibitor to an enzyme is the net result of a complex interplay of solvation, entropy, and enthalpy and is therefore difficult to predict in the general case.

The computer graphics studies with thermolysin inhibitors demonstrated that the ability to dock inhibitors in the active site of an enzyme in a way that would seem to increase the number of attractive interactions does not ensure that the new inhibitor will be more active. The free energy of binding changes may not be visually obvious except in special cases such as when hydrophobic binding is increased. One may have to rely on computational estimates of binding free energy changes in the general case. Remarkable progress has recently been made in this area. Bash and co-workers (53) and Wong and McCammon (54) have successfully calculated the relative free energy of binding for a pair of inhibitors of thermolysin and trypsin, respectively, with impressive accuracy using the thermodynamic cycle-perturbation method. The scope and practicality of this method need to be evaluated, but the prospect of being able to estimate free-energy changes, even qualitatively, offers exciting possibilities for the future.

NOTE ADDED IN PROOF

A recent report has appeared [D. Mayer et al., *J. Computer-Aided Mol. Design 1*: 3–16 (1987)] presenting a more rigorous mapping of the ACE active site. Two additional reports have appeared [(H. Yanagisawa et al., *J. Med. Chem. 31*: 422–428 (1988) and H. Weller et al., *J. Enzyme Inhib. 2*: 183–193 (1988)] describing relevant conformationally restricted ACE inhibitors.

ACKNOWLEDGMENTS

I am indebted to Drs. E. Thorsett, A. Patchett, and W. Greenlee for their comments and to Professors P. A. Bartlett and B. W. Matthews for preprints of papers in press.

REFERENCES

1. Soffer, R. L., ed., *Biochemical Regulation of Blood Pressure.* John Wiley and Sons, New York, 1981.
2. Horovitz, Z. P., ed., *Angiotensin Converting Enzyme Inhibitors: Mechanisms of Action and Clinical Implications.* Urban and Schwarzenberg, Baltimore, 1981.
3. Wyvratt, M. J., and A. A. Patchett, Recent developments in the design of angiotensin-converting enzyme inhibitors. *Med. Res. Rev. 5*:483–531 (1985).
4. Patchett, A. A., and E. H. Cordes, The design and properties of N-carboxyalkylpeptide inhibitors of angiotensin converting enzyme. *Adv. Enzymol. 57*:1–84 (1985).
5. Ondetti, M. A., and D. W. Cushman, Angiotensin-converting enzyme inhibitors: Biochemical properties and biological actions. *CRC Crit. Rev. Biochem. 16*:381–411 (1984).
6. Petrillo, E. W. Jr., and M. A. Ondetti, Angiotensin-converting enzyme inhibitors: Medicinal chemistry and biological actions. *Med. Res. Rev. 2*:1–41 (1982).
7. Ondetti, M. A., and D. W. Cushman, Enzymes of the renin-angiotensin system and their inhibitors. *Annu. Rev. Biochem. 51*:283–308 (1982).
8. Cushman, D. W., and M. A. Ondetti, Inhibitors of angiotensin-converting enzyme. *Prog. Med. Chem. 17*:42–104 (1980).
9. Cushman, D. W., H. S. Cheung, E. F. Sabo, and M. A. Ondetti, Design of potent competitive inhibitors of angiotensin-converting enzyme. Carboxyalkanoyl and mercaptoalkanoyl amino acids. *Biochemistry 16*:5484–5495 (1977).
10. Byers, L. D., and R. Wolfenden, A potent reversible inhibitor of carboxypeptidase A. *J. Biol. Chem. 247*:606–608 (1972).
11. Byers, L. D., and R. Wolfenden, Binding of the by-product analog benzylsuccinic acid by carboxypeptidase A. *Biochemistry 12*:2070–2078 (1973).
12. Monzingo, A. F., and B. W. Matthews, Structure of a mercaptan-thermolysin complex illustrates mode of inhibition of zinc proteases by substrate-analogue mercaptans. *Biochemistry 21*:3390–3394 (1982).
13. Gardell, S. J., C. S. Craik, D. Hilvert, M. S. Urdea, and W. J. Rutter, Site-directed mutagenesis shows that tyrosine 248 of carboxypeptidase A does not play a crucial role in catalysis. *Nature 317*:551–555 (1985).
14. Christianson, D. W., and W. N. Lipscomb, The complex between carboxypeptidase A and a possible transition-state analogue: Mechanistic inferences from high-resolution x-ray structures of enzyme-inhibitor complexes. *J. Am. Chem. Soc. 108*:4998–5003 (1986).
15. Page, M. I., Entropy, binding energy, and enzyme catalysis. *Angew. Chem. Int. Ed. Engl. 16*:449–459 (1977).
16. Klutchko, S., M. L. Hoefle, R. D. Smith, et al., Synthesis and angiotensin-converting enzyme inhibitory activity of 3-(mercaptomethyl)-2-oxo-1-pyrrolidineacetic acids and 3-(mercaptomethyl)-2-oxo-1-piperidineacetic acids. *J. Med. Chem. 24*:104–109 (1981).
17. Condon, M. E., E. W. Petrillo Jr., D. E. Ryono, et al., Angiotensin-converting enzyme inhibitors: Importance of the amide carbonyl of mercaptoacyl amino acids for hydrogen bonding to the enzyme. *J. Med. Chem. 25*:250–258 (1982).

18. Thorsett, E. D., E. E. Harris, S. Aster, et al., Dipeptide mimics. Conformationally restricted inhibitors of angiotensin-converting enzyme. *Biochem. Biophys. Res. Commun. 111*:166–171 (1983).

19. Gund, P., J. D. Andose, J. B. Rhodes, and G. M. Smith, Three-dimensional molecular modeling and drug design. *Science 208*:1425–1431 (1980).

20. Weller, H. N., E. M. Gorden, M. B. Rom, and J. Pluscec, Design of conformationally constrained angiotensin-converting enzyme inhibitors. *Biochem. Biophys. Res. Commun. 125*:82–89 (1984).

21. Patchett, A. A., E. Harris, E. W. Tristram, et al., A new class of angiotensin-converting inhibitors. *Nature 288*:280–283 (1980).

22. Patchett, A. A., The design of enalapril. In *Hypertension and the Angiotensin System: Therapeutic Approaches*, A. E. Doyle and A. G. Bearn, eds. Raven Press, New York, pp. 155–163 (1984).

23. Thorsett, E. D., E. E. Harris, S. D. Aster, et al., Conformationally restricted inhibitors of angiotensin-converting enzyme. In *Peptides: Structure and Function, Proceedings of the Eighth American Peptide Symposium*, V. J. Hruby and D. H. Rich, eds. Pierce Chemical Co., Rockford, Ill., pp. 555–558 (1983).

24. Thorsett, E. D., E. E. Harris, S. D. Aster, et al., Conformationally restricted inhibitors of angiotensin converting enzyme: Synthesis and computations. *J. Med. Chem. 29*:251–260 (1986).

25. Still, W. C., and I. Galynker, Chemical consequences of conformation in macrocyclic compounds. *Tetrahedron 37*:3981–3996 (1981).

26. Thorsett, E. D., Conformationally restricted inhibitors of angiotensin-converting enzyme. *Actual. Chim. Ther. 13*:257–268 (1986).

27. Wyvratt, M. J., M. H. Tischler, T. J. Ikeler, et al., Bicyclic inhibitors of angiotensin converting enzyme. In *Peptides: Structure and Function, Proceedings of the Eighth American Peptide Symposium*, V. J. Hruby and D. H. Rich, eds. Pierce Chemical Co., Rockford, Ill., pp. 551–554 (1983).

28. Bull, H. G., N. A. Thornberry, M. H. J. Cordes, et al., Inhibition of rabbit lung angiotensin-converting enzyme by N-[(S)-1-carboxy-3-phenylpropyl]-L-alanyl-L-proline and N-[(S)-1-carboxy-3-phenylpropyl]-L-lysyl-L-proline. *J. Biol. Chem. 260*:2952–2962 (1985).

29. Hassall, C. H., A. Krohn, C. J. Moody, and W. A. Thomas, The design of a new group of angiotensin-converting enzyme inhibitors. *FEBS Lett. 147*:175–179 (1982).

30. Hassall, C. H., A. Krohn, C. J. Moody, and W. A. Thomas, The design and synthesis of new triazolo, pyrazolo-, and pyridazo-pyridazine derivatives as inhibitors of angiotensin-converting enzyme. *J. Chem. Soc. Perkin Trans. I*:155–164 (1984).

31. Attwood, M. R., R. J. Francis, C. H. Hassall, et al., New potent inhibitors of angiotensin-converting enzyme. *FEBS Lett. 165*:201–206 (1984).

32. Attwood, M. R., C. H. Hassall, A. Krohn, G. Lawton, and S. Redshaw, The design and synthesis of the angiotensin-converting enzyme inhibitor Cilazapril and related bicyclic compounds. *J. Chem. Soc. Perkin Trans. I*:1011–1019 (1986).

33. Gilbert, P. J., and W. A. Thomas, Nuclear magnetic resonance studies and conformations of bicyclic inhibitors of angiotensin-converting enzyme. 1.

Octahydropyridazo[1,2-a]-pyridizanediones as models for alanylproline and captopril. *J. Chem. Soc. Perkin Trans. II*:1077–1082 (1985).

34. Thomas, W. A., and I. W. A. Whitcombe, Nuclear magnetic resonance studies and conformational analysis of bicyclic inhibitors of angiotensin-converting enzyme. 2. The octahydro-6H-pyridazo[1,2-a][1,2]diazepines. *J. Chem. Soc. Perkin Trans. II*:747–755 (1986).

35. Monzingo, A. F., and B. W. Matthews, Binding of N-carboxymethyl dipeptide inhibitors to thermolysin determined by x-ray crystallography: A novel class of transition-state analogues for zinc peptidases. *Biochemistry 23*:5724–5729 (1984).

36. Andrews, P. R., J. M. Carson, A. Caselli, M. J. Spark, and R. Woods, Conformational analysis and active site modelling of angiotensin-converting enzyme inhibitors. *J. Med. Chem. 28*:393–399 (1985).

37. Tronrud, D. E., H. M. Holden, and B. W. Matthews, Structures of two thermolysin-inhibitor complexes that differ by a single hydrogen bond. *Science 235*:571–574 (1987).

38. Tronrud, D. E., A. F. Monzingo, and B. W. Matthews, Crystallographic structural analysis of phosphoramidates as inhibitors and transition-state analogs of thermolysin. *Eur. J. Biochem. 157*:261–268 (1986).

39. Gordon, E. M., S. Natarajan, J. Pluscec, et al., Ketomethyldipeptides. II. Effect of modifications of the alpha-aminoketone portion on inhibition of angiotensin-converting enzyme. *Biochem. Biophys. Res. Commun. 124*:148–155 (1984).

40. Grobelny, D., and R. Galardy, Inhibition of angiotensin-converting enzyme by aldehyde and ketone substrate analogues. *Biochemistry 25*:1072–1078 (1986).

41. Ciabatti, R., P. Giovanna, E. Bellasio, et al., Angiotensin-converting enzyme inhibitors as antihypertensive agents: 1-[(2-mercaptocycloalkyl)-carbonyl]-L-prolines. *J. Med. Chem. 29*:411–417 (1986).

42. Horrocks, W. D. Jr., and D. R. Sudnick, Lanthanide ion luminescence probes of the structure of biological macromolecules. *Acc. Chem. Res. 14*:384–392 (1981).

43. Holmes, M. A., and B. W. Matthews, Binding of hydroxamic acid inhibitors to crystalline thermolysin suggests a pentacoordinate zinc intermediate in catalysis. *Biochemistry 20*:6912–6920 (1981).

44. Holmes, M. A., D. E. Tronrud, and B. W. Matthews, Structural analysis of the inhibition of thermolysin by an active-site-directed irreversible inhibitor. *Biochemistry 22*:236–240 (1983).

45. Maycock, A. L., D. M. DeSousa, L. G. Payne, et al., Inhibition of thermolysin by N-carboxymethyl dipeptides. *Biochem. Biophys. Res. Commun. 102*:963–969 (1981).

46. Holmes, M. A., and B. W. Matthews, Structure of thermolysin refined at 1.6 Å resolution. *J. Mol. Biol. 160*:623–639 (1982).

47. Hangauer, D. G., A. F. Monzingo, and B. W. Matthews, An interactive computer graphics study of thermolysin-catalyzed peptide cleavage and inhibition by N-carboxymethyl dipeptides. *Biochemistry 23*:5730–5741 (1984).

48. Hangauer, D. G., P. Gund, J. D. Andose, et al., Modeling the mechanism of peptide cleavage by thermolysin. *Ann. N.Y. Acad. Sci. 439*:124–139 (1985).

49. Wolfenden, R., Transition state analog inhibitors and enzyme catalysis. *Annu. Rev. Biophys. Bioeng.* 5:271–306 (1976).

50. Hangauer, D. G., D. L. Ondeyka, A. A. Patchett, et al., Use of enzyme crystal structures and computer graphics for inhibitor design: Thermolysin as a model for angiotensin converting enzyme. Manuscript in preparation.

51. Greenlee, W. J., P. L. Allibone, D. S. Perlow, et al., Angiotensin-converting enzyme inhibitors: Synthesis and biological activity of acyl tripeptide analogues of enalapril. *J. Med. Chem.* 28:434–442 (1985).

52. Halgren, T. A., D. G. Hangauer, and B. L. Bush, Computational approaches to the binding of inhibitors to the active site of thermolysin. In *18th Middle Atlantic Regional Meeting of the American Chemical Society*, Newark, N.J. May 21–23 (1984).

53. Bash, P. A., U. C. Singh, F. K. Brown, et al., Calculation of the relative change in binding free energy of a protein-inhibitor complex. *Science* 235:574–575 (1987).

54. Wong, C. F., and J. A. McCammon, Dynamics and design of enzymes and inhibitors. *J. Am. Chem. Soc.* 108:3830–3832 (1986).

55. Holden, H. M., and B. W. Matthews, The binding of L-Valyl-L-tryptophan to crystalline thermolysin illustrates the mode of interaction of a product of peptide hydrolysis. *J. Biol. Chem.* 263: 3256–3260 (1988).

56. Holden, H. M., D. E. Tronrud, A. F. Monzingo, L. H. Weaver, and B. W. Matthews, Slow- and fast-binding inhibitors of thermolysin display different modes of binding: Crystallographic analysis of extended phosphonamidate transition-state analogs. *Biochemistry* 26: 8542–8553 (1987).

57. Barlett, P. A., and C. K. Marlowe, Phosphonamidates as transition-state analogue inhibitors of thermolysin. *Biochemistry* 22: 4618–4624 (1983).

58. Bartlett, P. A., and C. K. Marlowe, Possible role for water dissociation in the slow binding of phosphorous containing transition state analogue inhibitors of thermolysin. *Biochemistry* 26: 8553–8561 (1987).

8

Role of Computer-Aided Molecular Modeling in the Design of Novel Inhibitors of Renin

Giorgio Bolis* and Jonathan Greer
Abbott Laboratories, Abbott Park, Illinois

*Present affiliation: Computer Aided Molecular Design Department, Farmitalia Carlo Erba, Milan, Italy.

I. INTRODUCTION

A. Computer-Aided Approach in Modeling Proteins and Designing Drugs

In this chapter we will focus on the computer techniques of molecular modeling as they were used in our laboratory to show how information on the three-dimensional structure of molecular systems has greatly facilitated the process of designing renin inhibitors.

There are several methods by which the structure and function of biological systems are determined, and they are becoming more sophisticated in their usage in order to achieve greater precision and efficiency. X-ray crystallography is the tool that is providing the most accurate structural information about a molecule, and spectroscopic techniques are very efficacious for obtaining structural data of molecules that are not in crystallized form. Biological methods, like site-specific mutagenesis, are also becoming more widely used to characterize structure and function of proteins. Theoretical methods and the use of computers are becoming invaluable in the elucidation of molecular structures. Needless to say, close cooperation and coordination among all these methodologies will bring about the most fruitful results.

B. Renin-Angiotensin System

The renin-angiotensin system is one of the most important pathways in the body for the control of blood pressure. The clinical use of angiotensin-converting enzyme inhibitors, such as captopril (1) and enalapril (2) as antihypertensive agents shows clearly that this pathway can be successfully modulated to reduce blood pressure in a wide variety of hypertensive conditions (see Chapter 7). The enzyme renin is the first step in the pathway and appears to be highly specific in that its only known substrate is angiotensinogen. Therefore, many groups are currently trying to develop a renin inhibitor that will prove to be a useful and effective antihypertensive agent.

As long ago as 1982–83, very potent and highly specific inhibitors of renin were reported (Table 1) by several groups. Some of these were subnanomolar in their inhibition constant and thus easily potent enough to be useful. However, all these molecules were minimally modified peptides and thus suffered generically from the problem that they were all much too unstable metabolically to be useful clinical agents. Furthermore, although a new antihypertensive agent based on a different mechanism such as renin inhibition would be desirable, to be practical it was clear that such an agent needed to be orally active. None of the potent peptide inhibitors would be

Table 1 Potent Peptide Inhibitors of Renin

Source	Compound													Reference
	P_6	P_5	P_4	P_3	P_2	P_1		P'_1	P'_2	P'_3				
Burton	Pro	His	Pro	Phe	His	Phe	—	Phe	Val	Tyr				3
Szelke reduced H-142	Pro	His	Pro	Phe	His	Leu	R	Val	Ile	His	Lys			4
Szelke isostere H-261	Boc	His	Pro	Phe	His	Leu	OH	Val	Ile	His				5
Merck compound	Iva	His	Pro	Phe	His	Sta			Leu	Phe	NH$_2$			6
														7

absorbed after oral administration. Consequently, more work was needed to find a suitable renin inhibitor for clinical use. The goals that must be met by such a project are (1) high potency—i.e., in the nanomolar or subnanomolar range; (2) high specificity—the inhibitor must not inhibit any other enzymes to avoid side effects; (3) metabolic stability to give a reasonable half-life in vivo; (4) significant oral absorption; and (5) low toxicity.

The hallmark and virtue of a renin inhibitor project is the very high specificity of the renin molecule for its unique substrate. To properly understand the molecular basis of this high specificity requires knowledge of the three-dimensional structure of renin and its complex with substrate and inhibitors. Therefore, a number of groups set out early to try to produce crystals of renin for purposes of a full three-dimensional structure determination (8). Most efforts were focused on mouse submaxillary gland renin, which could be obtained in abundant quantities. Recently, an atomic resolution crystal structure was reported for human renin produced from recombinant DNA sources (44). So far, however, atomic coordinates are not available for this structure.

As an alternative, a number of groups have developed model three-dimensional structures of both mouse and human renin using comparative modeling techniques (9–13) that are based on the strong homology of the renins to the aspartic proteinase family of enzymes. In addition, the crystal structures of complexes of various inhibitors with the aspartic proteinases have elucidated the binding mode of peptide inhibitors to the active site. The ability to produce a model three-dimensional structure of renin together with the existence of very potent peptide renin inhibitors makes the renin inhibitor system an excellent candiate for the application of rational drug design methods.

C. Tools for Molecular Design

The work of designing renin inhibitors relies heavily on the enormous advances in molecular structure techniques and computer manipulation and elaboration of structural data in recent years. Nevertheless, the direct judgment and intuition of an expert medicinal chemist are still an irreplaceable tool. Detailed descriptions of the theoretical and computer techniques are given elsewhere in this book; here we would like to describe briefly the programs used in our laboratory for the molecular design work.

It is fair to say that a modeling endeavor like the one described in this chapter would be impossible without a good molecular graphics system. The molecular graphics program used in our laboratory is called Protein Display System (PDS) (see Chapter 2) and is run on an E&S MPS or PS300 and a host VAX 11/785. PDS was written at Abbott Laboratories, and, although it is costly to develop and sometimes bothersome to maintain a program in constant evolution, it has the advantage of offering the capability to implement particular features that would not otherwise be readily available in commercial products. PDS contains a number of routines that perform extremely useful operations in the process of modeling the structure of a protein from the known structures of homologous ones.

It is very important to have a flexible program that enables the manipulation of structures and the determination of the energetics of a molecular system (see Chapter 3). In our laboratory we use the molecular program DISCOVER from BIOSYM (14). We have also used its predecessor VFF developed by A. T. Hagler (15). The program is run on a FPS-164 array processor hosted by a VAX 11/785.

A good deal of the success in the process of modeling new compounds is due to the capability of organizing and analyzing the large amount of data, such as the chemical and molecular structure of all the synthesized compounds, their biological potency and metabolic stability, the computer calculations performed and their results, and so on. We found data base programs essential for these purposes; in particular, the program MACCS from MDL (16) allows storage and retrieval of molecular structures and also substructure searches. The general data base management system ORACLE (17) is used to store biological data and is interfaced by MACCS so that reports with structural and biological (or other types of) data can be generated; these reports are often used for structure-activity relationship analysis. Of critical importance was also the availability of the Brookhaven Protein Data Bank (23), which allowed us to construct the model of the renin molecule.

II. MODELING OF THE RECEPTOR AND SUBSTRATE

Several groups have used comparative modeling methods (18–21) to construct model structures for renin (9–13). Each group has performed the modeling in a somewhat different way. In particular, each group has used different members of the aspartic proteinase family as the basis for the modeling (Table 2). Nevertheless, because the aspartic proteinase structures are all quite similar, the overall renin structures produced are also very similar. However, the detailed conformations of the loops and chains in the critical active-site area can be quite different in the various models. This has important implications for the ability to design new compounds or to calculate and/or predict binding based on the modeled structures.

The comparative modeling techniques that were used to develop our model of renin have been described previously in detail (21,24,27,28). All the experimentally determined three dimensional structures for aspartic pro-

Table 2   Models of Renin Reported

Group	Structure used to build	Species built	Reference
Blundell	Endothiapepsin	Human/ mouse	9
Carlson	Rhizopuspepsin	Human	12
Akahane	Rhizopuspepsin	Human	11
Raddatz	Penicillopepsin	Human	13
Merck	Rhizopuspepsin[a]	—	22
Greer, Bolis	Pepsin, Penicillopepsin Rhizopus, Endothia	Human/ mouse	24

[a]Inhibitor modeling was performed directly on the Rhizopuspepsin structure.

teinases were assembled, including three fungal enzymes, penicillopepsin (35), rhizopuspepsin (36), and endothiapepsin (37) as well as the mammalian porcine pepsin (38). The structures were aligned onto each other in three-dimensional space so that their conserved structures were maximized. The overlapped structures show that there are structurally conserved regions (SCRs) among all the four structures and variable regions (VRs) which differ among the known structures. This is comparable to the situation found for the serine proteases (27) and anaphylatoxins (28,29). As might be expected, the three fungal enzymes are more closely related, but the mammalian pepsin structure differs somewhat from the others. Since the goal is to model human and mouse renin, which are both mammalian proteins, these relationships have considerable implications for the modeling.

When the immediate region of the active site of these aspartic proteinases is examined, the structures appear to be much more highly conserved, as expected. Pepsin still differs from the fungal enzymes; however, this may be due to the lesser degree of refinement of the pepsin structure than the other fungal proteases.

The sequences, as available, for these proteins were then compiled so that residues that occupied the same positions in the SCRs were aligned (Fig. 1). The two renin sequences were then aligned to those of the known structures. As previously described (27), the unambiguous sequence homologies that lie in the SCRs were aligned first. Then the rest of each of the SCRs were aligned without permitting any additions or deletions. The remaining portions of the sequence form the VRs. These sections were aligned to the known structure that best fit that sequence in terms of VR length and residue character. The resulting alignments appear in Figure 1.

If one examines the alignments in Figure 1, it is clear that the renin

```
PNO          1        5         10          15       20        25      30       35     PNO
PEP  A A A L I G D E P L E N Y L - - D T E Y F G T I G I G T P A Q D F T V I F D T G S  PEP
PEN  - - A A S G V A T N T P T A N - D E E Y I T P V T I G - - G T T L N L N F D T G S  PEN
RHI  - - A G V G T V P M T D Y G N - D I E Y Y G Q V T I G T P G K K F N L D F D T G S  RHI
END  - - - S T G S A T T T P I D S L D D A Y I T P V Q I G T P A Q T L N L D F D T G S  END
REN  - - - - - - - - - L T N Y L - - N S Q Y Y G E I G I G T P P Q T F K V V F D T G S  REN
HRN  L N G T T S S V I L T N Y M - - D T Q Y Y G E I G I G T D P Q T F K V V F D T G S  HRN
                      * *    *                        *  *

PNO        40          45            50          55        60         65         70    PNO
PEP  S N L W V P S V Y C S - S - L A C - S D H N Q F N P D D S S T F E A T S - Q E L S  PEP
PEN  A D L W V F S T E L P - A - S Q Q - S G H S V Y N P S - - A T G K E L S G Y T W S  PEN
RHI  S D L W V I A S T L C T - N - - - C G S G Q T K Y D P N Q S S T Y Q A D G - R T W S RHI
END  S A L W V F S S S E T T - A - S E V - D G Q T I Y T P S K S T T A K L L S G A T W S END
REN  A N L W V P S T K C S R L Y T A C - V Y H K L F D A S D S S S Y K H N G - D D F T  REN
HRN  S N V W V P S S K C S R L Y T A C - V Y H K L F D A S D S S S Y K H N G - T E L T  HRN
     *  * *        *                * *  * *  *   *   *   *            * *  *

PNO      75          80          85          90          95         100        105    PNO
PEP  I T Y G - T G S M T G I L G Y D T V Q V G G I S D T N Q I F G L S E T E P G S F L  PEP
PEN  I S Y G D G S S A S G N V F T D S V T V G G V T A H G Q A V Q A A Q Q I S A - Q F  PEN
RHI  I S Y G D G S S A S G I L A K D N V N L G G L L I K G Q T I E L A K R E A A - S F  RHI
END  I S Y G D G S S A S G I L A K D T V T V G G L T V T G Q A V E S A L K V S - S S F  END
REN  I H Y G - S G R V K G F L S Q D S V T V G G I T V T Q T F G E V T E L P L - - I P  REN
HRN  L R Y S - T G T V S G F L S Q D I I T V G G I T V T Q M F G E V T E M P A - - L P  HRN
     * *    *     *  *     * *          *  *  *           *                       *

PNO     115         120         125         130         135         140        145    PNO
PEP  Y Y - A P F D G I L G L A Y P S I S A S - - - G A T P V F D N L W D Q G L V S Q    PEP
PEN  Q Q D T N N D G L L G L A F S S I N T V Q P S Q T T F F D T V K S - S - L A Q      PEN
RHI  A S - G P N D G L L G L G F D T I T T V - - R G V K T P M D N L I S Q G L I S R    RHI
END  T E - D S T I D G L L G L A P S T L N T V S P T Q Q K T F F D N A K A - S - L D S  END
REN  F M L A Q - F D G V L G M G F P A Q A V G - - - G V T P V F D H I L S Q G V L K E  REN
HRN  F M L A E - F D G V V G M G F I E Q A I G - - - R V T P I F D N I I S Q G V L K E  HRN
     * *     *   *  *  * *  *               *        *             *    *       *

PNO  150         155         160         165         170         175        180   185 PNO
PEP  D L F S V Y L S S - N - D - D - S G S V V L L G G I D S S Y Y T G S L N W V P V S  PEP
PEN  P L F A V A L K H - - - - - Q - Q P G V Y Y D F G F I D S S K Y T G S L T Y T G V D PEN
RHI  P I F G V Y L G K - A - K N G - G G G E Y I F G G Y D S T K F K G S L T T V P I D  RHI
END  P V F T A A L G Y - H - A - - - P G T Y A F G F I D T T A Y T G S I T Y T A V S    END
REN  K V F S V Y Y N R - G - P H L - L G G E V V L G G S D P E H Y Q G D F H Y V S L S  REN
HRN  D V F S F Y Y N R D S E N S Q S L G G Q I V L G G S D P Q H Y E G N F H Y I N L I  HRN
     *   *  *  *                        * *                              *

PNO           190         195         200         205         210        215        220 PNO
PEP  V E - G Y W Q I T L D S I T M D G - E T I A C S G G C Q A I V D T G T S L L T G P  PEP
PEN  N S Q G F W S F N V D S Y T A G S - Q S G D G - - - F S G I A D T G T T L L L L D  PEN
RHI  N S R G W W G I T V D R A T V G T S T V A - - S - - F D G I A D T G T T L L Y L P  RHI
END  T K Q G F W E W T S T G Y A V G S - G T F L S - T S I D G I A D T G T T L L Y L P  END
REN  K T - D S W Q I T M K G V S V G S - S T L L C E D G C L A L V D T G A S F I S A P  REN
HRN  K T - G V W Q I Q M K G V S V G S - S T L L C E D G C L A L V D T G A S Y I S G S  HRN
         *  *                               *     *                         *

PNO  225      230         235         240         245       250         255      260  PNO
PEP  T S A I A - N I Q S D I G A - S E N S D - - G R M V I S - C S S I D S L P D I V F  PEP
PEN  D G V V S - Q Y Y S Q V S G - A Q Q D S N A G G Y V F D - C S T N - - L P D F S V  PEN
RHI  N N I A A - S V A R A Y G G A - S D N G D - - G T Y V V S - C D - - T S A F K P L V I RHI
END  A T V V S - A Y W A Q V S G - S G S K S S - - S V G G Y V F P C S A T L P S F T V  END
REN  T S S I E - L I M Q A L G A - K - K - R L F D Y V V K - C N E G P T L P D I S F    REN
HRN  T S S I E - K L M E A L G A - K - K - R L F D Y V V K - C N E G P T L P D I S F    HRN
     *  *  *                                                *

PNO  265         270         275         280         285         290         295      PNO
PEP  T I D G V Q Y P L S P S Y Y I L Q D D D - - - - S C T S G F E G M - D V P T S S G  PEP
PEN  S I S G Y T A T V P G S L I N Y G P S G - D G S T C L G G I Q S N S G I - - - -    PEN
RHI  S I N G A S F Q V S P G S L V F - E F - Q G Q - C I A G F G Y G - N W - - - -      RHI
END  G V G S A R I V I P G D Y I D - Q Y P I S T S S S C F G G I Q S - A G I - - - -    END
REN  N L G G R A Y T L S S T D Y V L Q Y P N R R D K L C T V A L H A M - D I P P P T G  REN
HRN  H L G G K E Y T L T S A D Y I F Q E S Y S S K K L C T L A I H A M - D I P P P T G  HRN
                                             *  *              *  *  *  *  *  *  *  *  *

PNO  300         305         310         315         320         325                   PNO
PEP  E L W I L G D V F I R Q Y Y T V F D R A - N N K V G L A P V A                      PEP
PEN  G F S I F G D I F L K S Q Y V V F D S D - G P Q L G F A P Q A                      PEN
RHI  G F A I I G D T F L K N N Y V V F N Q G - V P E V Q I A P V A E                    RHI
END  G I N I F G D V A L K A A F V V F N G A T T P T L G F A S L                        END
REN  P V W V L G A T F I R K F Y T E F D R H - N N R V G F A L A R                      REN
HRN  P T W A L G A T F I R K F Y T E F D R R - N N R I G F A L A R                      HRN
     *              *  *  *  *  *  *  *  *   *  *  *  *  *  *
```

Figure 1 Sequence alignment of the aspartic proteinases. Boxes enclose the SCRs. The sequence numbering is that of porcine pepsin. The sequences are labeled as follows: PEN — penicillopepsin, RHI = rhizopuspepsin, END = endothiapepsin, PEP = porcine pepsin, REN = mouse submaxillary gland renin, and HRN = human renin. The asterisks mark the residues that were included in the active-site region for the energy calculations.

sequences are much closer to porcine pepsin than they are to any of the fungal enzymes in terms of sequence homology as well as similarity of VRs. For the VRs around residues 196–210 and 286–300, as well as for the long region from 252 through 283 where the pepsin structure differs from the fungal enzymes, sequence length and homology, show a closer relationship of the renins to pepsin than to the fungal proteases. Most importantly, two loops in the immediate active site region—the so-called "flap" which includes residues 70–80, and residues 295–300—are very similar in pepsin and the renins but quite different in the fungal enzymes. In the latter case, the occurrence of a relatively unique Pro–Pro–Pro sequence in both human and mouse renins indicates that while the pepsin conformation of this loop was a more useful guide than the fungal enzymes, it had to be modified to accommodate the renin sequence. For this purpose, all the known structures in the Brookhaven Data Bank were examined for similar Pro–Pro–Pro sequences, which were then used to guide the modeling of this loop. The above considerations suggest that the pepsin structure should be weighted more heavily in the modeling process. However, since the pepsin structure has not been as fully refined as the other aspartic proteinase structures, it was not used exclusively.

Using this sequence alignment for the renins, the three-dimensional model can be constructed. In general, the main-chain coordinates for the SCRs were taken from the pepsin structure with the exception of the immediate active-site area, which was taken from the better-refined penicillopepsin structure. This consisted of the stretch from residues 30 through 38 and 210 through 222 including the two active-site aspartates, 32 and 215. The VRs were chosen from among the known structures so that the best-fitting structure for the respective renin sequence was obtained (Fig. 1).

Having produced a tentative model for the renin enzyme, the next step was to model the interaction between the substrate and the enzyme. For this task we made use of two experimental crystal structures that were available: a complex of pepstatin with the rhizopus enzyme (36), and a pepstatin fragment on the penicillopepsin molecule (39,40). The sequence of pepstatin is Iva–Val–Val–Sta–Ala–Sta, but the sequence of the fragment of the substrate of renin which we want to model into the active site is Phe–His–Leu–Val–Ile–His, where the scissile bond is found between the Leu and Val residues. The crystal structures clearly indicate the interactions between the portion of the inhibitor N-terminal to the scissile bond, Phe–His–Leu (P$_3$–P$_1$), and the enzyme; thus the main-chain coordinates for this part of the inhibitor were used directly, and the angiotensinogen sequence "mutated" onto this main chain. However, the unusual main chain of the statine residue did not allow the conformation of the C-terminal portion of the inhibitor, Val–Ile–His (P$_1'$–P$_3'$) to be modeled directly. This portion was modeled by exploring all possible conformations for the Val–Ile–His on the enzyme surface that were

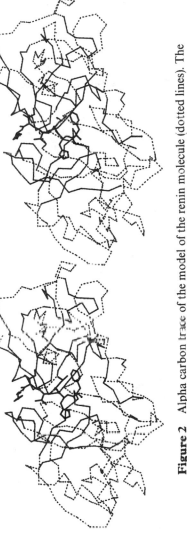
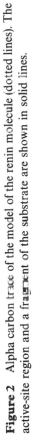

Figure 2 Alpha carbon trace of the model of the renin molecule (dotted lines). The active-site region and a fragment of the substrate are shown in solid lines.

similar to the binding conformation of the pepstatin molecule. One unique conformation was found for the Val P_1' and Ile P_2' positions (Fig. 2). However, for His P_3', several possible conformations were accessible.

The model renin structure with the substrate bound was modified by hand to remove bad inter-side-chain contacts by rotating about the respective side chain χ angles. Because of limited computer resources and the increased approximation of the model away from the active site, initial energy refinement was performed on the active-site region of the model structure. The active site region was defined as all residues that lay within 7 Å of any atom of the hexapeptide parent compound. Additional residues were added to complete a disulfide bridge around residues 45 and 52. The resulting active site contained nine fragments of the renin molecule; the residues included are noted in Figure 1 and depicted in Figure 2. The N- and C-terminal residues of each fragment, which lay outside the volume, were kept close to their original position by using a harmonic term added to the potential function during the minimization in order to avoid any significant departures from the model, because the rest of the protein was not included. Because of the close proximity of Asp 32 and Asp 215 and current proposals for the aspartic proteinase mechanism of action (37,40,41), Asp 215 was protonated for the energy calculations. The total structure, including the inhibitor, contained 1650 atoms.

The minimization process was performed in two steps. In the first step, consisting of 200–300 cycles, every atom of the system was constrained with a forcing potential to remain in close proximity to the starting structure. This technique allows relaxation of close contacts without introducing drastic distortions into the structure. In the second step, the system was allowed to relax (forcing only the terminal residues to their original position). A typical minimization required 2500–3000 iterations to bring the system to a stable minimization defined by the maximum derivative of the potential function being <0.01. This required about 30 hr computing time on a FPS-164 array processor. The resulting structure was used for model building.

III. WORKING WITH THE RECEPTOR–INHIBITOR MODEL

As mentioned in the Introduction, there are a number of requirements necessary to obtain a useful drug—high potency, specificity, metabolic stability, bioavailability, and low toxicity. The assembling of all these conditions in a single molecule is definitely not a simple task; oftentimes we find ourselves in the frustrating situation of having a potent compound that is rapidly degraded, or, in the feverish pursuit of increased transport properties, we lose potency. It is therefore necessary to continuously modify the structure of the molecule until an optimum compromise among all the requirements is achieved. Whenever any of the above requirements can be addressed using knowledge of the structure, we find that use of the model of the receptor-inhibitor can contribute to facilitate this process of optimization.

Computerized molecular modeling is a relatively recent phenomenon. The techniques associated with it can be very powerful and efficient, but they have to be used appropriately, and the results must be evaluated with care. This implies that we must always be aware of the approximations and limitations of the model and also remember that the experimental data used to construct the model have a certain degree of reliability. It is therefore very important to approach the model just described with the proper attitude in order to obtain the best results.

The most important point to keep in mind is that the model represents the present status of our understanding, our current working hypothesis. It is therefore subject to modifications as we gather more information about the system. These data may come from experiments like x-ray crystallography (see Chapter 4) or NMR (see Chapter 5), or from calculations or molecular simulations (see Chapters 2 and 3). The flexibility of the tools at our disposal allows us to explore many modifications of the structure and, to a good extent, visualize the consequences of these modifications.

In this way, the computer model can be approached as a very creative environment which serves a multiple purpose: it is a way of devising design strategies, a stimulus for new ideas, a field in which to test different hypotheses in the process of predicting new inhibitors, and a means for understanding or rationalizing experimental data.

As a first step, it is very useful to take a global view of the model just built. The first thing we observe in our model (Fig. 2) is the way in which the substrate fits into the active site: we notice that the main chain of the peptide is lying in a near extended fashion with the P_3, P_1, P_2' side chains on one side of the backbone and the P_2, P_1', P_3' side chains on the other side. This observation already gives us an indication of a general strategy of how to develop new inhibitors. First we choose an appropriate substitute for the scissile bond: either a reduced bond (5) or a hydroxy isostere (6). Then we can modify the segment P_3-P_1 of the peptide almost independently of the second segment $P_1'-P_3'$ and expect the effects to be almost additive (Fig. 3).

We can take into account the detailed interactions that occur between the inhibitor and the enzyme (Fig. 4). For example, there are a number of hydrogen bonds between the enzyme and the P_1-P_3 segment of the inhibitor. On the other hand, the $P_1'-P_3'$ part seems to be less tightly bound by hydrogen bonds; this immediately suggests that it will be more difficult to make substitutions in the main chain of the first part of the peptide because of the necessity of maintaining the specific binding functions, while the second

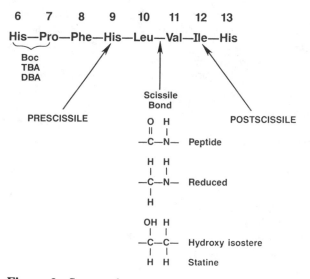

Figure 3 Strategy for modeling renin inhibitors.

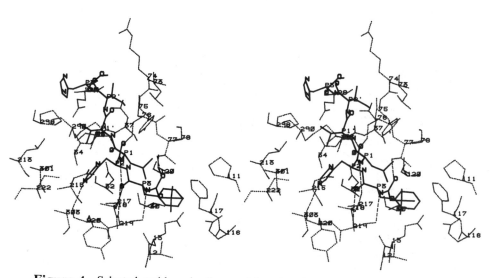

Figure 4 Selected residues in the model active site of renin (dotted lines). The fragment of the natural substrate with blocking groups at both ends of the peptide is shown in solid lines. Hydrogen bonds between the substrate and the enzyme appear as dashed lines.

part will lend itself to more extensive modifications. Other types of important interactions are the electrostatic and hydrophobic interactions, the latter being characterized by the fact that the parts of the interacting molecules that are hydrophobic in character tend to associate owing to the attractive dispersion forces.

The model of the complex (Fig. 4) can be a powerful tool when we want to design cyclic compounds or conformationally restricted analogs. Thus, it would be unlikely that we would consider a cyclization of the inhibitor from the N terminus of P_3 to the C terminus of P'_3, because that would distort the linearity of the inhibitor. Groups that are close in space can be chosen and connected by a bridge that is carefully selected to avoid perturbing or colliding with the surrounding enzyme. Examples of this approach will be given later.

With the aid of a molecular mechanics program we could also determine the relative flexibility of different parts of the active site. This type of information is relevant when we want to make modifications to a compound so that it will become bulkier or smaller: If the modified part of the inhibitor is interacting with a flexible section of the enzyme, some residues of the enzyme will probably move and accommodate the new molecule. On the other hand, if the inhibitor interacts with a rigid section, it will form steric hindrances or unfavorable interactions.

It is often useful to model compounds that have already been synthesized into the enzyme whether they are good or bad inhibitors. This process allows better understanding of the interactions of the complex and could eventually provide information about the enzyme itself. The visualization of a particular compound in the active site superimposed upon, for example, the parent compound of that series, permits us to characterize the weak or strong points of this new molecule and hence to improve its design.

A number of laboratories have already successfully used computer-modeling techniques to model inhibitors of aspartic proteinases (11,13,22). In the following section we will illustrate with examples from the work in our laboratory, and we will discuss the use of the model of the renin-inhibitor complex in designing novel inhibitors, rationalizing experimental data, and understanding the interaction of compounds with the enzyme.

IV. APPLICATIONS AND EXAMPLES

A. Improved Inhibitory Potency

The first task in developing a renin inhibitor is, of course, to obtain a compound that would bind to the enzyme strongly and with good specificity. The logical procedure is to start with the fragment of the natural substrate described in the previous section and make modifications to it so as to make it an inhibitor and then improve its binding and/or specificity. At this point we have to note that our capability in predicting quantitative binding energy for such a large molecular system as the renin-inhibitor complex is limited. Part of the reason is that the methodologies for determining the entropic contribution to the binding energy are still in the developmental stage, although some successes have been achieved on some molecular systems (30, 34). With the tools at our disposal we can often predict when a compound is not active, or we can point to new directions while maintaining good potency, and this is indeed of great value in terms of saving time and resources at the experimental stage.

Our model substrate was easily turned into an inhibitor by reducing the carbonyl function between the Leu and the Val residues (5). This compound, when synthesized, showed an IC_{50} of 300 nM and was considered the parent compound for the subsequent modeling work. By making modifications to this basic inhibitor, we can work toward improving its binding and its stability against metabolic degradation, or we can change its chemicophysical properties as needed. The changes are basically aimed at improving the hydrogen bonding and the electrostatic and hydrophobic interactions between the inhibitor and the enzyme. The first example, showing improvement of binding through hydrogen bonding, is taken from the literature. Based on the transition state analog inhibitor hypothesis and the utility of statine-based inhibitors in the aspartic proteinases, Szelke et al. (6) proposed the replacement of the peptide bond of the substrate with a hydroxy isostere which enhanced the binding of the corresponding inhibitor in the reduced form by over an order of magnitude. The presence of a hydroxyl group between residues P_1 and P_1' enhances binding by hydrogen bonding with the two aspartates, 32 and 215, of the enzyme. Figure 5 shows how the binding would take place in our model active site with a typical fragment of residues P_1 and P_1': Asp 215, which is protonated, is hydrogen bonding with the lone pair of the oxygen in the hydroxyl group whose hydrogen in turn forms a hydrogen bond with the charged aspartate group of Asp 32. The hydroxyl group is so optimally positioned in the active site that this functional group has been used in many of our series of compounds.

Wherever specific hydrogen bonding or polar sites are not available in the active site, improvement in the binding can be achieved by optimizing the hydrophobic interaction between the inhibitor and the enzyme. One such instance of a hydrophobic environment is found in the S_1 subsite of the active site of renin. A major gain in potency was obtained by the Merck group by modifying the side chain at position P_1 in their series of octapeptide renin inhibitors (42). As mentioned before, the group at Merck Sharp & Dohme used the structure of rhizopuspepsin for their modeling studies (Table 2). Having observed a large hydrophobic pocket in the proximity of the P_1 site

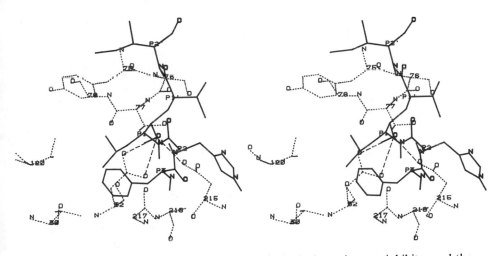

Figure 5 Detail of the interactions between the hydroxy-isostere inhibitor and the active site of renin near aspartates 32 and 215. One of the oxygens of the side chain of Asp 215 is protonated (labeling scheme as in Fig. 4).

and inferring a similar situation at the corresponding position of human renin, an attempt was made to better fill that pocket by replacing the leucyl side chain with a cyclohexylalanyl group. This modification brought an improvement in renin inhibition of about 70-fold compared to the corresponding compound with the leucyl side chain. Ironically, the same substitution on their original model structure, rhizopuspepsin, caused little improvement (42).

In the subsection on optimization of a binding site, further examples will be given describing the effects of modifying the side chain at position P_1 in two series of compounds.

B. Increased Metabolic Stability

It is well known that a peptide is easily subject to metabolic degradation by a host of hydrolase enzymes: in particular, when considering our hexapeptide parent compound, it was noted that the Phe–His peptide bond is subject to hydrolysis by the enzyme chymotrypsin (24). In addressing this problem, we will show in the following example the process of devising protection from proteolytic degradation and the methods used to elucidate biological data associated with the compounds thus synthesized.

There are basically three ways to stabilize a compound from the action of peptidase enzymes: (1) Change the character of the peptide bond. This method is useful in cases in which the functional groups of the peptide bond are not involved in hydrogen bond interactions. (2) Changing the amino acid recognized by the cleaving enzyme, an amino acid replacement, or even a change from L to D form, could be sufficient to avoid cleavage, but, again, the replacement could be detrimental if the amino acid in question is important for binding or specificity to renin. (3) Protect the peptide bond. This method requires structural modification of the peptide so that access to the peptide bond by the cleaving agent is inhibited.

To choose a method of stabilizing the peptide bond, we turned our attention to the model and observed that the carbonyl function of Phe P_3 is involved in a hydrogen bond with NH of Ser 219 of the enzyme. We also knew that a replacement of the Phe side chain diminished the potency and specificity of the parent inhibitor. We concluded, then, that modifications of the Phe residue would be too detrimental to binding, while a possibility remained to operate on the NH of His P_2 in order to bring about a good protection of the Phe–His peptide bond.

As we can see in Figure 4, the side chain of residue P_1 lies in reasonable proximity of the main-chain NH of residue P_2 to permit these two groups to be bridged. This structure would restrict the conformation of the inhibitor and at the same time protect the peptide bond between P_3 and P_2. We then modeled onto the active site a series of these compounds with different macrocycle size and minimized the structure of the complexes. Analyzing the latter, we noticed that all the important interactions remained intact except a possible hydrogen bond between the NH of His P_2 to the flap and some minor changes of conformation that occur in the flap to accommodate part of the methylene bridge. On the practical side, His P_2 was replaced by an Ala residue to simplify the chemical synthetic work. To verify that potency was not badly diminished by the elimination of the NH functional group at position P_2, an N-methyl Ala version of the parent compound was prepared and found to be equally active (Table 3). The cyclic compounds (see scheme I) were then synthesized, and the results are reported in Table 3. The potency of the 14-member ring compound was half that of the N-methylated and parent versions of the parent compound; but the 10-member ring compound

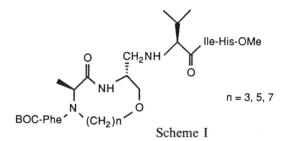

Scheme I

Table 3 Properties of the Cyclic Renin Inhibitors

Compound	IC$_{50}$ (μM)[a]			NMR conf.		Chymotrypsin Cleavage t$_{\frac{1}{2}}$ (min)
	Human renin	Porcine pepsin	Cathepsin D	% trans	% cis	
Boc-Phe-His-Leu^{R}Val-Ile-His-OMe	0.25	>10(10)	>10(6)	—	—	—
Boc-Phe-Ala-Leu^{R}Val-Ile-His-OMe	1.4	>10(0)	>10(0)	100	0	10-15
Boc-Phe$_T$Ala-Leu^{R}Val-Ile-His-OMe $\rvert$ CH$_3$	1.2	>10(0)	>10(24)	100	0	—
Boc-Phe$_T$Ala-Ser^{R}Val-Ile-His-OMe $\rvert\_$(CH$_2$)$_3$	>100(23)	>10(0)	>10(0)	0	100	—
Boc-Phe-Ala-Ser^{R}Val-Ile-His-OMe $\rvert\_$(CH$_2$)$_5$	69	>10(0)	>10(0)	20	80	—
Boc-Phe$_C$Ala-Ser^{R}Val-Ile-His-OMe $\rvert\_$(CH$_2$)$_7$	2.7	>10(0)	>10(0)	50	50	Not cleaved

[a]Numbers in parentheses are the percent inhibition at 10^{-5}M. These are reported when the inhibition was too weak to calculate an IC$_{50}$ value.

313

was completely inactive. The 14-membered ring compound was shown to be stable to cleavage by chymotrypsin. All the cyclic inhibitors maintained high specificity for renin.

The fact that the 12- and 14-member ring compounds displayed significant inhibition after such a drastic modification to the parent compound reinforced our confidence in the validity of the renin-inhibitor model. Nevertheless, we were puzzled as to why the 10-member ring compound was inactive, since from modeling it also seemed to fit into the renin model active site satisfactorily. Consequently, we decided to analyze the structural properties of the cyclic inhibitors in solution. A detailed structural analysis by NMR of the cyclic compounds was performed (24,26) including two-dimensional NOE experiments for the 10-member ring compound which yielded a number of interproton distances that allowed us, by means of constrained molecular dynamics calculations, to determine the exact pucker of the macrocycle and the conformation of the Phe–Ala segment of the inhibitor. It was found that in these cyclic compounds the Phe–Ala peptide bond exists as cis and trans isomers in various percentages (Table 3). We tried, then, to place into our model structure of the active site the cis isomers of the cyclic inhibitors. We found that major collisions occurred between the Boc and Phe

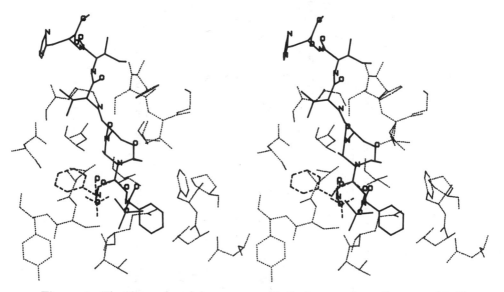

Figure 6   The 10-membered ring compound in the trans conformation as modeled in the active site of renin (——). The Boc–Phe segment of the inhibitor in the cis conformation is shown (-------)with bad steric hindrances with residues 218–219 of renin.

P_3 of the inhibitor and residues 217 219 of renin (Fig. 6). It was therefore clear that only the trans form can bind to the enzyme. This discovery of an inactive cis form of the inhibitors allows the complete rationalization of the inhibition of human renin by the cyclic compounds. The 10-membered ring is inactive because it is entirely cis. The 12-membered ring shows a little activity, since it is partially in the trans form. Very significant activity is found in the 14-membered ring, since it is 50% in the trans form. When corrected for being only 50% in the active form, the 14-membered ring is just as active as the unsubstituted parent molecule.

C. Bioavailability

When modifying compounds to obtain higher potency, effort should also be invested in reducing its size as much as possible. In fact, in analyzing the problem of gastrointestinal transport and absorption from the structural perspective, we realize that the molecular size and shape of a peptidic substance are important physical properties that affect the above phenomena. For example, passive diffusion, a pathway by which many drug substances are absorbed from the intestinal tract, is directly related to molecular weight (43). We may conclude, therefore, that size reduction represents an important strategy in peptide and peptidomimetic drug discovery.

Analyzing, once again, the model of the renin active site with the hexapeptide parent compound (Fig. 4) and with the perspective of decreasing its size, it appears that shortening the chain length of the inhibitor has sharply different effects whether residues are removed from the N terminus or the C terminus. There is a network of hydrogen bonds between the main chain of the N-terminal half of the reduced inhibitor and the enzyme, but none seem to be present in the other half. The carbonyl function of Phe P_3 and the NH of His P_2 are hydrogen bonding with the NH of Ser 219 and the carbonyl of Gly 217, respectively. This configuration of antiparallel pleated sheet appears in all reported instances of aspartic proteinases–inhibitor structures (36,39,40) and is important for proper alignment of the substrate (or the inhibitor) into the crevice of the active site. We should expect, therefore, a great loss of binding by removing the residues at positions P_3 and P_2. The binding of the C terminal half of the inhibitor to the enzyme seems to be dominated by less specific hydrophobic forces, suggesting that this segment is more amenable to reduction in size or to modification than the first half of the inhibitor.

A number of compounds were synthesized to verify this hypothesis, and the results are reported in Table 4. As can be seen from this table, the compounds with no P_2 or P_3 residues are inactive, but compounds in which residues were deleted from the C terminus showed only small loss of activity.

Table 4 Reduced Size Renin Inhibitors

No.				Structure						$IC_{50}(nM)$
	P_3	P_2	P_1		P'_1	P'_2	P'_3			
1	Boc	His	Leu	R	Val	Ile	His	OMe		300
2	Boc	His	Leu	R	Val	Ile	His	OMe		No inhibition
3	Boc	—	Leu	R	Val	Ile	His	OMe		No inhibition
4	Boc	His	Leu	R	Val	Ile	—	OMe		2300
5	Boc	His	Leu	R	Val	$NHCH_2Ph$	$NHCH_2Ph$			370
6	Boc	His	Cal[a]	R	Val	$NHCH_2Ph$	$NHCH_2Ph$			34

[a]Cal = cyclohexylalanine.

This loss could be regained by replacing the eliminated residues with an appropriate smaller hydrophobic group that can add a significant amount of dispersion energy (32).

Further reduction in size without losing or actually increasing potency was obtained in a series of compounds in which a hydroxyl group was used between residues P_1 and P'_1, as discussed at the beginning of this section. Analyzing an energy-minimized structure of the hexapeptide in which a hydroxyl group has been inserted between residues P_1 and P'_1, we observe that, in addition to the interactions of the hydroxyl moiety with the two aspartates already described, the side chain of residue Val P'_1 lies in the vicinity of Leu 213, Asp 215, and Pro 298, and Ile P'_2 is in a pocket lined by residues Tyr 75, Leu 73, Gln 128, and Asn 37. Also notable is the close proximity of the Val P'_1 carbonyl oxygen to the α-NH of Ser 76, suggesting the possible formation of a hydrogen bond at this position. Therefore, as a replacement of the Leu–Val–Ile–His segment of the hexapeptide parent inhibitor, the hydroxy ketone, scheme II, was designed in order to shorten the C-terminal portion of the inhibitor while maintaining the maximum number of possible interactions between the inhibitor and the enzyme.

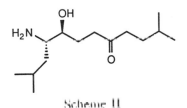

Scheme II

When modeled into the active site appended to a Boc-Phe-Ala group (see Table 5, compound 1, and Fig. 7), we notice that the hydroxy ketone fragment superimposes nicely upon the backbone of Val P'_1 and Ile P'_2, with the isopentyl group fitting into the pocket at position P'_2. In this conformation, the pocket for the side chain of position P'_1 would remain empty. The ketone function is found to be hydrogen bonding with the α-NH of Ser 76. From Table 5 we also notice that a replacement of the ketone with a sulfone moiety yielded a compound with similar activity. Modifications on the C-terminus did not bring large variations in activity, but further improvement was obtained by replacement of the P_1 and P_2 side chains (31).

One last example of a short and yet very potent compound is given in Figure 8. This compound, whose structure is shown in scheme III, with an IC_{50} of 0.4 nM, maintains the strong hydrogen bonds of the Phe P_3 carbonyl with the NH of Ser 219 and the NH of cyclohexyl alanyl P_1 residue with the carbonyl of Gly 217. In addition, the diols at position P'_1 hydrogen bond with

Table 5 Dipeptide Renin Inhibitions with a Hydroxy Ketone

No	A	B	R1	X	R2	$IC_{50}(\mu M)$
1	Boc Phe	Ala	Isobutyl	CO	$i\text{-}C_5H_{11}$	2.4
2	Boc Phe	Ala	Isobutyl	SO_2	$i\text{-}C_5H_{11}$	2.4
3	Boc Phe	Ala	Isobutyl	SO_2	$i\text{-}CH_2CH_2Ph$	1.8
4	Boc Phe	Ala	Cyclohexylmethyl	SO_2	$i\text{-}C_3H_7$	0.076
5	Boc Phe	His	Cyclohexylmethyl	SO_2	$i\text{-}C_3H_7$	0.0076

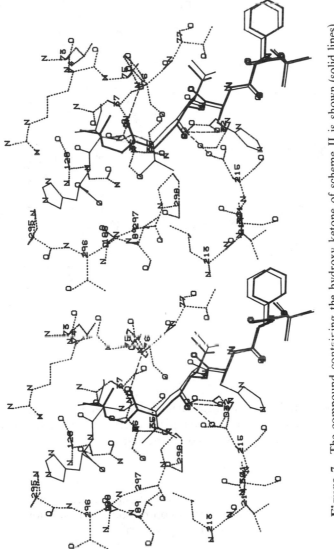

Figure 7 The compound containing the hydroxy ketone of scheme II is shown (solid lines) superimposed on the parent compound (dotted lines).

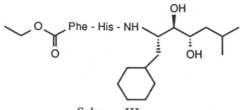

Scheme III

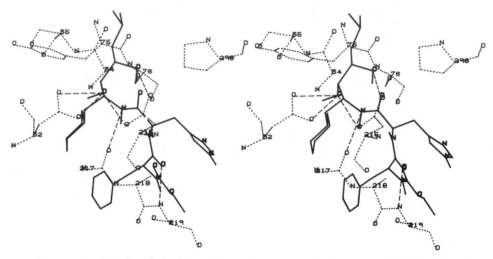

Figure 8 Details of the interactions of a very potent compound with selected residues of the renin molecule.

the two aspartates Asp 32 and 215. The first hydroxyl group binds to Asp 32 in a similar fashion as in the hydroxyl isostere shown in Figure 5, and the second one appears to bind strongly to the Asp 215 (33).

D. Optimization of a Binding Site

The following example illustrates the effect of systematically varying the side chain at P_1 in two different series of compounds (25) and how, with our model, we could rationalize the biological data.

From Figure 9 (see Plate III, after p. 16) we can see that the P_1 residue is found in a hydrophobic pocket formed by residues Val 30, Phe 117, Val 120, and Tyr 75. In the same pocket is also found the side chain of Phe P_3. The series of compounds for this example are illustrated in scheme IV, in which the variable R group is reported in the first columns of Table 6.

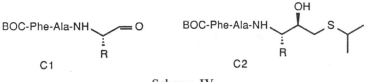

Scheme IV

Table 6 Side Chain Substitutions at the P_1 site

| | IC_{50}, nM or (Inhib. at 10^{-5}M) | |
R	C1	C2
(a) Isobutyl[a]	20,000	700
(b) (Cyclohexyl)methyl[a]	460	9
(c) Cyclohexyl[a]	1,000	1,500
(d) (Cyclohexyl)ethyl[a]	55,000	(45%)
(e) (Dicyclohexyl)methyl	40,000	—
(f) (Adamantyl)methyl	35,000	—
(g) Benzhydryl	—	(11%)
(h) (2,4,6-Trimethyl)benzyl	—	(5%)
(i) Benzyl	—	170

[a]Compounds for which energy calculations were performed.

Using the structure of the renin-inhibitor complex as a guide, we modeled the compounds listed in Table 6 by superimposing the main chain of residues Phe and Ala onto the main chain of the Phe P_3 and His P_2 residues of the parent compound. The compounds in series C1 were modeled in the form of hydrated aldehydes. For eight of the complexes thus obtained, energy calculations were performed, both energy minimizations and molecular dynamics simulations, in order to better understand the interactions of these inhibitors with renin. The compounds selected for analysis were the ones having as R: (a) isobutyl, (b) (cyclohexyl)methyl, (c) cyclohexyl, and (d) (cyclohexyl)ethyl (see Table 6).

The common features of all the structures after being subjected to energy calculations were as follows. The hydrogen bond between the carbonyl of Phe P_3 and the NH of Ser 219 was retained, and the side chains of residues P_1 (the variable R) and P_3 remained close to one another in the same hydrophobic pocket. The largest changes in the active site occurred in the regions near the C terminus of the inhibitors including loop 290–300 and the segment of residues 72–80. Other parts of the enzyme moved to a lesser degree.

Comparing the complexes containing compounds within each series, we observed that the backbone at position P_1 in compounds with R = cyclohexyl, (cyclohexyl)methyl, and (cyclohexyl)ethyl retained a similar position relative to the active site, whereas the compounds with R = isobutyl showed a displacement that caused a readjustment of the active site mainly in the loop 290–300. A reason for such a displacement is that the isobutyl group, the smallest of the side chains, moves deeper into the large hydrophobic pocket to fill it more completely. The difference between the two series is found in the degree of displacement. Taking the compound with R = (cyclohexyl)methyl as reference, we found that in series C1 and Cα connected to the isobutyl group is 0.7 Å away from the Cα of the reference, whereas the Cα's of the compounds with R = cyclohexyl and (cyclohexyl)ethyl are found at a distance less than 0.3 Å to the Cα of the reference. In series C2, on the other hand, the corresponding distances are 0.9 Å and 0.5 Å; the changes in structure are therefore more pronounced in series C2. The extent to which the enzyme can accommodate different inhibitors is shown in Figure 10 (see Plate III, after p. 16), where the Cα trace of the active site residues is displayed when bound to inhibitors with a small (R = isobutyl) and a large (R = (cyclohexyl)ethyl) P_1 side chain. The root mean square (r.m.s.) difference of the enzyme structures containing the two compounds is 0.9 Å; the largest deviation from one structure to the other is 2.3 Å at residue Pro 294.

When we compare compounds with the same R group from two different series, C1 and C2, we observed that the largest changes in the enzyme structure also occur in the loop segment of residues 290–300 and in residues 74–79. This appears to be primarily due to the difference in the size of the C-terminal group in the two series. A significant difference in the contact surfaces (which can be taken as approximately representing the dispersion energy) between the inhibitors and the enzyme can be observed in Figure 11 (see Plate IV, after p. 16) where the R group is (cyclohexyl)methyl and the C terminus of the inhibitors of the two different series C1 and C2 are displayed with their van der Waals surfaces in contact with the surface of the neighboring residues of the active site. It is apparent that the extended C terminus of series C2 compounds restricts the mobility of the inhibitor in the active site and improves binding relative to series C1.

Using the above modeled and energy-determined structures we can explain qualitatively the very different potencies reported in Table 6 for the different R substituents at position P_1. Compounds with (cyclohexyl)methyl are seen to fill the hydrophobic pocket optimally, maximizing the dispersion energy. Compounds with R = benzyl were analyzed by model-building techniques, and it was observed that the benzyl structure was very similar to and was occupying the same space as the (cyclohexyl)methyl, but the complementarity of the phenyl ring to the hydrophobic pocket was not as adequate as the cyclohexyl ring. The smaller isobutyl side chain, despite conformational changes, still does not fill the pocket and therefore binds more weakly. Cyclohexyl, by virtue of the ring's being situated closer to the main chain, not only fails to fill the pocket but also imposes quite different conformational changes in the P_1 binding pocket. Both of these effects can be expected to diminish binding. Larger side chains containing (cyclohexyl)ethyl fit the hydrophobic pocket with difficulty. In series C1, the ring of this side chain is accommodated by displacing the phenyl ring of Phe P_3, which is lying in the same pocket; in series C2, the ring has bad steric interactions with residues Tyr 75, Gly 78, and Phe 117 of the active site. Complexes with inhibitors having larger P_1 side chains, such as (e), (f), (g), (h) (Table 6; Fig. 12 [see Plate IV, after p. 16]), showed such large overlaps and bad steric interactions when modeled that molecular mechanics calculations were not feasible. The generally better binding showed by compounds of series C2 compared to series C1 can be accounted for by the presence of the longer C-terminal group in series C2 which provides these compounds with more dispersion energy interaction with the enzyme.

V. CONCLUSIONS

Since the renin inhibitor project started at Abbott Laboratories, much has been learned about designing renin inhibitors. The modeling of the renin enzyme provided the framework for designing inhibitors and for studying the interactions of the enzyme with different compounds. The increased understanding of the mode of interaction between the enzyme and the inhibitors, as derived from experimental results, modeling work, and cal culations, stimulated more ideas for designing new inhibitors. Drastic departures from the basic substrate structure have been attempted, and the ability to suggest new directions has been proved in several instances.

At the same time, methodologies for modeling and energy calculations have been refined and improved. Much work is still ongoing in attempting to quantitate the energetics of molecular systems for a better determination of enthalpic and entropic energies Also, more sophisticated molecular graphic programs are becoming available, making some of the modeling tasks easier to perform.

The most important result derived from this work is that a close collaboration among crystallographers, NMR spectroscopists, biologists, and synthetic and theoretical chemists brought about a comprehensive picture of the renin-inhibitor complex, making the tasks of designing new compounds and interpreting experimental data more efficient. There is, of course, much room for improvement in all areas of expertise, but we feel that the key to success lies in the further evolution of this interdisciplinary collaboration.

REFERENCES

1. Cushman, D. W., and M. A. Ondetti, Inhibitors of angiotensin-converting enzyme. *Prog. Med. Chem. 17*:41–104 (1980).
2. Patchett, A. A., E. Harris, E. W. Tristram, M. J. Wyvratt, M. T. Wu, D. Taub, E. R. Peterson, T. J. Ikeler, J. ten Broeke, L. G. Payne, D. L. Ondeyka, E. D. Thorsett, W. J. Greenlee, N. S. Lohr, R. D. Hoffsommer, H. Joshua, W. V. Ruyle, J. W. Rothrock, S. D. Aster, A. L. Maycock, F. M. Robinson, R. Hirschmann, C. S. Sweet, E. H. Ulm, D. M. Gross, T. C. Vassil, and C. A. Stone, A new class of angiotensin-converting enzyme inhibitors, *Nature 288*:280–283 (1980).
3. Schechter, I., and A. Berger, On the size of the active site in proteases. I. Papain. *Biochem. Biophys. Res. Commun. 27*:157–162 (1967).
4. Burton, J., R. J. Cody Jr., J. A. Herd, and E. Haber, Specific inhibition of renin by an angiotensinogen analog: Studies in sodium depletion and renin-dependent hypertension. *Proc. Natl. Acad. Sci. USA 77*:5476–5479 (1980).
5. Szelke, M., B. Leckie, A. Hallett, D. M. Jones, J. Sueiras, B. Atrash, and A. F. Lever, Potent new inhibitors of human renin. *Nature 299*:555–557 (1982).
6. Szelke, M., D. M. Jones, B. Atrash, A. Hallett, and B. Leckie, Novel transition-state analogue inhibitors of renin. In *Peptides: Structure and Function. Proceedings of the Eighth American Symposium*, V. J. Hruby and D. H. Rich, eds. Pierce Chemical Co., Rockford, Ill., pp. 579–582 (1983).
7. Boger, J., N. S. Lohr, E. H. Ulm, M. Poe, E. H. Blaine, G. M. Fanelli, T.-Y. Lin, L. S. Payne, T. W. Schorn, B. I. LaMont, T. C. Vassil, I. I. Stabilito, D. F. Veber, D. H. Rich, and A. S. Bopari, Novel renin inhibitors containing the amino acid statine. *Nature 303*:81–84 (1983).
8. Navia, M. A., J. P. Springer, M. Poe, J. Boger, and K. Hoogsteen, Preliminary x-ray crystallographic data on mouse submaxillary gland renin and renin-inhibitor complexes. *J. Biol. Chem. 259*:12714–12717 (1984).
9. Blundell, T., B. L. Sibanda, and L. Pearl, Three-dimensional structure, specificity and catalytic mechanism of renin. *Nature 304*:273–275 (1983).
10. Sibanda, B. L., T. Blundell, P. M. Hobart, M. Fogliano, J. S. Bindra, B. W. Dominy, and J. M. Chirgwin, Computer graphics modelling of human renin. Specificity, catalytic activity and intron-exon junctions. *FEBS Lett. 174*:102–111 (1984).
11. Akahane, K., H. Umeyama, S. Nakagawa, I. Moriguchi, S. Hirose, K. Iizuka, and K. Murakami, Three-dimensional structure of human renin. *Hypertension 7*:3–12 (1985).
12. Carlson, W., M. Karplus, and E. Haber, Construction of a model for the three-dimensional structure of human renal renin. *Hypertension 7*:13–26 (1985).
13. Raddatz, P., C. Schittenhelm, and G. Barnickel, Computer-graphics methods in pharmaceutical research: Visualization of renin–inhibitor complexes. *Kontakte 3*: 3 (1985).
14. Biosym Technologies, 10065 Barnes Canyon Road, San Diego, Calif. 92121.
15. Dauber, P., D. Osguthorpe and A. T. Hagler, Structure energetics and dynamics of ligand binding to dihydrofolate reductase. *Biochem. Soc. Trans. 10*:312–318 (1982).

16. Molecular Design Limited, 1122 B Street, Hayward, Calif. 94541.

17. Oracle Corporation, 20 Davis Drive, Belmont, Calif. 93002.

18. Browne, W. J., et al., A possible three-dimensional structure of bovine alpha-lactalbumin based on that of hen's egg-white lysozyme. *J. Mol. Biol. 42*:65–86 (1969).

19. Shotton, D. M., and H. C. Watson, Three-dimensional structure of tosylelastase. *Nature 225*:811–816 (1970).

20. Blundell, T. L., B. L. Sibanda, M. J. E. Sternberg, and J. M. Thornton, Knowledge-based prediction of protein structures and the design of novel molecules. *Nature 326*:347–352 (1987).

21. Greer, J., Model for haptoglobin heavy chain based upon structural homology. *Proc. Natl. Acad. Sci. USA 77*:3393–3397 (1980).

22. Boger, J., In *Third SCI-Rsc Medicinal Chemistry Symposium*, R. W. Lambert, ed. Cambridge University Press, London (1986).

23. Bernstein, F. C., T. F. Koetzle, G. J. Williams, E. E. Meyer Jr., M. D. Brice, J. R. Rodgers, O. Kennard, T. Shimanouchi, and M. Tasumi, The protein data bank: A computer-based archival file for macromolecular structures. *J. Mol. Biol. 112*:535–542 (1977).

24. Sham, H. L., G. Bolis, H. H. Stein, S. W. Fesik, P. A. Marcotte, J. J. Plattner, C. A. Rempel, and J. Greer, Renin inhibitors. Design and synthesis of a new class of conformationally restricted analogues of angiotensinogen. *J. Med. Chem. 31*:284–295 (1988).

25. Luly, J. R., G. Bolis, N. BaMaung, J. Soderquist, J. F. Dellaria, H. Stein, J. Cohen, T. J. Perun, J. Greer, and J. J. Plattner, New inhibitors of human renin that contain novel Leu–Val replacements. Examination of the P_1 site. *J. Med. Chem. 31*:532–539 (1988).

26. Fesik, S. W., G. Bolis, H. L. Sham, and E. T. Olejniczak, Structure refinement of a cyclic peptide from two-dimensional NMR data and molecular modeling. *Biochemistry 26*:1851–1859 (1987).

27. Greer, J., Comparative model-building of the mammalian serine proteases. *J. Mol. Biol. 153*:1027–1042 (1981).

28. Greer, J., Model structure for the inflammatory protein C5a. *Science 228*:1055–1060 (1985).

29. Greer, J., Comparative structural anatomy of the complement anaphylatoxin proteins C3a, C4a, and C5a. *Enzyme 36*:150–163 (1986).

30. Singh, U. S., F. K. Brown, P. A. Bash, and P. A. Kollman, An approach to the application of free energy perturbation methods using molecular dynamics. *J. Am. Chem. Soc. 109*:1607–1614 (1987).

31. Bolis, G., A. K. L. Fung, J. Greer, H. D. Kleinert, P. A. Marcotte, T. J. Perun, J. J. Plattner, and H. H. Stein, Renin inhibitors. Dipeptide analogues of angiotensinogen incorporating transition-state, nonpeptidic replacements at the scissile bond. *J. Med. Chem. 30*:1729–1737 (1987).

32. Plattner, J. J., J. Greer, A. K. L. Fung, H. Stein, H. D. Kleinert, H. L. Sham, J. R. Smital, and T. J. Perun, Peptide analogues of angiotensinogen. Effect of peptide chain length on renin inhibition. *Biochem. Biophys. Res. Commun. 139*:982–990 (1986).

33. Kleinert, H. D., J. R. Luly, P. A. Marcotte, T. J. Perun, J. J. Plattner, and H. Stein, Renin inhibitors. Improvements in the stability and biological activity of small peptides containing novel Leu–Val replacements. *FEBS Lett.* *230*:38–42 (1988).

34. Wong, C. F., and J. A. McCammon, Dynamics and design of enzymes and inhibitors. *J. Am. Chem. Soc.* *108*:3830–3832 (1986).

35. James, M. N. G., and A. R. Sielecki, Structure and refinement of penicillopepsin at 1.8 Å resolution. *J. Mol. Biol.* *163*:299–361 (1983).

36. Bott, R., E. Subramanian, and D. R. Davies, Three-dimensional structure of the complex of the *Rhizopus chinensis* carboxyl proteinase and pepstatin at 2.5 Å resolution. *Biochemistry* *21*:6956–6562 (1982).

37. Pearl, L., and T. Blundell, The active site of aspartic proteinases. *FEBS Lett.* *174*:96–101 (1984).

38. Andreeva, N. S., A. S. Zdanov, A. E. Gustchina, and A. A. Fedorov, Structure of ethanol-inhibited porcine pepsin at 2 Å resolution and binding of the methyl ester of phenylalanyl-diiodotyrosine to the enzyme. *J. Biol. Chem.* *259*:11353–11365 (1984).

39. James, M. N. G., A. Sielecki, F. Salituro, D. H. Rich, and T. Hofmann, Conformational flexibility in the active sites of aspartyl proteinases revealed by a pepstatin fragment binding to penicillopepsin. *Proc. Natl. Acad. Sci. USA* *79*:6137–6141 (1982).

40. James, M. N. G., and A. R. Sielecki, Stereochemical analysis of peptide bond hydrolysis catalyzed by the aspartic proteinase penicillopepsin. *Biochemistry* *24*:3701–3713 (1985).

41. Boger, J., Renin inhibition. *Annu. Rep. Med. Chem.* *20*:257–266 (1985).

42. Boger, J., L. S. Payne, D. S. Perlow, N. S. Lohr, M. Poe, E. H. Blaine, E. H. Ulm, T. W. Schorn, B. I. LaMont, T.-Y. Lin, M. Kawai, D. H. Rich, and D. F. Veber, Renin inhibitors. Syntheses of subnanomolar, competitive, transition-state analogue inhibitors containing a novel analogue of statine. *J. Med. Chem.* *28*:1779–1790 (1985).

43. Diamond, J. M., and E. M. Wright, Biological membranes: The physical basis of ion and nonelectrolyte selectivity. *Annu. Rev. Physiol.* *31*:581–646 (1969).

44. James, M. N. G., A. R. Sielecki, M. Fujinaga, A. K. Muir, M. E. P. Murphy, C. T. Carilli, and J. Shine, The molecular structure of recombinant human renin. Abstracts of the 18th Linderstøm-Lang Conference on Aspartic Proteinases, p. 68.

9

Inhibitors of Dihydrofolate Reductase

Lee F. Kuyper
Wellcome Research Laboratories, Research Triangle Park,
North Carolina

I. INTRODUCTION

The usefulness of several drugs important in the treatment of cancer, bacterial infections, and malaria stems from the inhibition of the enzyme dihydrofolate reductase (DHFR). Examples include methotrexate (structure 1; MTX), a close analog of folic acid that is widely used in cancer chemotherapy (1);

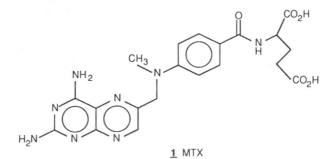

<u>**1**</u> MTX

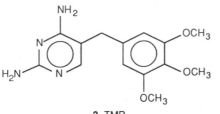

<u>**2**</u> TMP

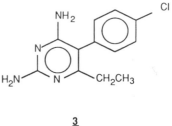

<u>**3**</u>

trimethoprim (structure 2; TMP), an antibacterial agent that is uniquely selective for DHFR from bacteria (2); and pyrimethamine (structure 3), a potent inhibitor of DHFR from the malarial organisms (3). As a drug "receptor," DHFR has been much studied during the past three decades, and a vast amount of information about this protein has been published and recently reviewed (4–11). Among the more recent developments, the determination of the three-dimensional molecular structure of the enzyme is clearly the one of great interest to the drug designer. This chapter will emphasize our interest in using that structural information to understand protein-ligand interactions and ultimately to rationally design novel ligands that might be therapeutically useful. As will be discussed, knowledge of the DHFR structure has permitted the successful design of novel inhibitors.

II. THE ENZYME

A. Role in Cellular Metabolism

The role of DHFR in cellular metabolism and the biochemical basis for its position as a drug target are reasonably well understood and have been described in detail elsewhere (12,13). Only the more salient aspects of the subject warrant discussion here.

DHFR catalyzes the NADPH-dependent reduction of the 5,6 double bond of dihydrofolate (FH_2) to produce tetrahydrofolate (FH_4) as shown in Figure 1. (DHFR from some sources is also capable of reducing folate to dihydrofolate.) Derivatives of FH_4 in which one carbon functions have been enzymatically added to the 5 or 10 positions or both serve as one-carbon donors in the biosynthesis of purines, pyrimidines, and several amino acids.

Of the many transformations involving FH_4, the one that appears most important to DHFR-related chemotherapy is the biosynthesis of thymidylate (dTMP), as illustrated in Figure 2. In that process FH_4 is first converted to the active cofactor 5,10-methylenetetrahydrofolate by serine hydroxy-methylene transferase, an enzyme that uses a serine-donated methylene group to bridge the 5 and 10 positions of FH_4. That cofactor is then employed by thymidylate synthase in the conversion of deoxyuridylate (dUMP) to dTMP. The 5,10-methylene group and the hydrogen at position 6 of the cofactor form the 5-methyl group of the nucleotide product. Notably, the by-product is FH_2. This reaction is the only known use of a tetrahydrofolate cofactor in which the cofactor is oxidized to the dihydro form and is also the only

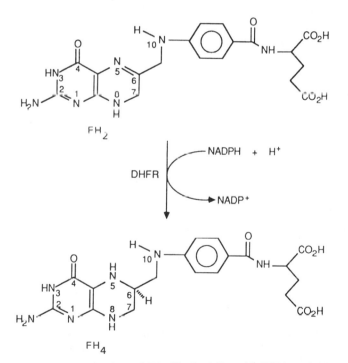

Figure 1 Reduction of 7,8-dihydrofolic acid (FH_2) to 5,6,7,8-tetrahydrofolic acid (FH_4) by NADPH and hydrogen ion, catalyzed by dihydrofolate reductase (DHFR).

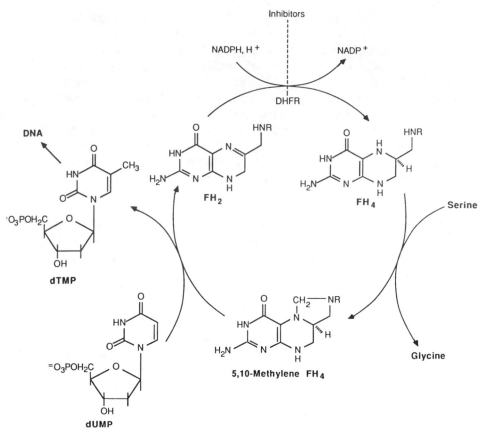

Figure 2   Role of DHFR in the biosynthesis of thymidylate (dTMP).

recognized de novo source of dTMP, an essential building block of DNA. Thus, for balanced cell growth, DHFR must be available to replenish the supply of FH_4 that is depleted in the biosynthesis of dTMP. Inhibition of DHFR leads to a cellular deficiency of tetrahydrofolate cofactors that disrupts the synthesis of purines, pyrimidines, and several amino acids and consequently results in cell death.

B.   Primary Structure

DHFR is a widely distributed enzyme that has been isolated from bacteria, bacteriophage, protozoa, fungi, plants, and animals. Amino acid sequences have been determined for DHFR from a number of organisms, and a representative set of those sequences is shown in Table 1 (see Ref. 6 for a more

Table 1 Amino Acid Sequences of DHFR from Selected Organisms

Ec	—	—	1M	2I	3S	4L	5I	6A	7A	8L	9A	10V	11D	12R	13V	14I	15G	16M	17E	18N	19A	20M	21P	22W	—	23N	24L	25P
Lc	—	—	—	1T	2A	3F	4L	5W	6A	7Q	8N	9R	10D	11G	12L	13I	14G	15K	16D	17G	18H	19L	20P	21W	—	22H	23L	24P
Ng	1M	2L	3K	4I	5T	6I	7I	0A	9A	10G	11A	12F	13N	14L	15C	16I	17G	18A	19G	20N	21A	20M	20P	24W	—	23H	26I	27P
Cl	1V	2R	3S	4L	5N	6S	7I	8V	9A	10V	11C	12Q	13N	14M	15G	16I	17G	18K	19D	20G	21N	22L	23P	24W	25P	26P	27L	28R
Hu	1V	2G	3S	4L	5N	6C	7I	8V	9A	10V	11S	12Q	13N	14M	15G	16I	17G	18K	19N	20G	21D	22L	23P	24W	25P	26P	27L	28R
Mo	1V	2R	3P	4L	5N	6C	7I	8V	9A	10V	11S	12Q	13N	14M	15G	16I	17G	18K	19N	20G	21D	22L	23P	24W	25P	26P	27L	28R

Ec	26A	27D	28L	29A	30W	31F	32K	33R	34N	35T	36L	—	—	—	—	—	37N	38K	39P	40V	41I	42M	43G	44H	45I	46T
Lc	25D	26D	27L	28H	29Y	30F	31R	32A	33Q	34T	35V	—	—	—	—	—	36G	37K	38I	39M	40V	41V	42G	43R	44R	45T
Ng	28E	29D	30F	31A	32F	33F	34K	35V	36Y	37T	38L	—	—	—	—	—	39G	40K	41P	42V	43I	44M	45G	46R	47K	48T
Cl	29N	30E	31Y	32K	33Y	34F	35Q	36R	37M	38T	39S	40T	41S	42H	43V	44E	45G	46K	47Q	48N	49L	50V	51I	52M	53G	54K	55K	56T
Hu	29N	30E	31F	32R	33Y	34F	35Q	36R	37M	38T	39T	40T	41S	42S	43V	44E	45G	46K	47Q	48N	49L	50V	51I	52M	53G	54K	55K	56T
Mo	29N	30E	31F	32K	33Y	34F	35Q	36R	37M	38T	39T	40T	41S	42S	43V	44E	45G	46K	47Q	48N	49L	50V	51I	52M	53G	54R	55K	56T

Ec	47W	48E	49S	50I	51G	—	—	—	52R	53P	54L	55P	56G	57R	58K	59N	60I	61I	62L	63S	64S	65Q	66P	—	67G	68T	69D	70D
Lc	46Y	47E	48S	49F	50P	—	—	51K	52R	53P	54L	55P	56E	57R	58T	59N	60V	61V	62L	63T	64V	65I	66S	67R	68Q	69A	70D	71Y	72C	73A	74A
Ng	49W	50E	51S	52L	53P	—	—	54V	55K	56P	57L	58P	59G	60R	61R	62N	63I	64V	65I	66S	67R	68Q	69A	70D	71Y	72C	73A	74A
Cl	57W	58F	59S	60I	61P	62E	63K	64N	65R	66P	67L	68K	69D	70R	71I	72N	73I	74V	75L	76S	77R	78E	79L	80K	81E	82A	83P	84K
Hu	57W	58F	59S	60I	61P	62E	63K	64N	65R	66P	67L	68K	69G	70R	71I	72N	73L	74V	75L	76S	77R	78E	79L	80K	81E	82P	83P	84Q
Mo	57W	58F	59S	60I	61P	62E	63K	64N	65R	66P	67L	68K	69D	70R	71I	72N	73I	74V	75L	76S	77R	78E	79I	80K	81E	82P	83P	84R

Ec	71R	—	72V	73T	74W	75V	76K	77S	78V	79D	80E	81A	82I	83A	84A	85C	86G	87D	88V	89P	—	—	—	—	—	90E	91I
Lc	72G	—	73A	74V	75V	76V	77H	78D	79V	80A	81A	82V	83F	84A	85Y	86A	87K	88Q	89H	90L	91D	92Q	—	—	—	93E	94L
Ng	75G	—	76A	77E	78T	79V	80A	81S	82L	83E	84V	85A	86L	87A	88L	89C	90A	91G	92A	93E	—	—	—	—	—	94E	95A
Cl	85G	86A	87H	88Y	89L	90S	91K	92S	93L	94D	95D	96A	97L	98A	99L	100L	101D	102S	103P	104E	105L	106K	107S	108K	109V	110D	111M	112V
Hu	85G	86A	87H	88F	89L	90A	91K	92S	93L	94D	95D	96A	97L	98R	99L	100I	101E	102Q	103P	104E	105L	106A	107N	108K	109V	110D	111M	112V
Mo	85G	86A	87H	88F	89L	90A	91K	92S	93L	94D	95D	96A	97L	98R	99L	100I	101E	102Q	103P	104E	105L	106A	107S	108K	109V	110D	111M	112V

Ec	92M	93V	94I	95G	96G	97G	98R	99V	100Y	101E	102Q	103F	104L	—	—	105P	106K	107A	108Q	109K	110L	111Y	112L	113T	114H	115I	116D	117A
Lc	95V	96I	97A	98G	99G	100A	101Q	102I	103Y	104T	105A	106F	107K	—	—	108D	109D	110V	111D	112T	113L	114L	115V	116T	117R	118I	119A	120G
Ng	96V	97I	98M	99G	100G	101A	102Q	103I	104Y	105G	106Q	107A	108M	—	—	109P	110L	111A	112T	113D	114L	115R	116I	117T	118E	119Y	120P	121L
Cl	113W	114I	115V	116G	117G	118T	119A	120V	121Y	122K	123A	124A	125M	126N	127H	128P	129G	130H	131L	132K	133L	134F	135V	136T	137R	138I	139L	140H
Hu	113W	114I	115V	116G	117G	118S	119S	120V	121Y	122K	123G	124A	125M	126N	127H	128P	129G	130H	131L	132K	133L	134F	135V	136T	137R	138I	139M	140Q
Mo	113W	114I	115V	116G	117G	118S	119S	120V	121Y	122K	123G	124A	125M	126N	127E	128P	129G	130H	131L	132K	133L	134F	135V	136T	137R	138I	139M	140Q

Ec	118Q	119H	120E	121G	122D	123T	124H	125F	126P	127D	128Y	129E	130P	131D	132D	133W	134E	135S	136V	137F	138S	—	—	—	—	—	139E
Lc	121S	122F	123E	124G	125D	126T	127K	128M	129I	130P	131L	132N	133W	134D	135D	136F	137T	138K	139V	140S	141S	—	—	—	—	—	142R
Ng	122S	123V	124E	125G	126D	127A	128E	129F	130P	131E	132I	133D	134P	135T	136H	137W	138P	139E	140A	141F	142P	143T	144E	—	—	—	145P
Cl	141E	142F	143L	144Q	145P	146T	147D	148D	149P	150E	151I	152I	153K	154V	155K	156P	157I	158L	159I	160L	161I	162N	163G	164V	165P	166E	167A	168D
Hu	141D	142F	143E	144S	145D	146I	147F	148E	149P	150E	151I	152D	153L	154E	155K	156Y	157K	158L	159L	160P	161E	162Y	163P	164G	165V	166L	167S	168D
Mo	141C	142F	143E	144S	145D	146I	147F	148E	149P	150E	151I	152D	153L	154E	155K	156Y	157K	158L	159L	160P	161E	162Y	163P	164G	165V	166L	167S	168E

Ec	140F	141H	142D	143A	144D	145A	146N	147N	148S	149H	150S	151Y	152C	153F	154E	155I	156L	157E	158R	159R	—	—	—	
Lc	143T	144V	145F	146D	147T	148N	—	149P	150A	151L	152T	153H	154T	155Y	156E	157V	158W	159Q	160K	161K	162A	—	—	
Ng	146A	147V	148S	149S	150K	151G	—	—	152V	153A	154V	155T	156F	157V	158H	159V	160L	161G	162K	—	—	—	
Cl	169I	170Q	171E	172E	173D	174G	—	—	175I	176Q	177Y	178K	179F	180E	181V	182Y	183Q	184K	185S	186V	187L	188A	189Q
Hu	169V	170Q	171E	172E	173K	174G	—	—	175I	176K	177Y	178K	179F	180E	181V	182Y	183E	184K	185N	186D	—	—	
Mo	169V	170Q	171E	172E	173D	174G	—	—	175I	176K	177Y	178K	179F	180E	181V	182Y	183E	184K	185K	186D	—	—	

Ec = *E. coli* (ref 14), Lc = *L. casei* (ref 15), Ng = *N. gonorrhoeae* (ref 16). Cl = Chicken Liver (ref 17), Hu = Human (ref 10), Mo = Mouse (ref 19)
A - Alanine, R - Arginine, N - Asparagine, D - Aspartic Acid, C - Cysteine, Q - Glutamine, E - Glutamic Acid, G - Glycine, H - Histidine, I - Isoleucine, L - Leucine, K - Lysine, M - Methionine, F - Phenylalanine, P - Proline, S - Serine, T - Threonine, W - Tryptophan, Y - Tyrosine, V - Valine.
Sequence alignment for the Ec, Lc, and Cl enzymes follows that of ref 20 which was based on the corresponding three-dimensional structures. Alignment of the Ng, Hu, and Mo sequences were based on maximal homology.

complete tabulation). The linear alignment of protein sequences in Table 1 is based on superposition of corresponding three-dimensional structures (20), except for the sequences of DHFR from *Neisseria gonorrhoeae* and human.

Relatively high homology (75–90%) is found between pairs of enzymes of animal origin, whereas bacterial species show only 25–40% homology. Sequence homology between the bacterial and animal enzymes is 20–30%.

The enzymes from vertebrates are generally about 25 residues longer than the bacterial proteins, and, as seen in Table 1, those extra residues are accommodated as insertions at various locations throughout the sequence. In spite of low homology, the three-dimensional architectures of the bacterial and animal enzymes are very similar, as will be discussed in more detail below. Most of the insertions are found at the protein surface and appear to have no major influence on the overall geometry of the enzyme. In addition to backbone similarities, a significant number of residues in the substrate binding cleft are highly conserved. Linear sequence comparison of DHFR from 11 different sources shows that 12 residues are strictly conserved and that each of them is located in or near the active site. Suggested functions for each of these residues are discussed in detail by Kraut and Matthews (4). Such a detailed analysis of differences and similarities between DHFR from various sources is extremely important to inhibitor design. The selectivity of an inhibitor for the enzyme of a disease-causing organism (versus human DHFR) is crucial to the usefulness of a compound. If the two enzymes in question are similar, it may be difficult to devise an inhibitor that is appropriately selective.

Despite the similarities observed for isozymes of DHFR, highly selective inhibitors are known. The antibacterial agent TMP, for example, binds tightly to DHFR from most bacterial species but binds weakly to the human enzyme. The current understanding of the basis for that differential binding will be discussed later.

C. Three-Dimensional Structure

Detailed x-ray crystal structures of several species of DHFR in complex with a variety of ligands have been reported during the past 10 years by the group led by Kraut and Matthews and also by Wellcome Research Laboratories. A compilation of those structures is given in Table 2. (The structure of a plasmid-encoded DHFR has also been reported (34), but that class of DHFR is beyond the scope of this chapter.)

Classified by Richardson as a doubly wound mixed β-sheet (35), the structure of DHFR is dominated by a central eight-stranded β-sheet that is flanked on either side by two alpha helices. That architecture is illustrated by a ribbon representation of *Lactobacillus casei* DHFR in Figure 3. Following the nomenclature of Matthews et al. (24), the individual strands of the β-sheet are labeled alphabetically in order of occurrence in the linear protein sequence. Each helix is assigned the letter of the β-strand that it precedes in the sequence.

Each of the four different isozymes for which three-dimensional structures are now known shows the same general folding pattern in spite of low

Table 2 A Listing of Reported X-Ray Structures of DHFR

Enzyme Source	Ligands Binary[a]	Ligands Ternary[b]	References
L. casei	—	MTX	21–23
E. coli	MTX	—	22–24, 27
	TMP	—	25, 26
	TMP analogs	—	27–29
	Pyrimethamine	—	27
	—	TMP	30
Chicken liver	NADPH	—	20
	—	TMP	26
	—	Dihydrotriazines	20, 31
	—	TMP analogs	31
	—	Adamantylpyrimidine	31
Mouse L1210	—	TMP	32, 33
	—	MTX	32, 33

[a]Enzyme is complexed with listed ligand only.
[b]Enzyme is complexed with listed ligand and cofactor NADPH.

sequence homologies and the occurrence of residue insertions and deletions. The manner in which insertions and deletions are accommodated is illustrated in Figure 4 for the structures of the *Escherichia coli* and chicken enzymes.

A striking feature of the enzyme structure is a deep cleft that exists between the B and C helices. This large cavity serves as the binding site for diaminopyrimidine-type inhibitors, as illustrated in Figure 5 for the *L. casei* DHFR complex with MTX (21–23). The lower half of the cleft is occupied by the nicotinamide portion of NADPH. The adenosine moiety of the cofactor binds in a shallow niche on the opposite side of the β-sheet, with the diphosphate bridge draped over the edge of the sheet in an apparently favorable position for stabilization by the dipoles of helices C and F (36). For additional details of the interactions between cofactor and enzyme, see Ref. 23.

The core of the inhibitor-binding site is hydrophobic and is composed primarily, for example, of Leu-19, Leu-27, Phe-30, Phe-49, and Leu-54 in *L. casei* DHFR, as shown in Figure 6. At either end of this hydrophobic core is a polar region with hydrogen-bonding sites. At one end, deep within the cleft, the carboxylic acid side chain of an aspartate (or glutamate in the enzyme of vertebrate origin) provides a key interaction for inhibitor binding and

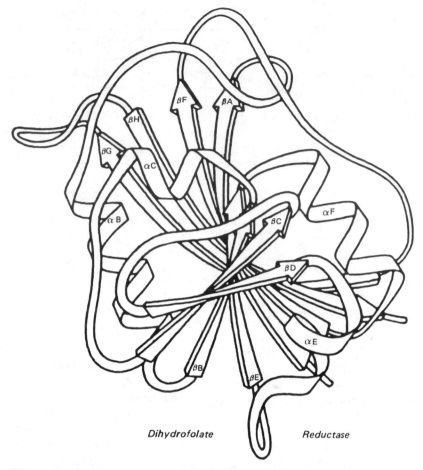

Figure 3 A ribbon representation of *L. casei* DHFR from Ref. 35 showing the central eight-stranded β-sheet and the flanking alpha-helices. Reproduced by permission of J. S. Richardson and Academic Press.

appears to play an important functional role in the reduction of substrate (37). At the other end of the hydrophobic core, the guanidinium moiety of a strictly conserved arginine residue is buried in a hydrophobic pocket. The sequestered nature of these two readily ionizable groups suggests functional importance to ligand binding, which will be discussed further in later sections of this chapter.

Crystal structures of human DHFR have not been reported, although the enzyme has been crystallized (38). Molecular models of that protein have

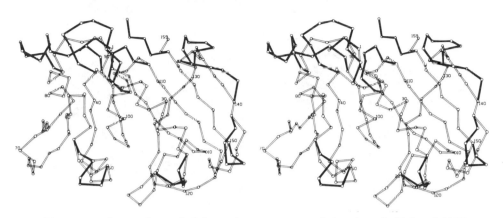

Figure 4 Comparison of alpha-carbon structures of *E. coli* and chicken DHFR. The complete *E. coli* enzyme skeleton is shown with open bonds, and the chicken DHFR structure is included as filled bonds in regions of insertions and deletions. Every 10th residue of the *E. coli* enzyme structure is numbered.

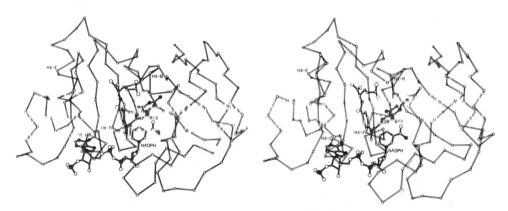

Figure 5 An alpha-carbon backbone representation of the *L. casei* DHFR ternary complex with MTX and NADPH. Ligand atoms are shown as follows: carbon, small open circle; oxygen, larger open circle; nitrogen, blackened circle; phosphorus, larger blackened circle. The four alpha-helices B, C, E, and F are labeled.

been constructed from crystal structures of the chicken (4) and mouse (33) enzymes. As shown in Table 1, those three proteins are highly homologous, with no insertions or deletions, and are therefore assumed to have very similar backbone structures. Indeed, the modeling transformations required to convert the mouse or chicken DHFR crystal structures into the human

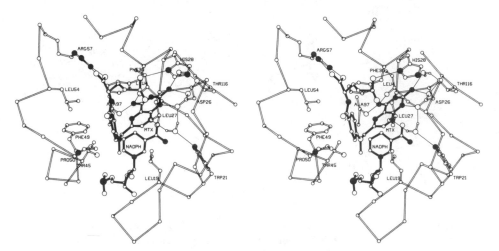

Figure 6 Binding site of MTX in the *L. casei* DHFR ternary complex. The protein is represented by an alpha-carbon backbone with a selected set of amino acid side chains and is shown with open bonds. Two backbone carbonyl groups that hydrogen bond to the 4-amino group of MTX are also included. MTX and NADPH are depicted with filled bonds. Hydrogen atoms, shown only for the two water molecules, are represented by very small open circles, carbon atoms by small open circles, oxygens by larger open circles, nitrogens by blackened circles, and phosphorus by larger blackened circles. Several hydrogen bonds between MTX, protein, and two water molecules are shown as single lines between atoms.

DHFR models were straightforward. In other words, residue differences were easily accommodated by the three-dimensional structures. This is important, because, in the past, DHFR from vertebrate sources such as mouse, chicken, rat, or pigeon has been used as a convenient surrogate for the more difficult to obtain human enzyme. In discussions of the structural origins of the DHFR selectivity of TMP in a later section of this chapter, we assume that relevant features of the chicken DHFR structure will also be found in the structure of human DHFR.

D. Stereochemistry of Reduction

Although no crystal structure has been reported for a DHFR complexed with substrate, either folate or dihydrofolate, a plausible model for the stereochemistry of dihydrofolate binding was recently proposed (4). Our rendering of that model is depicted in Figure 7. The model is consistent with structural features of a complex between chicken DHFR and a folate-related compound, biopterin, that has not yet been published in detail. It is also

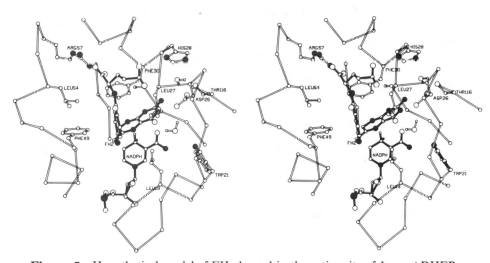

Figure 7   Hypothetical model of FH$_2$ bound in the active site of *L. casei* DHFR. The protein is represented by an alpha-carbon backbone with a selected set of amino acid side chains and is shown with open bonds. FH$_2$ and NADPH are shown with filled bonds. Hydrogen atoms, shown only for the two water molecules and the 4-carbon of NADPH, are represented by very small open circles. Carbon atoms are shown as small open circles, oxygen atoms as larger open circles, nitrogen atoms as blackened circles, and phosphorus as larger blackened circles. The 4-pro-R hydrogen of NADPH is the closer, more visible hydrogen of the 4-CH$_2$ group.

consistent with known stereochemical facts concerning the substrates, in particular the absolute configuration of the product tetrahydrofolate and the stereospecificity of hydride transfer from NADPH. The x-ray crystal structure of 5,10-methenyltetrahydrofolate (39) and its configurational relationship with tetrahydrofolate (40) recently established the absolute configuration of carbon-6. The ability of DHFR to catalyze the transfer of the 4-pro-R hydrogen of NADPH has been known since the early 1960s (41,42).

An interesting aspect of the model for substrate binding is the orientation of the pteridine ring system of dihydrofolate. This mode of binding is dictated by the known position of binding of NADPH and the observed stereochemistry of the catalyzed reduction reaction, but it is intriguingly different from the observed binding of the inhibitor MTX, a close structural analog.

The pteridine rings of the two molecules are related by a 180° rotation about an axis roughly coincident with the C6—C9 and C2—NH$_2$ bonds. MTX apparently prefers the flipped orientation primarily because of an ionic interaction that can be made between the protonated pteridine ring of MTX and the carboxylate anion of Asp-26 in the *L. casei* enzyme, an interaction that presumably contributes significantly to the difference in enzyme affinity between MTX and dihydrofolate. The ratio of binding constants is greater than 5 orders of magnitude, in favor of MTX (43).

Further details of this model and a thorough discussion of its mechanistic implications can be found in the excellent review by Kraut and Matthews (4).

E. Inhibitor–Binding Constants

One key ingredient in a program for inhibitor design is a simple and accurate method for measuring the affinity between enzyme and inhibitor. A number of methods have been devised for DHFR including those that make use of NMR (44), fluorescence titrations (45), and equilibrium dialysis (46). However, the simplest and most common is a spectrophotometric method that provides an I_{50} value, which is the concentration of inhibitor that slows the normal rate of enzyme-catalyzed reaction by half. In most cases, I_{50} values provide an accurate picture of relative DHFR affinities for a series of inhibitors. An I_{50} value is not, however, a true inhibition constant, and it can be misleading in certain circumstances. For example, the selectivity of an inhibitor for a bacterial DHFR versus the human enzyme, as measured by the ratio of I_{50}'s for the two isozymes, will be accurate only if the two enzymes show identical affinity for the substrate FH_2. Reported values of the FH_2-binding constant, measured as Michaelis constants, for various bacterial and animal DHFR exhibit a 300-fold range (8). Therefore, selectivity should be measured from more rigorous types of inhibitor-binding constant, such as K_i or K_d, that are independent of the FH_2 Michaelis constant.

The I_{50} method is also inadequate for treating inhibitors that exhibit very high affinity (approximately subnanomolar K_i) for the enzyme (47). Reported I_{50} values in such cases should be viewed with caution.

III. ENZYME–INHIBITOR INTERACTIONS

A. General Background

Thousands of inhibitors of DHFR have been reported over the past 30 years, and most are included in a useful compilation recently published by Blaney et al. (48). From among those thousands of compounds have emerged several important drugs, as mentioned in the Introduction.

A detailed understanding of how these drugs interact with DHFR should enhance the possibilities of designing more effective inhibitors. Most of the currently available information on DHFR-drug interactions at the molecular level comes from x-ray crystallography, and much of that work has recently been thoroughly reviewed (4,9). In the following sections only the salient structural features of the MTX and TMP complexes with DHFR will be discussed.

B. X-Ray Crystal Structures of DHFR–Drug Complexes

1. Methotrexate

Two different DHFR complexes with MTX have been reported in highly refined form (22,23): the binary complex with *E. coli* DHFR, and the ternary complex with *L. casei* DHFR and NADPH. A preliminary report of a third structure with mouse L1210 DHFR and NADPH has also appeared (32,33). We will focus on the structure of the *L. casei* DHFR ternary complex that was briefly referred to in Section II.

A multitude of enzyme-inhibitor interactions govern the stability and the geometry of association of the MTX-DHFR complex. The pteridine ring of MTX binds deep in the enzyme cleft, making a number of nonpolar and hydrogen-bonding interactions (see Figs. 3, 6). Although the pKa of N-1 of MTX is only 5.3 (49), a host of data suggests that it is fully protonated in the enzyme complex (50). Perhaps the most convincing data is from a series of ^{13}C-NMR experiments in which the pKa of MTX bound to DHFR was shown to be > 10 (51). The protonated pyrimidine binds ionically to the carboxyl group of Asp-26 through two hydrogen bonds, one from protonated N-1 and the other from the 2-NH$_2$ group, as shown in Figure 6. The second hydrogen of the 2-NH$_2$ group forms a hydrogen bond with a buried water molecule at the back of the cleft, and the 4-NH$_2$ group donates hydrogen bonds to the backbone carbonyl oxygens of Leu-4 and Ala 97. In addition, N-5 of MTX can apparently hydrogen-bond to a fixed water molecule that is held in place via hydrogen bonds to Trp-21 and Asp-26.

Nonpolar contacts of the pteridine ring involve backbone or side-chain atoms of Leu-4, Trp-5, Ala-6, Leu-19, Leu-27, Phe-30, and Ala-97. Contacts also occur with the nicotinamide ring of NADPH. The p-aminobenzoic acid unit of MTX is located in the hydrophobic core of the enzyme active site, with the phenyl ring close to the side chains of Leu-27, Phe-30, Phe-49, and Leu-54. The alpha-carboxyl group of the glutamate moiety of MTX is ionically associated with the sequestered guanidinium group of Arg-57. The geometry of that ion pair allows for two hydrogen bonds. The gamma-carboxyl group appears to interact ionically with His-28 via a single hydrogen bond.

The dissociation constant of MTX from its ternary complex with DHFR is on the order of 10^{10} (43) and represents about 14 kcal/mol of binding energy. This binding energy appears to result from a large number of relatively small contributions that arise not only from many different kinds of direct interaction between inhibitor and protein but also from interactions with water molecules. Entropy must also play a role in binding (52), and energies associated with conformational properties of both inhibitor and protein cannot be ignored. Clearly inhibitor binding to DHFR is complex.

2. Trimethoprim

The effectiveness of TMP as an antibacterial agent is due in part to its differential affinity for bacterial DHFR versus human DHFR. The estimated ratio of TMP affinity constants for these two species of enzyme, based on K_i values for the *E. coli* and mouse enzymes (46), is about 3000:1, which is equivalent to approximately 5 kcal/mol in binding energy. Such selectivity is a property that is generally crucial to the usefulness of antimicrobial DHFR inhibitors, and an understanding of that trait of TMP would be expected to aid in the design of novel, selective inhibitors.

A great deal is now known about TMP binding to DHFR. Structures of TMP bound to DHFR from various sources have been solved by x-ray crystallography (see Table 2) and have also been studied in solution by NMR spectroscopy (53, 54). Detailed investigations of DHFR affinity using kinetic and equilibrium techniques have also been reported (46).

The first crystal structure of DHFR containing bound TMP was reported for the binary complex between TMP and the enzyme from *E. coli* bacteria by a group from Wellcome Research Laboratories in the U.K. The active site of that structure in its refined form is shown in Figure 8. The diaminopyrimidine ring of TMP is associated with the *E. coli* enzyme in a manner completely analogous to the binding of that ring in MTX to *L. casei* DHFR. The 4-amino group of TMP is hydrogen-bonded to the backbone carbonyl oxygens of Ile-5 and Ile-94, and the 2-amino donates hydrogen bonds to a buried water molecule and the carboxyl group of Asp-27. The pyrimidine ring of TMP is protonated at N-1 when bound to DHFR, as shown unambiguously by ^{15}N NMR experiments in which the signal from the ^{15}N-labeled N-1 appears as a proton-coupled doublet in the TMP-DHFR complex (55). That N-1 hydrogen is hydrogen-bonded to the carboxyl group of Asp-27. Clearly the ionic interaction with the active-site acidic residue is a key feature of binding for the diaminopyrimidine-type inhibitor.

The trimethoxyphenyl group of TMP is located in the hydrophobic core of the protein active site, similar to the p-aminobenzoic acid unit of MTX, and is close to the side chains of Leu-28, Phe-30, Ile-50, and Leu-54. The conformation of TMP in its DHFR-bound state is similar to that observed in a crystal structure of TMP as its hydrobromide salt (56). This indicates that the DHFR-bound form is a low-energy conformation. The conformational energy surface of TMP, produced from full relaxation molecular mechanics calculations (57, 58), shows an extended low-energy valley that includes the

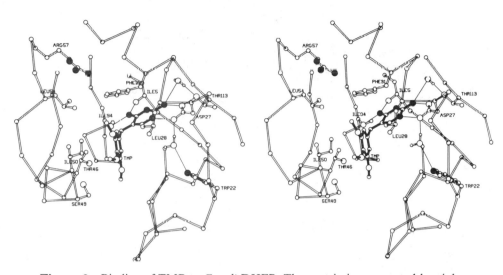

Figure 8 Binding of TMP to *E. coli* DHFR. The protein is represented by alpha-carbon backbone and selected amino acid side chains and is depicted with open bonds. The bonds of TMP are filled. Hydrogen atoms, included only for the two water molecules, are represented by very small open circles; carbon atoms, by small open circles; oxygen atoms, by larger open circles; and nitrogen atoms, by blackened circles. A set of selected hydrogen bonds is shown by single lines between atoms.

form from the *E. coli* DHFR complex. That energy surface is shown in Figure 9. These data suggest that the conformational properties of TMP are compatible with the active-site geometry of *E. coli* DHFR and that little strain is induced upon binding.

Informative as it was, the structure of the *E. coli* DHFR-TMP binary complex left questions about the potential structural effects of cofactor binding. The binding of cofactor and TMP, as well as various other inhibitors, has been shown to be cooperative. That is, the affinity of either ligand is enhanced by the presence of the other. In addition, the binding cooperativity between TMP and cofactor is known to play a significant role in the preferential affinity of TMP for bacterial DHFR (46). Baccanari et al. have shown that TMP has much greater affinity for the cofactor-containing complex of DHFR from *L. casei* or *E. coli* than for the corresponding enzyme alone (46). In contrast, only a small difference in TMP affinity was observed between the binary and ternary complexes of mouse DHFR. The mouse enzyme is presumably a good model for human DHFR because of the 89% sequence homology between the two proteins (see Table 1). Thus the presence of NADPH has a marked effect on the therapeutically crucial, relative affinity of bacterial and mammalian DHFR for TMP.

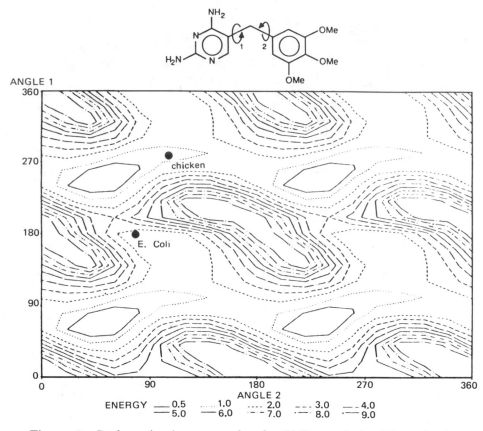

Figure 9 Conformational energy surface for TMP as calculated· by molecular mechanics. The surface points representing the conformations of TMP observed in the *E. coli* and chicken DHFR complexes are indicated.

The Wellcome group has recently reported the x-ray crystal structure of TMP bound in a ternary complex with *E. coli* DHFR and cofactor, providing a basis for at least beginning to understand the origins of cooperativity at the molecular level. A comparison of that ternary complex and the corresponding binary complex is shown in Figure 10. The geometry of binding of TMP and the conformation of most of the protein are essentially the same in the two complexes. The major difference is found in a flexible loop, formed by residues 15–21, that joins β-strand A to alpha-helix B. In the binary complex, that loop adopts a conformation that orients its residues well away from

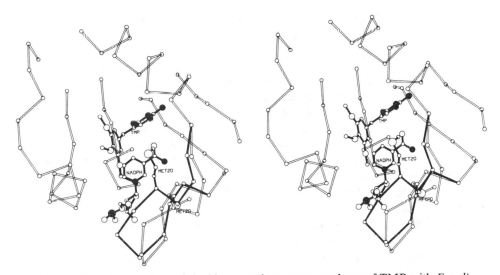

Figure 10   Comparison of the binary and ternary complexes of TMP with *E. coli* DHFR. Protein is represented only by alpha-carbon backbone, except for the side chain of Met-20. Protein from the binary complex is shown with open bonds; that from the ternary complex, with filled bonds. TMP, from the binary structure, and NADPH are shown with filled bonds. Carbon atoms are represented by small open circles, oxygen atoms by larger open circles, sulfur atoms by the largest open circles, nitrogen atoms by blackened circles, and the phosphorus atom by the larger blackened circle.

TMP, apparently providing little or no favorable interaction with the inhibitor. The conformation of that loop is significantly different in the cofactor-bound complex. The cofactor-induced conformation permits a number of favorable interactions between the loop and the ribose portion of the nicotinamide half of the cofactor and also positions the side chain of Met-20 into juxtaposition with the trimethoxyphenyl group of TMP. The latter interaction may be partly responsible for the cooperativity of the two ligands. Direct contact between TMP and cofactor may also contribute to the cooperative binding. These two effects are the most obvious ones that can be gleaned from the x-ray structures, but there may be other contributions to cooperativity from more subtle conformational differences and also differences in solvation.

The observation of differences in conformation between the binary and ternary complexes of TMP and *E. coli* DHFR illustrates a point relevant to the design of novel DHFR inhibitors: the cofactor should be considered an important and integral part of the enzyme active site. The structure of the ternary complex appears to be the biologically relevant form of the enzyme and is therefore probably the structure of choice for inhibitor design purposes.

As mentioned above, very little cooperativity between TMP and NADPH is observed in complexes with vertebrate DHFR. Again x-ray crystal structure data have provided a basis for understanding that lack of cooperativity. Although no crystal structure of a TMP-vertebrate DHFR binary complex has been reported, a refined crystal structure of TMP bound in ternary complex with chicken DHFR has been reported (26) and is illustrated in Figure 11. Interestingly, the conformation of TMP in that complex is much different from that observed in the corresponding ternary complex of *E. coli* DHFR. In the chicken enzyme complex, TMP adopts a low-energy conformation (see Fig. 9) that limits direct interaction with bound cofactor, in contrast to the *E. coli* DHFR case. Perhaps this simple observation sufficiently explains the difference in cooperativity for the two systems.

A structural explanation of the differential affinity of TMP for bacterial versus vertebrate DHFR has been proposed by Matthews et al. (31). Thorough analysis of the differences between the chicken DHFR-NADPH-

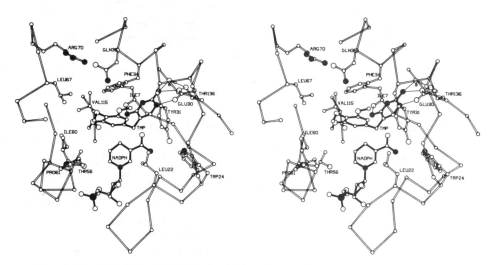

Figure 11   Binding of TMP in the chicken liver DHFR ternary complex. Protein is represented by alpha-carbon backbone and selected amino acid side chains and is shown with open bonds. TMP and NADPH are depicted with filled bonds. Hydrogen atoms, shown only for the one water molecule, are represented by very small open circles; carbon atoms, by small open circles; oxygen atoms, by larger open circles; nitrogen atoms, by blackened circles; and the phosphorus atom, by the larger blackened circle. Selected hydrogen bonds are shown as single lines between atoms.

TMP and *E. coli* DHFR-TMP structures revealed that the active site cleft in the chicken enzyme is 1.5–2.0 Å wider than the cleft of the *E. coli* enzyme. This structural difference is illustrated in Figure 12. Although the difference is relatively subtle, it appears to play a significant role in the way TMP binds differently to the two proteins. In the *E. coli* enzyme, the cleft width is well suited for binding TMP; favorable contacts for the trimethoxyphenyl ring are provided from both sides of the cleft (Ile-50 on the left side and Leu-28 on the right).

TMP is not so favorably accommodated in the larger active site of chicken DHFR. Model-building experiments by Matthews et al. show that positioning of the trimethoxyphenyl ring of TMP for favorable contact with the left side of the cleft (Ile-60) in the chicken enzyme leaves a gap between TMP and the right side of the cleft (Tyr-31) (31). In that hypothetical model, favorable hydrophobic interactions analogous to those between TMP and Leu-28 in the *E. coli* DHFR complex are absent, regardless of the orientation of the side chain of Tyr-31. As shown in Figure 11, the trimethoxyphenyl group of TMP does not bind in the (apparently unfavorable) lower region of the chicken DHFR cleft but binds instead in a niche at the upper end of the cavity that appears to provide a more favorable environment. However, the geometry of

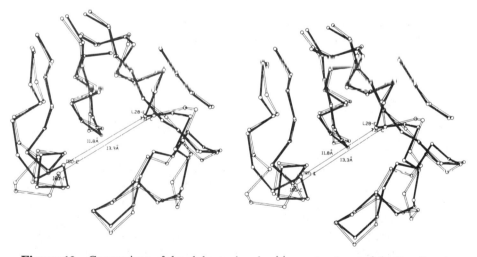

Figure 12 Comparison of the alpha-carbon backbone structures of the *E. coli* and chicken ternary complexes with TMP. The *E. coli* protein is shown with filled bonds, and chicken DHFR with open bonds. The two proteins were superimposed by the least-squares procedure in MacroModel (61) using the alpha-carbons of the B and C helices. The distances between Leu-28 and Ile-50 of the *E. coli* enzyme and Tyr-31 and Ile-60 of the chicken protein are shown.

TMP is such that to position its trimethoxyphenyl ring in that upper binding site requires placing the pyrimidine ring in a less than optimal location. Compared to other diaminopyrimidine-containing complexes, the pyrimidine ring of TMP in the chicken DHFR complex is located about 1 Å closer to the B-helix, and in contrast to those other complexes, the 4-amino group is too distant (4 Å) from the carbonyl oxygen of Val-115 for a hydrogen bond. The lack of that hydrogen bond in the chicken enzyme complex is one relatively clear-cut structural detail that contributes to the differential affinity of TMP, although it probably is not the only cause of the 5 kcal/mol difference in binding energy. A combination of many subtle differences in intermolecular interactions, including those of water molecules, probably accounts for the selectivity of TMP. A complete understanding of those differences remains a challenge to experimentalists and theoreticians alike.

IV.   INHIBITOR DESIGN

The three-dimensional structures of DHFR offer the medicinal chemist an unusual opportunity to learn about drug-receptor interactions and to explore the possibilities of rational inhibitor design. Although the number of examples of successful inhibitor design based on DHFR structure is still somewhat small, the cases published are encouraging, especially because the DHFR active site has already been probed by thousands of known inhibitors (48). A few examples of how the DHFR structure can be used to model the interactions of active-site-directed, irreversible inhibitors are discussed below, followed by illustrations of receptor-based design of reversible DHFR inhibitors.

A.   Active-Site-Directed, Irreversible Inhibitors

1.   Example 1

The dihydrotriazine DHFR inhibitor 4, which arose from the pioneering work of Baker on the design of active-site-directed, irreversible enzyme inhibitors (59), has been shown to bind specifically to the hydroxyl group of Tyr-31 of DHFR from chicken liver by amino acid sequence studies of the covalently bound enzyme (60). Although the compound was designed a number of years ago without the aid of enzyme structure, it might be instructive for future design of irreversible inhibitors to use the three-dimensional structure of chicken DHFR for modeling the covalent complex of compound 4.

Figure 13 depicts one possible model of that covalent complex that we constructed using the computer program MacroModel (61). The covalent

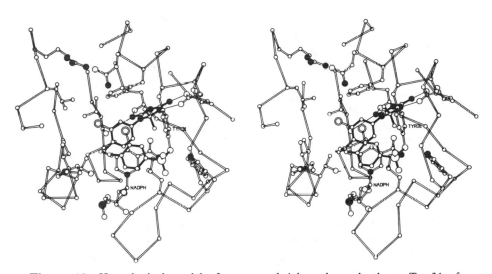

Figure 13 Hypothetical model of compound 4 bound covalently to Tyr-31 of chicken DHFR. Protein is represented by alpha-carbon backbone and selected amino acid side chains and is shown with open bonds. NADPH is also shown with open bonds, and the bonds of compound 4 are filled. Carbon atoms are represented by small open circles, oxygen atoms by larger open circles, the sulfur by the largest open circle, nitrogen by blackened circles, the phosphorus atom by the larger blackened circle, and chlorine atoms by two concentric circles. Selected hydrogen bonds are shown as single lines between atoms.

bond to the phenol oxygen atom of Tyr-31 can be formed from a conformation of compound 4 that appears to be relatively free of strain. The diaminodihydrotriazine ring is favorably positioned for donating hydrogen bonds to the now well-established acceptor oxygen atoms of the protein active site, and the lengthy aryl substituent appears to be sterically compatible with the active site geometry.

2. Example 2

An irreversible analog of MTX has been reported by Rosowsky et al. (62) in which the gamma-carboxy function was modified for potential covalent attachment to His-28 of *L. casei* DHFR. His-28 is the binding site for the gamma carboxyl group of MTX as shown by x-ray crystallography (see Fig. 6). The inhibitor, compound 5, does show irreversible inhibition of the *L. casei* enzyme, and sequence analysis of the covalent complex confirmed the involvement of His-28 (63). Interestingly, detailed analysis of the labeled histidine residue showed equivalent amounts of the two isomeric forms of the histidine derivative: alkylation of His-28 occurred nonselectively on both the delta and epsilon nitrogens. The noncovalent form of the enzyme-inhibitor complex must be sufficiently mobile in the region of His-28 to allow formation of the two isomeric species of the covalent complex.

3. Example 3

Johanson and Henkin have designed and synthesized an arginine-specific irreversible inhibitor based on the x-ray crystal structures of *E. coli* and *L. casei* DHFR bound to MTX (64). Molecular modeling led to the prediction that the alpha-diketone functionality of compound 6 would interact covalently with *E. coli* and *L. casei* DHFR but with nonhomologous arginine residues in the two enzymes. In the *E. coli* DHFR-MTX structure, Arg-52 is hydrogen-bonded to the amide carbonyl oxygen of MTX, as shown in Figure 14, and would presumably be well positioned for reaction with the alpha-diketone function of compound 6. In contrast, the side chain of Arg-52 in the *L. casei* DHFR-MTX-NADPH complex does not associate with MTX but is folded back to hydrogen-bond to a backbone carbonyl oxygen (see Fig. 6).

A one-residue insertion preceding Arg-52 in the *L. casei* enzyme amino acid sequence, compared to the *E. coli* DHFR sequence (see Table 1), is probably responsible for this difference in the orientation of Arg-52 in the two structures. Molecular modeling suggested that conformational adjustment of the arginine side chain in the *L. casei* DHFR structure for interaction with the diketone group of compound 6 was not possible because of steric interactions

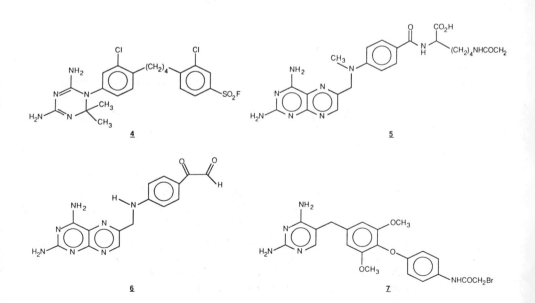

with adjacent side chains. The side chain of Arg-31, on the other hand, can be readily positioned close to the diketone of compound 6 and was therefore predicted to be the site of covalent interaction in the *L. casei* enzyme. Arg-31 of *L. casei* DHFR corresponds in sequence to Lys-32 of the *E. coli* enzyme. Compound 6 irreversibly inactivated the two species of DHFR under appropriate conditions, and analysis of peptide fragments from the two covalent complexes was consistent with the modeling predictions.

4. Example 4

One last example of covalently bound inhibitors is the trimethoprim analog 7, another compound that was prepared prior to the availability of DHFR structures. The inhibitor irreversibly inactivates DHFR from *L. casei* and *N. gonorrhoeae* but binds only reversibly to the enzyme from chicken and *E. coli* (65). Molecular modeling of compound 7 in the *L. casei* DHFR crystal structure has been used to predict the site of covalent attachment of compound 7 to that enzyme (66).

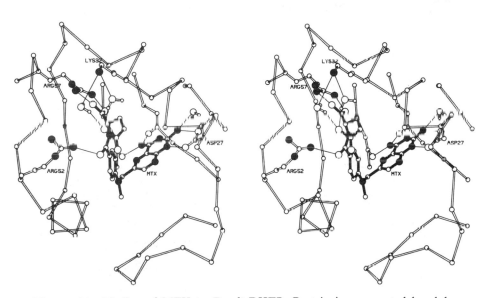

Figure 14 Binding of MTX to *E coli* DHFR. Protein is represented by alpha-carbon backbone, selected amino acid side chains, and two backbone carbonyl groups that hydrogen-bond to MTX. The protein is shown with open MTX with filled bonds. Hydrogen atoms, included only for the water molecule, are represented by very small open circles; carbon atoms, by small open circles; oxygen atoms, by larger open circles; and nitrogen atoms, by blackened circles. Selected hydrogen bonds are shown by single lines between atoms.

The active site of the *L. casei* enzyme contains three histidine residues that appeared to be potential sites for alkylation by compound 7. A molecular model of each of the six possible isomeric covalent complexes (one for each histidine side-chain nitrogen) was constructed and energy-minimized using the molecular mechanics software package called AMBER (58). The hypothetical structure with compound 7 linked to the delta-nitrogen of His-22 was significantly lower in energy than any of the other five model complexes, and subsequent sequence analysis of the covalently labeled enzyme confirmed the linkage to His-22 (67), although verification of the predicted selectivity for the delta nitrogen was not attempted. The hypothetical model of compound 7 bound to His-22 is shown in Figure 15. As in the case of the chicken DHFR–compound 4 covalent complex, modeling suggests that compound 7 can bind covalently in a low-energy conformation and with reasonable complementarity to the enzyme active site.

In agreement with studies on the irreversibility of compound 7, the structural equivalent of His-22 exists in *N. gonorrhoeae* DHFR (His-25) but not in DHFR from *E. coli* (Asn-23) or chicken (Pro-26), as shown in Table 1. Sequence studies of the *N. gonorrhoeae* DHFR covalent complex show that

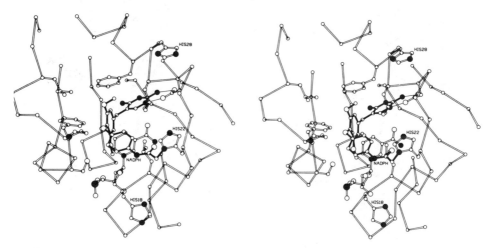

Figure 15 Hypothetical model of compound 7 bound covalently to His-22 of *L. casei* DHFR. Compound 7 is shown with filled bonds, and protein and NADPH are shown with open bonds. Only side chains of the three active-site histidines are labeled. Carbon atoms are represented by small open circles, oxygen atoms by larger open circles, nitrogen atoms by blackened circles, and the phosphorus atom by the larger blackened circle. Selected hydrogen bonds are shown as single lines between atoms.

His-25 of that enzyme is indeed modified by compound 7 (65). The success of this semiquantitative modeling study suggests that methodology of this type might be useful to de novo design of irreversible inhibitors.

B. Reversible, Competitive Inhibitors

1. Example 1

The first example of successful receptor-based design of reversible DHFR inhibitors was published in 1982 (68). In that work the structure of *E. coli* DHFR in complex with MTX was used to design analogs of TMP. Because the mode of TMP binding to DHFR was not known at that time, the design goals of that effort were to prepare analogs of TMP that would not only exhibit very strong affinity for *E. coli* DHFR but that might also provide some insight into the geometry of DHFR binding of TMP and related inhibitors. The result of that study was a series of TMP analogs that incorporated carboxyl functionalities designed to interact ionically with an active-site cation.

The active site of *E. coli* DHFR contains three positively charged residues—Lys-32, Arg-52, and Arg-57. In the *E. coli* DHFR-MTX crystal structure, each of those residues is associated with MTX but in different ways, as shown in Figure 14. The gamma-carboxy group of MTX interacts with the side chain of Lys-32; however, that interaction appears to be weak and is actually mediated through intervening water molecules at the exposed surface of the protein. The side chain of Arg-52 is also solvent-exposed and forms a hydrogen bond to the carbonyl oxygen of the p-aminobenzoic acid unit of MTX. In contrast to the solvent-accessible environment of Lys-32 and Arg-52, the local surroundings of Arg-57 are hydrophobic. Only the diamino edge of the guanidinium group is exposed to solvent, and the group is located in a recessed pocket composed of several lipophilic residues. The alpha-carboxy group of MTX is linked to Arg-57 through two hydrogen bonds in what appears to be a strong interaction (69). That interaction and the buried location of Arg-57 made that potential binding site for TMP analogs stand out among the three residues in question.

A series of carboxy-containing analogs of TMP, compounds 8a–f, were prepared with the purpose of probing for a favorable ionic interaction. The observed DHFR affinity data for those compounds and their ester derivatives, shown in Table 3, strongly suggest that the desired interaction does occur. All but one of the acidic analogs are significantly more active than TMP and also more active than the corresponding neutral esters.

Based on the affinity data and molecular modeling experiments, a hypothetical model for the binding of TMP and those acidic analogs was proposed. With the pyrimidine ring of TMP modeled to bind to *E. coli*

Table 3   Affinity Data from a Series of Acid and Ester
Analogs of TMP and *E. coli* DHFR

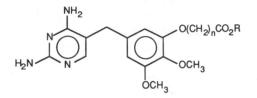

10^9 K_i, M

n	Acid (R=H)	Ester (R=Me, Et)
TMP	1.3	
1	2.6	11.
2	0.37	—
3	0.035	0.47
4	0.066	0.76
5	0.024	0.86
6	0.050	1.9

DHFR in a manner identical to that observed for that ring of MTX, the
trimethoxybenzyl group appeared to be sterically compatible with the active-
site geometry when oriented in the low-energy conformation that had been
found in the crystal structure of TMP hydrobromide (56). This model for
TMP binding positioned one of the metamethoxy groups so that the
carboxyalkyl substituents of the acidic analogs projected directly toward the
guanidinium group of Arg-57. The distance between the methoxy group and
Arg-57 was consistent with the relatively weak binding of the carboxymeth-
oxy analog and the intermediate activity of the carboxyethoxy analog.
Neither substituent was sufficiently long to place the carboxy group into
optimal juxtaposition with Arg-57.

This model for TMP binding was confirmed by the x-ray crystal structure
of the *E. coli* DHFR-TMP complex discussed above, and the proposed
interaction of the acidic analogs with Arg-57 was also verified by x-ray
crystallography (29). The structures of the carboxypentoxy and carboxyethoxy analogs in complex with *E. coli* DHFR are shown in Figures 16
and 17, respectively. The carboxyl group of the former compound is closely
associated with Arg-57, consistent with its exceptionally strong affinity for the
enzyme. Conversely, the shorter-chain analog of intermediate activity positions its carboxyl farther from Arg-57, engaging in only one hydrogen bond.

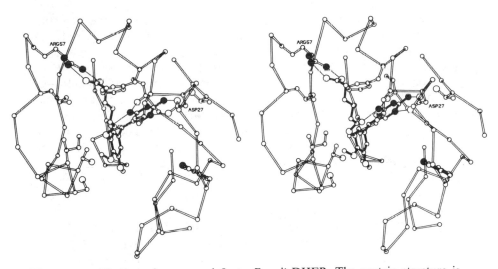

Figure 16 Binding of compound 8e to *E. coli* DHFR. The protein structure is shown with open bonds, and bonds of compound 8e are filled. Carbon atoms are represented by small open circles, oxygen atoms by larger open circles, and nitrogen atoms by blackened circles. Selected hydrogen bonds are depicted by single lines between atoms.

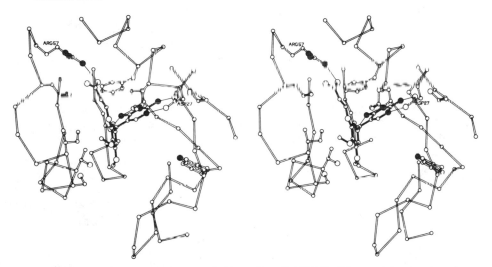

Figure 17 Binding of compound 8b to *E. coli* DHFR. The protein structure is shown with open bonds, and bonds of compound 8b are filled. Carbon atoms are represented by small open circles, oxygen atoms by larger open circles, and nitrogen atoms by blackened circles. Selected hydrogen bonds are depicted by single lines between atoms.

   This successful example of inhibitor design, synthesis, and structure
determination of the enzyme-inhibitor complex should illustrate the potential
of this approach to drug design. One can imagine performing this sequence of
steps in an iterative fashion to fine-tune the desired properties of the inhibitor.
For example, in the case above the carboxylic acid functionalities enhanced
enzyme affinity but also caused a decrease of antibacterial activity, presumably because of barriers to penetration of the bacterial cell wall by negatively
charged groups. We have searched for substituents that interact with the
arginine-binding site but do not impede cell penetration. Molecular modeling
of those hypothetical inhibitors into the DHFR active site was used to assess
the potential for binding to Arg-57. A sample of that work has been reported
(28) and is illustrated by compound 9, in which an acyl sulfonamide unit
serves as the anionic partner for Arg-57. Exceptional enzyme affinity
suggested that the sulfonamide was indeed capable of binding to the arginine
side chain, and x-ray crystallography of the *E. coli* DHFR-9 complex
confirmed that. The structure of that complex is shown in Figure 18.
However, that compound too was found to be relatively inactive against
bacterial cell cultures.

2.   Example 2

Independent of the above work, a similar study was subsequently reported in
which acidic analogs of brodimoprim (structure 10) were designed to interact
with Arg-57 and also His-28 of *L. casei* DHFR (70, 71). Analogs of compound
10 that correspond to those of TMP discussed above were prepared and
found to inhibit DHFR in a manner similar to that observed for the TMP
analogs. These workers also synthesized analogs of compound 10 with two
carboxylic acid substituents, one to interact with Arg-57 and another to bind
to His-28 in analogy to the interactions observed for the glutamate moiety of
MTX. An impressive 3000-fold increase in affinity over that of parent
inhibitor 10 for *L. casei* DHFR was found for compound 11, and the

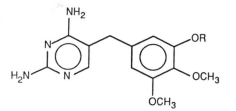

8: R = -(CH$_2$)$_n$CO$_2$H
 a-**f**: n = 1-6, respectively

9: R = -CH$_2$CONHSO$_2$—⬡—NH$_2$

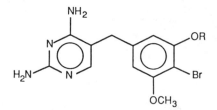

10: R = CH$_3$

11: R = -(CH$_2$)$_3$CH(CH$_2$)$_2$CO$_2$H
                    |
                 CO$_2$H

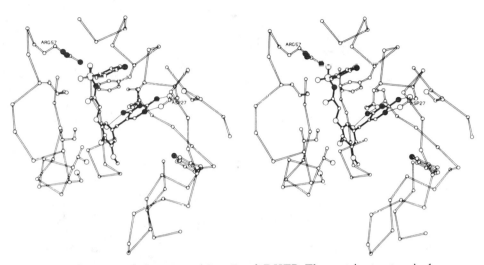

Figure 18   Binding of compound 9 to *E. coli* DHFR. The protein structure is shown with open bonds, and bonds of compound 9 are filled. Carbon atoms are represented by small open circles, oxygen atoms by larger open circles, the sulfur atom by the largest open circle, and nitrogen atoms by blackened circles. Selected hydrogen bonds are depicted by single lines between atoms.

association with His-28 was confirmed by NMR studies (72). The two examples of inhibitor design described above take advantage of electrostatic interactions. The following two examples focus instead on the hydrophobic core of the active site.

3.   Example 3

Maag et al. recently reported the design of novel DHFR inhibitors based primarily on structural matching to MTX in its complex with *E. coli* DHFR (73). Hypothetical inhibitors were constructed to match the relative orientation of the diaminopyrimidine and phenyl rings of MTX and simultaneously minimize steric contacts between the enzyme active site and those parts of the inhibitor that do not correspond to MTX. The results of that study are exemplified by compound 12, a very potent inhibitor of DHFR from *E. coli* as well as other sources, in which a nortropan moiety serves to hold the phenyl and pyrimidine rings in the desired relative orientation. Figure 19 shows MTX in the conformation found in its complex with *E. coli* DHFR superimposed with a model of compound 12 that was generated using MacroModel. Our version of a hypothetical model of inhibitor 12 bound to the *E. coli* enzyme is presented in Figure 20.

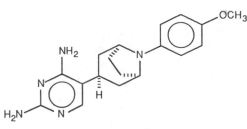

12

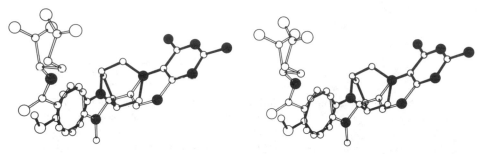

Figure 19 A hypothetical model of compound 12 matched to MTX from its complex with *E. coli* DHFR. The diaminopyrimidine rings were superimposed, and the conformation of compound 12 was then adjusted for optimal matching of the two phenyl rings. Carbon atoms are represented by small open circles, oxygen atoms by larger open circles, and nitrogen atoms by blackened circles.

4. Example 4

In another study, conformationally restricted analogs of TMP were designed in an attempt to furnish inhibitors of superior DHFR selectivity (74). The concept and usefulness of conformationally restricted analogs of drug molecules are well recognized, but that type of compound is normally prepared in attempts to define the unknown, active conformation of the parent drug. That conformational information is known and can be used for analog design with TMP. As discussed in an earlier section of this chapter, the conformation of TMP bound to *E. coli* DHFR is very different from that of the chicken DHFR-TMP complex, and we have attempted to enhance the differential affinity for these two enzymes by altering the TMP structure to favor the conformation of the *E. coli* enzyme complex. Compounds 13–16 were designed with that purpose.

Linking carbon-6 of the pyrimidine ring of TMP to the ortho position of the trimethoxyphenyl ring by a three-carbon bridge produces a tricyclic

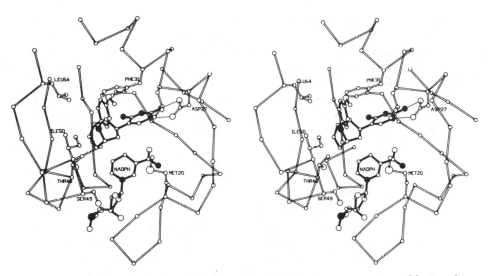

Figure 20 Hypothetical model of compound 12 in ternary complex with *E. coli* DHFR. Protein structure is shown with open bonds and NADPH, and compound 12 is shown with filled bonds. Carbon atoms are represented by small open circles, oxygen atoms by larger open circles, and nitrogen atoms by blackened circles.

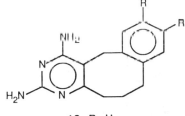

13: R = H
14: R = OCH₃

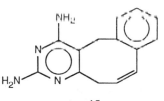

15

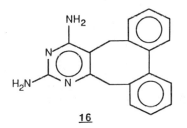

16

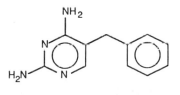

17

structure with a central eight-membered ring of limited conformational flexibility. Compound 13, for example, appears to have four low-energy conformations based on molecular mechanics calculations and NMR data. The conformations, two sets of mirror-image pairs, are shown in Figure 21. Similar to dibenzocyclooctane (75), compound 13 can adopt a twist-boat conformation, forms A and A' in Figure 21, or a chair conformation, forms B and B'. The chair conformation of the free base of compound 13 in methanol is somewhat more stable than the twist-boat conformation, as shown by NMR studies.

Compound 13 was designed to mimic the conformation of TMP in the *E. coli* DHFR complex, and as shown in Figure 22, the twist-boat form A of compound 13 matches that TMP conformation relatively well. The overall compatibility of form A of compound 13 with the active-site geometry of *E. coli* DHFR was evaluated using molecular mechanics modeling in a manner similar to that used by Blaney et al. (76). Although that type of calculation is generally inadequate for quantitative estimates of enzyme-inhibitor inter-

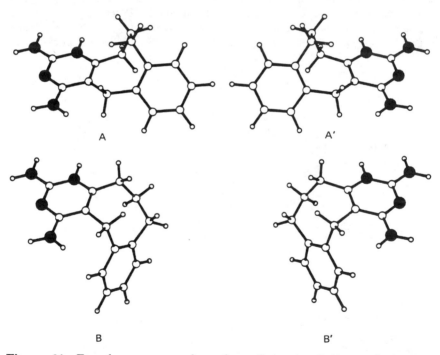

Figure 21 Four low-energy conformations of compound 13 as calculated by molecular mechanics. Forms A and A' are twist-boat conformations, and B and B' are chair conformations.

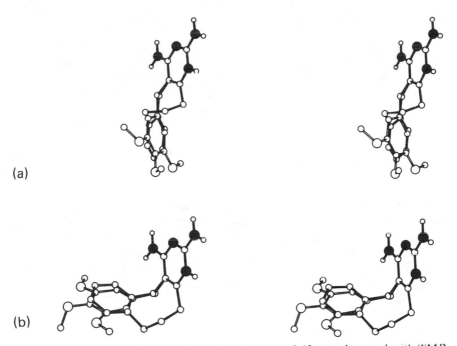

Figure 22 (a) Stereo image of form A of compound 13 superimposed with TMP from its *E. coli* DHFR ternary complex. Carbons are shown as small open circles, oxygens as larger open circles, and nitrogens as blackened circles. (b) Stereo image of form B′ superimposed with TMP from its chicken DHFR ternary complex.

action energies, primarily because it does not address the effects of solvent and entropy, we have found reasonable agreement between differences in calculated interaction energies and differences in observed binding constants for *E. coli* DHFR and a series of closely related analogs of TMP (77). Comparison of the calculated interaction energy of forms A and A′ with those obtained for the series of TMP analogs suggested that the geometry of A and A′, including the three-carbon bridge, was compatible with the binding cleft of the *E. coli* enzyme. As shown in Table 4, the measured activity of compound 13 against *E. coli* DHFR exceeds that of the unsubstituted benzylpyrimidine 17, in agreement with the modeling predictions.

Inhibitor 13 was designed prior to the availability of the x-ray crystal structure of TMP bound to chicken DHFR and was based only on the *E. coli* DHFR-bound conformation of TMP and the hope that conformational restriction would enhance selectivity. As shown in Table 4, the selectivity of 13 for *E. coli* DHFR versus rat liver DHFR is disappointingly low, but that

Table 4 DHFR Inhibition Data for TMP and Several Analogs

Compound No.	*E. coli* $10^8 I_{50}$, M	Rat liver $10^8 I_{50}$, M	Selectivity ratio
1 (TMP)	0.7	35,000	50,000.
17	340.	15,000	44.
13	17.	67	3.9
14	1.3	1,660	1,277.
16	8.	1,800	225.

was subsequently rationalized by the observation that the conformation adopted by TMP in its complex with chicken DHFR is similar to conformation B′ of compound 13, as illustrated in Figure 22. Much to our chagrin, the conformational limitations imposed by the three-carbon bridge of compound 13 precisely selected both of the conformations observed for TMP in its DHFR complexes and actually decreased the differential affinity for the two species of enzyme.

Analysis of the geometry of the A and B types of conformation of compound 13 suggested that for an analog containing a double bond in the

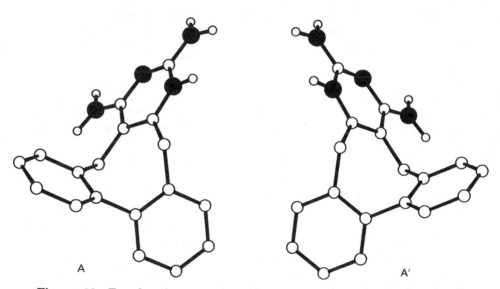

Figure 23 Two low-energy conformations of compound 16 as calculated by molecular mechanics. Carbon atoms are represented by small open circles, and nitrogen atoms by larger blackened circles.

three-carbon linkage, such as structure 15, the B type of conformation would be greatly disfavored because of geometry requirements of the double bond. Molecular mechanics calculations indicated that structure 15 would be capable of adopting only one pair of mirror-image conformations similar to the A-type pair of compound 13, the two that closely match the conformation of TMP in its *E. coli* DHFR complex. Based on conformational studies, one would predict that structure 15 would exhibit greater DHFR selectivity than compound 13. Unfortunately, we encountered difficulties in the synthesis of compound 15 and opted for an alternative target with similar conformational characteristics.

Conformational properties of structure 16, as calculated by molecular mechanics, were very similar to those of structure 15, and the mirror-image pair of calculated conformations of structure 16 are shown in Figure 23. This

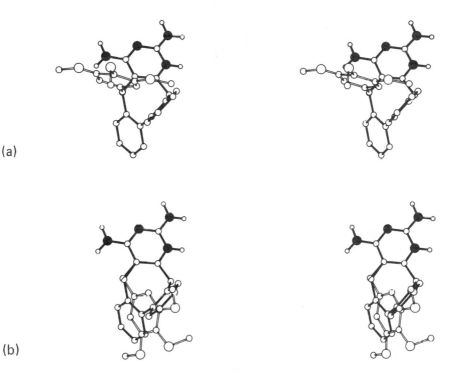

(a)

(b)

Figure 24 (a) Stereo image of form A′ of compound 16 superimposed with TMP from its chicken DHFR ternary complex. Carbons are represented as small open circles, oxygens as larger open circles, and nitrogens as blackened circles. (b) Stereo image of form A′ of compound 16 superimposed with TMP from its *E. coli* DHFR ternary complex.

biphenyl derivative was also relatively easy to synthesize. As illustrated in
Figure 24, form A of compound 16 superimposes reasonably well with the *E.
coli* DHFR-bound form of TMP but does not match the chicken DHFR-
bound conformation. Similar differentiation was found for form A' of
structure 16. The degree of complementarity of 16 with the active site of *E.
coli* DHFR appeared high, according to molecular mechanics calculations, in
spite of the extra bulk of the additional phenyl group. A hypothetical model
of compound 16 bound to *E. coli* DHFR is shown in Figure 25. Similar
calculations on the corresponding chicken DHFR complex are of obvious
interest but have not yet been done.

Consistent with our expectations, compound 16 did exhibit high affinity
for the *E. coli* enzyme and was 50-fold more selective than compound 13.
Presumably the selectivity of structure 16 could be further improved with
appropriate substitution. The effect on selectivity of methoxy groups, for
example, can be significant, as shown by the comparison of activities in Table
3 for compounds 13 and 14 and also benzylpyrimidine 17 and TMP.
Structure 16 offers a number of sites for such substitution.

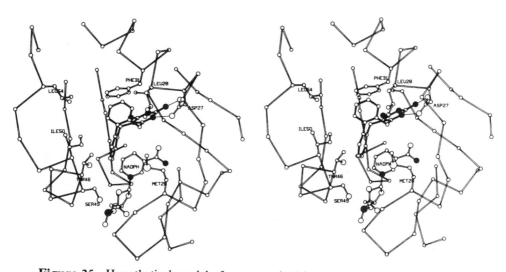

Figure 25 Hypothetical model of compound 16 in ternary complex with *E. coli*
DHFR. Protein and NADPH structure are represented by open bonds, and
compound 16 by filled bonds. Carbon atoms are shown as small open circles, oxygen
atoms as larger open circles, the sulfur atom as the largest open circle, nitrogen atoms
as blackened circles, and the phosphorus atom as the larger blackened circle. Selected
hydrogen bonds are shown as single lines between atoms.

III. CONCLUSIONS

Recently a variety of experimental methods, especially protein crystallography, have dramatically increased our understanding of the molecular interactions that control the affinity between DHFR and various ligands. The examples of inhibitor design described above show how that information has begun to lead to ligands of novel structure. Knowledge of receptor structure clearly provides a logical basis for the design of unique ligands and, coupled with luck and design strategies based on factors associated with metabolism, pharmacokinetics, distribution, toxicity, etc., will very likely lead to novel and useful drugs in the near future.

The binding of an inhibitor to an enzyme is a very complex process that involves not only interactions between enzyme and inhibitor but also interactions of the inhibitor and enzyme, both free and complexed, with solvent molecules. Additionally, entropic contributions to the overall process can be very important. In the evaluation of hypothetical ligands, that is, potential targets for synthesis, one would like to be able to predict accurately DHFR binding constants, and to do that in a general way, the full complexity of the problem must be addressed. Exciting new computational methods (78–81), together with ever-increasing computer power, may soon make that kind of prediction practical. However, even without such accurate predictions, the three-dimensional structure of DHFR has permitted the successful design of novel compounds with potent activities.

ACKNOWLEDGMENTS

Various sets of x-ray coordinates of DHFR were generously provided by Drs. David Matthews and Joseph Kraut, whom we also thank for a preprint of their review article (4). We are grateful to Jim Bentley for valuable assistance with the computer-related activities necessary to this chapter and to Drs. Mike Cory and David Henry for their continued interest and support of this approach to drug design. Drs. David Baccanari and Robert Ferone have provided DHFR-related data and insight, and their suggested changes to this manuscript are appreciated. Dr. Chris Beddell is acknowledged for originally suggesting compound 13 as a conformationally constrained analog of TMP. Computer programs TEXSAN GRAPHICS from Molecular Structure Corp., College Station, TX, and MacroModel (61) were used to compose and plot the figures presented in this chapter.

REFERENCES

1. Roth, B., and C. C. Cheng, Recent progress in the medicinal chemistry of 2,4-diaminopyrimidines. In *Progress in Medicinal Chemistry*, Vol. 19, C. P. Ellis and G. B. West, eds. Elsevier Biomedical Press, Amsterdam, pp. 269–331 (1982).

2. Salter, A. J., Trimethoprim-sulfamethoxazole: An assessment of more than 12 years of use. *Rev. Infect. Dis. 4*:196–236 (1982).

3. Hitchings, G. H., The metabolism of plasmodia and the chemotherapy of malarial infections. In *Tropical Medicine from Romance to Reality*, C. Wood, ed. Academic Press, London, pp. 79–98 (1978).

4. Kraut, J., and D. A. Matthews, Dihydrofolate reductase. In *Biological Macromolecules and Assemblies*, Vol. III. F. Jurnak and A. McPherson, eds. John Wiley and Sons, New York, pp. 1–71 (1987).

5. Hitchings, G. H., L. F. Kuyper, and D. P. Baccanari, Selective inhibitors of dihydrofolate reductase. In *Design of Enzyme Inhibitors as Drugs*, M. Sandler and H. J. Smith, eds. Oxford University Press, New York (in press).

6. Champness, J. N., L. F. Kuyper, and C. R. Beddell, Interaction between dihydrofolate reductase and certain inhibitors. In *Topics in Molecular Pharmacology*, Vol. 3, A. S. V. Burgen, G. C. K. Roberts, and M. S. Tute, eds. Elsevier, New York, pp. 335–362 (1986).

7. Roth, B., Design of dihydrofolate reductase inhibitors from x-ray crystal structures. *Fed. Proc. 45*:2765–2772 (1986).

8. Blakley, R. L., Dihydrofolate reductase. In *Folates and Pterins*, Vol. 1, R. L. Blakley and S. J. Benkovic, eds. John Wiley and Sons, New York, pp. 191–253 (1984).

9. Freisheim, J. H., and D. A. Matthews, The comparative biochemistry of dihydrofolate reductase. In *Folate Antagonists as Therapeutic Agents*, Vol. 1, F. M. Sirotnak, J. J. Burchall, W. D. Ensminger, and J. A. Montgomery, eds. Academic Press, New York, pp. 69–131 (1984).

10. Beddell, C. R., Dihydrofolate reductase: Its structure, function, and binding properties. In *X-Ray Crystallography and Drug Action*, A. S. Horn and C. J. DeRanter, eds. Oxford University Press, New York, pp. 169–193 (1984).

11. Roth, B., Selective inhibitors of bacterial dihydrofolate reductase: Structure-activity relationships. In *Handbook of Experimental Pharmacology*, Vol. 64, G. H. Hitchings, ed. Springer-Verlag, New York, pp. 107–127 (1983).

12. Hitchings, G. H., Functions of tetrahydrofolate and the role of dihydrofolate reductase in cellular metabolism. In *Handbook of Experimental Pharmacology*, Vol. 64, G. H. Hitchings, ed. Springer-Verlag, New York, pp. 11–23 (1983).

13. Blakley, R. L., and S. J. Benkovic, eds., *Folates and Pterins*, Vol. 1. John Wiley and Sons, New York (1984).

14. Baccanari, D. P., D. Stone, and L. Kuyper, Effect of a single amino acid substitution on *Escherichia coli* dihydrofolate reductase catalysis and ligand binding. *J. Biol Chem. 256*:1738–1747 (1981).

15. Bitar, K. G., D. T. Blankenship, K. A. Walsh, R. B. Dunlap, A. V. Reddy, and J. H. Freisheim, Amino acid sequence of dihydrofolate reductase from an amethopterin-resistant strain of *Lactobacillus casei*. *FEBS Lett. 80*:119–122 (1977).

16. Baccanari, D. P., R. L. Tansik, S. J. Paterson, and D. Stone, Characterization and amino acid sequence of *Neisseria gonorrhoeae* dihydrofolate reductase. *J. Biol. Chem. 259*:12291–12298 (1984).

17. Kumar, A. A., D. T. Blankenship, B. T. Kaufman, and J. H. Freisheim, Primary structure of chicken liver dihydrofolate reductase. *Biochemistry 19*:667–678 (1980).

18. Masters, J. N., and G. Attardi, The nucleotide sequence of the cDNA coding for the human dihydrofolic acid reductase. *Gene 21*:59–63 (1983).

19. Stone, D., S. J. Paterson, J. H. Raper, and A. W. Phillips, The amino acid sequence of dihydrofolate reductase from the mouse lymphoma L1210. *J. Biol. Chem. 254*:480–488 (1979).

20. Volz, K. W., D. A. Matthews, R. A. Alden, S. T. Freer, C. Hansch, B. T. Kaufman, and J. Kraut, Crystal structure of avian dihydrofolate reductase containing phenyltriazine and NADPH. *J. Biol Chem. 257*:2528–2536 (1982).

21. Matthews, D. A., R. A. Alden, J. T. Bolin, D. J. Filman, S. T. Freer, R. Hamlin, W. G. J. Hol. R. L. Kisliuk, E. J. Pastore, L. T. Plante, N. Xuong, and J. Kraut, Dihydrofolate reductase from *Lactobacillus casei*: X-ray structure of the enzyme-methotrexate-NADPH complex. *J. Biol. Chem. 253*:6946–6954 (1978).

22. Bolin, J. T., D. J. Filman, D. A. Matthews, R. C. Hamlin, and J. Kraut, Crystal structures of *Escherichia coli* and *Lactobacillus casei* dihydrofolate reductase refined at 1.7Å resolution. I. General features and binding of methotrexate. *J. Biol. Chem. 257*:13650–13662 (1982).

23. Filman, D. J., J. T. Bolin, D. A. Matthews, and J. Kraut, Crystal structures of *Escherichia coli* and *Lactobacillus casei* dihydrofolate reductase refined at 1.7Å resolution. II. Environment of bound NADPH and implications for catalysis. *J. Biol. Chem. 257*:13663–13672 (1982).

24. Matthews, D. A., R. A. Alden, J. T. Bolin, S. T. Freer, R. Hamlin, N. Xuong, J. Kraut, M. Poe, M. Williams, and K. Hoogsteen, Dihydrofolate reductase: X-ray structure of the binary complex with methotrexate. *Science 197*:452–455 (1977).

25. Baker, D. J., C. R. Beddell, J. N. Champness, P. J. Goodford, F. E. A. Norrington, D. R. Smith, and D. K. Stammers, The binding of trimethoprim to bacterial dihydrofolate reductase. *FEBS Lett. 126*:49–52 (1981).

26. Matthews, D. A., J. T. Bolin, J. M. Burridge, D. J. Filman, K. W. Volz, B. T. Kaufman, C. R. Beddell, J. N. Champness, D. K. Stammers, and J. Kraut, Refined crystal structures of *Escherichia coli* and chicken liver dihydrofolate reductase containing bound trimethoprim. *J. Biol Chem. 260*:381–391 (1985).

27. Baker, D. J., C. R. Beddell, J. N. Champness, P. J. Goodford, F. E. Norrington, B. Roth, and D. K. Stammers, X-ray studies of the binding of trimethoprim, methotrexate, pyrimethamine and two trimethoprim analogues to bacterial dihydrofolate reductase. In *Chemistry and Biology of Pteridines*, J. A. Blair, ed. Walter de Gruyter, New York, pp. 545–549 (1983).

28. Hyde, R. M., R. A. Paterson, C. R. Beddell, J. N. Champness, D. K. Stammers, D. J. Baker, P. J. Goodford, L. F. Kuyper, R. Ferone, B. Roth, and L. P. Elwell, The activity of sulfonamide-substituted benzylpyrimidines against dihydropteroate synthase, dihydrofolate reductase, and bacterial cell cultures. In *Chemistry and Biology of Pteridines*, J. A. Blair, ed. Walter de Gruyter, New York, pp. 505–509 (1983).

29. Kuyper, L. F., B. Roth, D. P. Baccanari, R. Ferone, C. R. Beddell, J. N. Champness, D. K. Stammers, J. G. Dann, F. E. A. Norrington, D. J. Baker, and P. J. Goodford, Receptor-based design of dihydrofolate reductase inhibitors: Comparison of crystallographically determined enzyme binding with enzyme affinity in a series of carboxy-substituted trimethoprim analogues. *J. Med. Chem.* 28:303–311 (1985).

30. Champness, J. N., D. K. Stammers, and C. R. Beddell, Crystallographic investigation of the cooperative interaction between trimethoprim, reduced cofactor and dihydrofolate reductase. *FEBS Lett.* 199:61–67 (1986).

31. Matthews, D. A., J. T. Bolin, J. M. Burridge, D. J. Filman, K. W. Volz, and J. Kraut, Dihydrofolate reductase. The stereochemistry of inhibitor selectivity. *J. Biol. Chem.* 260:392–399 (1985).

32. Stammers, D. K., J. N. Champness, J. G. Dann, and C. R. Beddell, The three-dimensional structure of mouse L1210 dihydrofolate reductase. In *Chemistry and Biology of Pteridines*, J. A. Blair, ed. Walter de Gruyter, New York, pp. 567–571 (1983).

33. Stammers, D. K., J. N. Champness, C. R. Beddell, J. G. Dann, E. Eliopoulos, A. J. Geddes, D. Ogg, and A. C. T. North, The structure of mouse L1210 dihydro-folate reductase-drug complexes, and the construction of a model of human enzyme. *FEBS Lett.* 218: 178–184 (1987).

34. Matthews, D. A., S. L. Smith, D. P. Baccanari, J. J. Burchall, S. J. Oatley, and J. Kraut, Crystal structure of a novel trimethoprim-resistant dihydrofolate re-ductase specified in *Escherichia coli* by R-plasmid R67. *Biochemistry* 25:4194–4204 (1986).

35. Richardson, J. S., The anatomy and taxonomy of protein structure. *Adv. Prot. Chem.* 34:167–339 (1981).

36. Hol, W. G. J., The role of the alpha-helix dipole in protein function and structure. *Prog. Biophys. Mol. Biol.* 45:149–195 (1985).

37. Howell, E. E., J. E. Villafranca, M. S. Warren, S. J. Oatley, and J. Kraut, Functional role of aspartic acid-27 in dihydrofolate reductase revealed by mutagenensis. *Science* 231:1123–1128 (1986).

38. Stuber, D., H. Bujard, E. Hochuli, H. P. Kocher, I. Kompis, K. Talmadge, E. K. Weibel, F. K. Winkler, and R. L. Then, Enzymatic characterization of recombi-nant human dihydrofolate reductase produced in *E. coli*. In *Chemistry and Biology of Pteridines 1986*, B. A. Cooper and V. M. Whitehead, eds. Walter de Gruyter, New York, pp. 839–842 (1986).

39. Fontecilla-Camps, J. C., C. E. Bugg, C. Temple Jr., J. D. Rose, J. A. Montgomery, and R. L. Kisliuk, Absolute configuration of biological tetrahydrofolates: A crystallographic determination. *J. Am. Chem. Soc.* 101:6114–6115 (1979).

40. Charlton, P. A., D. W. Young, B. Birdsall, J. Feeney, and G. C. K. Roberts, Stereochemistry of reduction of the vitamin folic acid by dihydrofolate reductase. *J. Chem. Soc. (Perkin Trans.)* I:1349–1353 (1985).

41. Pastore, E. J., and M. Friedkin, The enzymatic synthesis of thymidylate. II. Transfer of tritium from tetrahydrofolate to the methyl group of thymidylate. *J. Biol. Chem.* 237:3802–3810 (1962).

42. Blakley, R. L., B. V. Ramasastri, and B. M. McDougall, The biosynthesis of thymidylic acid. V. Hydrogen isotope studies with dihydrofolic reductase and thymidylate synthetase. *J. Biol. Chem. 238*:3075–3079 (1963).

43. Hood, K., and G. C. K. Roberts, Ultraviolet difference-spectroscopic studies of substrate and inhibitor binding to *Lactobacillus casei* dihydrofolate reductase. *Biochem. J. 171*:357–366 (1978).

44. Roberts, G. C. K., J. Feeney, A. S. V. Burgen, V. Yuferov, J. G. Dann, and R. Bjur, Nuclear magnetic resonance studies of the binding of substrate analogs and coenzyme to dihydrofolate reductase from *Lactobacillus casei*. *Biochemistry 13*:5351–5357 (1974).

45. Perkins, J. P., and J. R. Bertino, Dihydrofolate reductase from the L1210R murine lymphoma: Fluorometric measurements of the interaction of the enzyme with coenzymes, substrates, and inhibitors. *Biochemistry 5*:1005–1012 (1966).

46. Baccanari, D. P., S. Daluge, and R. W. King, Inhibition of dihydrofolate reductase: Effect of reduced nicotinamide adenine dinucleotide phosphate on the selectivity and affinity of diaminobenzylpyrimidines. *Biochemistry 21*:5068–5075 (1982).

47. Cha, S., Tight-binding inhibitors. I. Kinetic behavior. *Biochem. Pharmacol. 24*:2177–2185 (1975).

48. Blaney, J. M., C. Hansch, C. Silipo, and A. Vittoria, Structure-activity relationships of dihydrofolate reductase inhibitors. *Chem. Rev. 84*:333–407 (1984).

49. Poe, M., Acidic dissociation constants of folic acid, dihydrofolic acid, and methotrexate. *J. Biol. Chem. 252*:3724–3728 (1977).

50. Gready, J. E., Dihydrofolate reductase: Binding of substrates and inhibitors and catalytic mechanism. *Adv. Pharmacol. Chemother. 17*:37–102 (1980).

51. Cocco, L., B. Roth, C. Temple Jr., J. A. Montgomery, R. E. London, and R. L. Blakley, Protonated state of methotrexate, trimethoprim, and pyrimethamine bound to dihydrofolate reductase. *Arch. Biochem. Biophys. 226*:567–577 (1983)

52. Subramanian, S., and B. T. Kaufman, Interaction of methotrexate, folates, and pyridine nucleotides with dihydrofolate reductase: Calorimetric and spectroscopic binding studies. *Proc. Natl. Acad. Sci. USA 75*:3201–3205 (1978).

53. Cheung, H. T. A., M. S. Searle, J. Feeney, B. Birdsall, G. C. K. Roberts, I. Kompis, and S. J. Hammond, Trimethoprim binding to *Lactobacillus casei* dihydrofolate reductase: A ^{13}C NMR study using selectively ^{13}C-enriched trimethoprim. *Biochemistry 25*:1925–1931 (1986).

54. Birdsall, B., G. C. K. Roberts, J. Feeney, J. G. Dann, and A. S. V. Burgen, Trimethoprim binding to bacterial and mammalian dihydrofolate reductase: A comparison by proton and carbon-13 nuclear magnetic resonance. *Biochemistry 22*:5597–5604 (1983).

55. Bevan, A. W., G. C. K. Roberts, J. Feeney, and L. F. Kuyper, ^{1}H and ^{15}N NMR studies of protonation and hydrogen-bonding in the binding of trimethoprim to dihydrofolate reductase. *Eur. Biophys. J. 11*:211–218 (1985).

56. Phillips, T., and R. F. Bryan, The crystal structures of the antimalarial agents daraprim and trimethoprim. *Acta Crystallogr.* (Sect. A) A25:S200 (1969).

57. Kuyper, L., unpublished results from AMBER (58) calculations.

58. Weiner, P. K., and P. A. Kollman, AMBER: Assisted model building with energy refinement. A general program for modeling molecules and their interactions. *J. Comp. Chem. 2*:287–303 (1981).

59. Baker, B. R., *Design of Active-Site-Directed Irreversible Enzyme Inhibitors*, Wiley, New York (1967).

60. Kumar, A. A., J. H. Mangum, D. T. Blankenship, and J. H. Friesheim, Affinity labeling of chicken liver dihydrofolate reductase by a substituted 4,6-dia-minodihydrotriazine bearing a terminal sulfonyl fluoride. *J. Biol. Chem. 256*:8970–8976 (1981).

61. Guida, W., and N. Richards, unpublished.

62. Rosowsky, A., J. E. Wright, C. Ginty, and J. Uren, Methotrexate analogues. 15. A methotrexate analogue designed for active-site-directed irreversible inactivation of dihydrofolate reductase. *J. Med. Chem. 25*:960–964 (1982).

63. Freisheim, J. H., S. S. Susten, T. J. Delcamp, A. Rosowsky, J. E. Wright, R. J. Kempton, D. T. Blankenship, P. L. Smith, and A. A. Kumar, Structure, function and affinity labeling studies of dihydrofolate reductase. In *Chemistry and Biology of Pteridines*, J. A. Blair, ed. Walter de Gruyter, New York, pp. 223–227 (1983).

64. Johanson, R. A., and J. Henkin, Affinity labeling of dihydrofolate reductase with an antifolate glyoxal. *J. Biol. Chem. 260*:1465–1474 (1985).

65. Tansik, R. L., D. R. Averett, B. Roth, S. J. Paterson, D. Stone, and D. P. Baccanari, Species-specific irreversible inhibition of *Neisseria gonorrhoeae* dihy-drofolate reductase by a substituted 2,4-diamino-5-benzylpyrimidine. *J. Biol. Chem. 259*:12299–12305 (1984).

66. Chan, J., L. F. Kuyper, and B. Roth, Molecular mechanics modeling of a covalent complex between *L. casei* dihydrofolate reductase and an active-site directed irreversible inhibitor: Prediction of attachment site and three-dimensional structure. In *189th National Meeting of the American Chemical Society*, Miami Beach, Fla., April 28–May 3. See *Abstracts of Papers*; American Chemical Society, Washington, DC, 1985, abstract MEDI 87.

67. Joyner, S. S., B. Roth, and D. P. Baccanari, Irreversible inhibition of *L. casei* dihydrofolate reductase. *Fed. Proc. 44*:1620 (1985).

68. Kuyper, L. F., B. Roth, D. P. Baccanari, R. Ferone, C. R. Beddell, J. N. Champness, D. K. Stammers, J. G. Dann, F. E. A. Norrington, D. J. Baker, and P. J. Goodford, Receptor-based design of dihydrofolate reductase inhibitors: Comparison of crystallographically determined enzyme binding with enzyme affinity in a series of carboxy-substituted trimethoprim analogues. *J. Med. Chem. 25*:1120–1122 (1982).

69. Piper, J. R., J. A. Montgomery, F. M. Sirotnak, and P. L. Chello, Syntheses of α- and γ-substituted amides, peptides, and esters of methotrexate and their evaluation as inhibitors of folate metabolism. *J. Med. Chem. 25*:182–187 (1982).

70. Kompis, I., and R. L. Then, Rationally designed brodimoprim analogues: Synthesis and biological activities. *Eur. J. Med. Chem. Chim. Ther. 19*:529–534 (1984).

71. Müller, K., Computer-graphic examination of protein-molecule complexes. *Actual Chim. Ther. 11*:113–120 (1984).

72. Birdsall, B., J. Feeney, C. Pascual, G. C. K. Roberts, I. Kompis, R. L. Then, K. Müller, A. Kroehn, A ^{1}H NMR study of the interactions and conformations of rationally designed brodimoprim analogues in complexes with *Lactobacillus casei* dihydrofolate reductase. *J. Med. Chem. 27*:1672–1676 (1984).

73. Maag, H., R. Locher, J. J. Daly, and I. Kompis, 5-(N-Arylnortropan-3-yl)- and 5-(N-arylpiperidin-4-yl)-2,4-diaminopyrimidines. Novel inhibitors of dihydrofolate reductase. *Helv. Chim. Acta 69*:887–897 (1986).

74. Kuyper, L. F., S. E. Davis, and H. S. LeBlanc, unpublished.

75. Ollis, W. D., J. F. Stoddart, and I. O. Sutherland, The conformational behaviour of some medium-sized ring systems. *Tetrahedron 30*:1903–1921 (1974).

76. Blaney, J. M., P. K. Weiner, A. Dearing, P. A. Kollman, E. C. Jorgensen, S. J. Oatley, J. M. Burridge, and C. C. F. Blake, Molecular mechanics simulation of protein-ligand interactions: Binding of thyroid hormone analogues to prealbumin. *J. Am. Chem. Soc. 104*:6424–6434 (1982).

77. Kuyper, L. F., Molecular mechanics modeling of dihydrofolate reductase-inhibitor complexes: Correlation between calculated energy and observed affinity. In *189th National Meeting of the American Chemical Society*, Miami Beach, Fla., April 28–May 3. See *Abstracts of Papers*; American Chemical Society, Washington, DC, 1985, abstract MEDI 88.

78. Singh, U. C., F. K. Brown, P. A. Bash, and P. A. Kollman, An approach to the application of free energy perturbation methods using molecular dynamics: Applications to the transformations of $CH_3OH \rightarrow CH_3CH_3$, $H_3O + \rightarrow NH_4+$, glycine→alanine, and alanine→phenylalanine in aqueous solution and to $H_3O + (H_2O)_3 \rightarrow NH_4 + (H_2O)_3$ in the gas phase. *J. Am. Chem. Soc. 109*:1607–1614 (1987).

79. Wong, C. F., and J. A. McCammon, Dynamics and design of enzymes and inhibitors. *J. Am. Chem. Soc. 108*:3830–3832 (1986).

80. Tybrand, T. P., J. A. McCammon, and G. Wipff, Theoretical calculation of relative binding affinity in host-guest systems, *Proc. Natl. Acad. Sci. USA 83*:833–835 (1986).

81. Pettitt, M., and M. Karplus, Interaction energies: Their role in drug design. In *Topics in Molecular Pharmacology*, Vol. 3, A. S. V. Burgen, G. C. K. Roberts, and M. S. Tute, eds. Elsevier, New York, pp. 75–113 (1986).

10

Approaches to Antiviral Drug Design

Thomas J. Smith
Purdue University, West Lafayette, Indiana

I. INTRODUCTION

One of the most exciting recent advances in the field of virology has been the determination of the crystal structures of whole-virus capsids. Thus far the structures of the animal viruses [rhinovirus (1), poliovirus (2), and Mengo virus (3)], plant viruses [cowpea mosaic virus (4), tomato bushy stunt virus (5), southern bean mosaic virus (6), satellite tobacco necrosis virus (7), turnip crinkle virus (8)], and an insect virus [black beetle virus (9)] have been solved to high resolution. For the first time we have the capability to make comparisons of these picorna and "picornalike" viruses to better understand their evolution and different mechanisms of infection on a structural level. We are also now able to begin to design antiviral agents using the wealth of information contained in an atomic structure.

A. X-Ray Crystallography Principles

Since many crystallographic terms will be used in the following chapter, it is important to briefly review the general principles already discussed in this book. (For a more detailed description, see Chapter 4.) To give a conceptual understanding of x-ray crystallography, physical analogies will replace the more precise mathematical equations.

The first concept to be understood is how diffraction occurs. One way to explain diffraction is by reviewing an experiment performed in introductory physics labs. In this experiment, monochromatic light is passed through a grating of finely spaced lines. After waves pass through the gratings, they spread out and collide with those that have passed through neighboring gratings. As they collide, they add together to result in a single wave. If one wave is at its maximum while the other is at its minimum, the result is the cancellation of both waves. If both waves are at maximum, then the resultant wave is twice the height. The result of this experiment is that bands of light appear behind the grating, and the distance between these bands is related to the distance between the slits and the wavelength of light. Crystals are basically diffraction gratings except that the proteins are lined up in three dimensions, not just one. The result of taking the diffraction grating example from one to three dimensions is that the diffraction is no longer made up of bands of light but discrete spots, or maxima, in space. Like the diffraction grating example, though, the distance between spots is related to the distance between the repeating units (known as unit cells) and the light is now x-ray radiation. To summarize, the distance between reflections for a given crystal-to-film distance is related only to the dimensions of the unit cell and the wavelength of x-ray radiation. It is totally independent of what is in the unit cell.

Two terms will be used in the following chapter—structure amplitudes (F) and phases (α). The structure amplitudes are the intensities of the individual reflections, which can be easily measured using film or scintillation counters. The determination of the phases is much harder and represents the real problem in crystallography. As x-rays strike the atoms in the unit cell, they reflect off the different atoms at different points in space. These waves will add together in both positive and negative ways and yield a single new wave with possibly a new intensity and a new phase. The phase is the angular difference between the incident wave and the reflected wave. As the reflected waves from the atoms add together, the resultant wave may be translated compared to the incident wave so that the maximum is found at a different position in space—much like the difference between a sine and cosine wave. If one can determine the F and phase of each reflection, one can determine the atomic arrangement that produced such a pattern.

This relationship is similar to when one throws a handful of pebbles onto a calm pool, if one assumes that the waves generated by the pebbles are of the same wavelength. As one goes to different places in the pond, the waves from the individual pebbles will have added together to generate waves with different heights (F) and phases (α). If one samples enough points in the pond and determines the phase and height of the resultant waves, one can figure out where on the pond each pebble hit the surface. Using this analogy, one can explain the process of difference Fourier. If one adds one small pebble to the handful thrown into the pool, one will see a small change in the height of the resultant waves in the pond (as well as a small phase change). Since we now know the position of each of the other rocks, we can calculate what the wave should look like at every part of the pool, and by measuring the difference between the expected values and the values found when we add the additional rock, we can determine quickly where the new rock is striking the surface. The difference Fourier is like this. One knows what the F's and α's are for a native structure and measures the new F's when a drug is soaked into the crystal. Assuming that the α's have not changed a lot, one can quickly determine where the drug is by measuring the change in structure factors and applying the phases to find its position.

B. Technology Used for X-Ray Crystallographic Studies on Whole-Virus Capsids

The structure determination of large particles such as whole viruses has been a great achievement and has been made possible, in part, by technological advances in computational power and x-ray radiation sources. Since whole-virus studies have become so heavily dependent on these advances, it is useful to discuss the problems unique to these studies and how new technology has been used to solve them.

The angle between diffraction maxima, or the distance between the reflections, is inversely proportional to the unit cell lengths of the crystal. Since intact picornavirus capsids have molecular weights of about 10×10^6, they necessarily pack into very large unit cells. It therefore follows that a full set of x-ray diffraction data for virus crystals will be enormous.

To exemplify the magnitude of this problem, let us say that one had a "typical" protein of about 30,000 molecular weight packed into a monoclinic $P2_1$ cell. To collect a full data set, to 3-Å data set resolution, one would need to measure the intensity of about 20,000–40,000 reflections. In the case of virus capsids, a full 3-Å data set is composed of over 1 million reflections, with 30,000–40,000 reflections on each 0.3° oscillation photograph (Fig. 1). To compound this seemingly monumental task of collecting data, most virus crystals are very sensitive to x-ray radiation, and each oscillation photograph therefore requires a fresh crystal.

In the case of radiation sensitivity, one solution has been to use intense x-ray radiation from a synchrotron. A synchrotron is a large magnetic ring of oscillating polarity. Inside this football stadium-sized ring is a thin vacuum chamber. Electrons and their antimatter counterpart positrons are injected into the ring with a linear accelerator, and their velocity is then increased and maintained with the synchronized oscillation of the magnetic field. These particles are accelerated to speeds approaching the speed of light and therefore require huge amounts of energy to maintain their circular movement. What has been a serious problem for particle physicists and subsequently a huge benefit to crystallographers was that some of this energy is released as x-rays tangent to the ring. The power of these x-rays is enormous. The unfocused beam at the Cornell High Energy Synchrotron Source can quickly burn holes through lead bricks and shatter uncooled focusing mirrors, but most importantly, the strong, focused beam can reduce the exposure time of 17 hr on the conventional rotating anode x-ray generator to a mere 2 min. This factor of 1000 allows one more freedom to survey various compounds or conditions of interest with a much smaller commitment of time.

A valuable companion to virus crystallography has been the supercomputer. In the frantic process of synchrotron data collection, where beam- time is at a premium, there is little time to properly orient the crystals, or as was the case of the highly radiation-sensitive Mengo crystals, it is impossible to take setting photographs. It is therefore a formidable task to index the 30,000–40,000 reflections on these films, since little is known of the crystal's orientation. The "American method" of shooting first and asking questions later has worked well using Purdue University's Cyber 205 Supercomputer by estimating by hand the orientations of the crystal either from the position and angles of the major zone axis or with a program called "zones." The

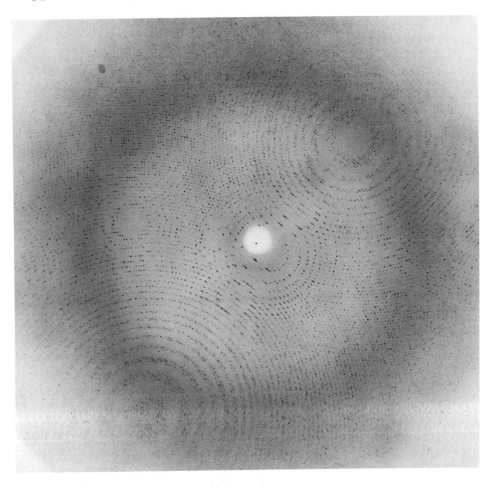

Figure 1 A 0.3° oscillation photograph of Mengo virus taken at the Cornell High Energy Syncrotron Source (CHESS). Such films typically contain 30,000–40,000 reflections.

zones program compares the measured angles between the various crystal axes on the film (as made evident by different sets of concentric ellipses) and matches them to the set of theoretical axes to determine what crystal orientation was necessary to produce such a pattern on the film (10). This requires the sorting of thousands of permutations and then going to the film to use hundreds of reflections to refine the initial estimate of the orientation. Before the supercomputer, it would have required months to process a full

data set. It is also important to note that the advent of the huge computational power of computers such as the Cyber 205 has allowed the
application of molecular replacement to be tested and then used for phasing
the human rhinovirus 14 (HRV 14) structure. With conventional computers,
such a method would have been used with great caution because of the
magnitude of the problem and a failure in the method or a mistake in its
application would have meant a huge delay in the solution of the HRV 14
structure.

A project where the culmination of all of these crystallographic advances
has yielded rapid and exciting results is in the study of the interaction
between antiviral agents (WIN compounds) and HRV 14 (11,33). For the first
time, we have the capability to examine the interactions between an antiviral
agent and a whole capsid to learn more about both the capsid function and
drug design.

II. RHINOVIRUS AS A DRUG RECEPTOR

A. Process of Picornavirus Infection

Rhinovirus, poliovirus, hepatitis A, Mengo virus, and Coxsackie virus are
among the smallest RNA-containing animal viruses (12) and belong to the
picornavirus family. They have a molecular weight of approximately
8.5×10^6, and their external shells have icosahedral symmetry with dia-
meters of about 300 Å. Each capsid is composed of 60 copies of four different
viral proteins VP_1, VP_2, VP_3, and VP_4.

Picornavirus infection can be divided into at least four steps, with each
being a possible target for antiviral drug design. The first stage in viral
infection is cellular recognition. In the case of rhinovirus, it has been shown
that the numerous serotypes bind to one of two cell surface proteins (13),
suggesting that although there are many amino acid differences between the
different serotypes, they exhibit very conservative binding interactions with
their cellular receptors.

After binding to the cell receptors, the virions enter the cell via an
endosomal vesicle. This stage of infection is one of the most poorly
understood. Somehow, the RNA from the virions must travel from the inside
of the capsid through the endosomal vesicle wall and into the cytoplasm.
Although the exact process is not known, it is believed that binding to the cell
surface receptor itself causes large conformational changes in the capsid (14).
This has been shown by the finding that when poliovirus binds to the cell
surface but disassociates before it can enter the cell, the resultant particle has
an altered PI and is no longer infectious. It is also known that endosomal
vesicles activate their proton pumps once in the cytoplasm, causing a pH

drop inside the vesicle, and that such low pH's cause conformational changes in both poliovirus and rhinovirus (15). These processes may alone or together cause the capsid to inject the RNA into the cytoplasm (uncoating). Nothing is known about the structural changes that are necessary, however.

Once the RNA is released into the cytoplasm, the cellular ribosomes read the viral message. This RNA is translated as a single polypeptide representing coat proteins, RNA polymerase, and highly specific proteases required to cleave this polypeptide into its proper components (15–17) (Fig. 2). Interestingly, there have not yet been any agents targeted to these specific proteases in any viral system.

The last stage of infection involves viral assembly and subsequent release of the virus. The coat proteins VP_0, VP_1, and VP_3 assemble as individual 6S protomer units, and then five such units come together as 14S pentameric units (18). In order for 12 copies of these pentameric units to encapsidate the viral RNA (16), VP_0 maybe autocatalytically cleaved into VP_2 and VP_4 with RNA possibly acting as the base for the reaction (19). Finally, new virions are released from the cell. In the case of poliovirus, this is thought to be mediated via a rather nonspecific vesicle mechanism rather than simply cell lysis, since most of the synthesized virus is released before cell death (14).

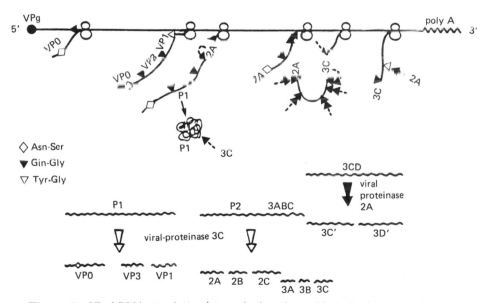

Figure 2 Viral RNA translation into a single polypeptide and subsequent cleavage by viral proteases 2A and 3C.

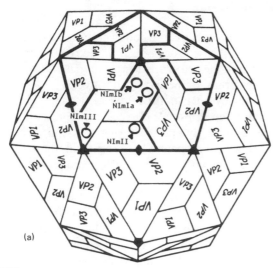

(a)

SBMV

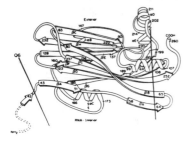

HRV14

VP1

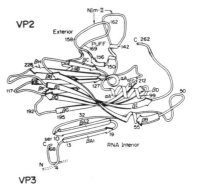

(b)

Figure 3 (a) Icosahedral arrangement of the viral proteins with the neutralizing immunogen sides (NIm) labeled. Triangles represent threefold axis, elipses represent twofold axis, and pentamers represent fivefold axis. (b) Ribbon drawings of the various human rhinovirus 14 (HRV 14) proteins and southern bean mosaic virus (SBMV) protein for comparison.

378

B.   Structure of Rhinovirus

As previously mentioned, the structure of rhinovirus has been determined to
3-Å resolution (1). Perhaps the most striking finding was that the basic
structural motif of the capsid was 60 copies of eight-stranded β-barrels
(Fig. 3), just as was found previously with the small spherical RNA plant
viruses (5–7) and was found subsequently with other animal (2,3), plant (4,8),
and insect viruses (9).

Interestingly, a 25-Å-deep canyon was found around each icosahedral
five-fold axis. Around the rim of these canyons there are four different
antigenic sites. Because of the dimensions of the canyon, the bottom of the
canyon is inaccessible to antibodies and therefore does not need to change to
avoid immunological recognition. For this reason, it was postulated that the
canyon may play a role in receptor recognition (Fig. 4).

If the cell surface protein (receptor) binds in the deep portion of the
canyon, then the virus can mutate its "face" to ward off antibody recognition
without changing the interactions with the cell receptor. Therefore, if one
were to target a compound to the capsid, one would try to design it in such a
way that it would bind to either the canyon floor or to the β-barrels, since
these regions are resistant to change because of their important roles in
cellular recognition and capsid structure (1).

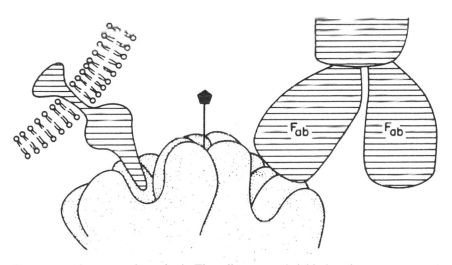

Figure 4   The canyon hypothesis. The cell receptor may bind to the canyon around
the icosahedral fivefold axis, but its dimensions do not permit access to antibodies.

THE CANYON HYPOTHESIS

III. DESIGNING ANTIVIRAL DRUGS

A. Lead Structures Based on the Oxazoline–Phenoxy Ring Structures

Since there are over 100 different serotypes of rhinovirus, and because the virus can easily mutate its antigenic surface, development of a vaccine for the common cold has been impractical. Despite the rhinoviruses' rather dynamic and diverse capsid structures, the Sterling-Winthrop Research Institute has synthesized a series of effective antiviral agents that have a broad serotype specificity (20–23).

This family of antiviral agents has been developed over the past 10 years from the initial lead compound arildone (24–27). Arildone was found to have limited antiviral activity in cell culture, but subsequent changes in the chemical structure led to compounds with about a 1000-fold increased activity. Hundreds of such compounds were made and tested, and QSAR activity correlation studies directed them to the present structures. Since no structural information was available, this family was refined purely from activity assays. This family of antiviral agents inhibit the infection of several picornaviruses including all strains of rhinovirus and certain strains of poliovirus and Coxsackie viruses.

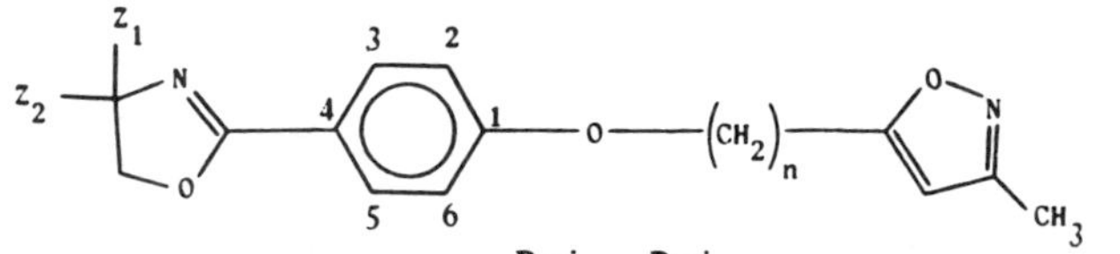

Compound	Z_1	Z_2	Position 2	Position 3	n	HRV14	HRV2
Optimum length of aliphatic chain							
WIN 53670	H	H	H	H	4	Inactive	7.3
WIN 52035	H	H	H	H	5	0.7	1.1
WIN 53337	H	H	H	H	6	2.9	2.1
WIN 51711	H	H	H	H	7	0.4	3.5
WIN 53455	H	H	H	H	8	3.9	5.9
Substitution on the oxazoline group							
WIN 51711	H	H	H	H	7	0.4	3.8
WIN 52084 *S/R*	H	CH_3	H	H	7	0.06	0.11
WIN 52084 *S*	H	CH_3	H	H	7	0.04	0.08
WIN 52084 *R*	H	CH_3	H	H	7	0.4	1.7
WIN 52193	CH_3	CH_3	H	H	7	0.1	1.5
Substitutions on the phenolic group							
WIN 52035	H	H	H	H	5	1.2	1.0
WIN 54089	H	H	CH_3	H	5	0.8	0.09
WIN 53338	H	H	Cl	H	5	2.5	0.06
WIN 54274	H	H	H	CH_3	5	1.6	1.2
WIN 54090	H	H	H	Cl	5	0.3	0.9

Figure 5 Effectiveness of a variety of antiviral compounds. MIC values (μM). (Adopted from Ref. 11.)

The basic structure of these compounds is an oxazoline ring attached to a phenoxy ring which is in turn connected to an isoxazole ring via an aliphatic chain (Fig. 5). They are quite hydrophobic and have been shown to inhibit the uncoating of the viruses rather than viral attachment to the cell membrane or membrane penetration (23). These compounds have been shown to prevent the loss of VP_4 and stabilize the virion against alkaline and thermal denaturation (20).

B. Locating the Drug-Binding Site on Human Rhinovirus 14

Since the crystal structure of HRV 14 had been solved, it was a rather straightforward task to soak a drug into the crystal and use the difference Fourier technique to find the drug-binding site. The drug WIN 52,084 was chosen for further study.

As with any difference Fourier experiment, a series of control experiments were performed before data collection to ensure that it would be possible to bind drugs to virions while in a crystalline form. It was first found that, if a concentrated solution of WIN compound in dimethyl sulfoxide was added to HRV 14 crystals soaking in TRIS buffer containing polyethylene glycol, the crystals could sustain large concentrations of drugs for 1 week and still diffract x-rays. This result was interesting, since isoelectric point focusing experiments showed that these compounds (uncharged at neutral pH's) caused a pI change in the capsids from 6.9 to 7.2. This suggested that either there was a conformational change that is not involved in particle packing or that the drugs covered charges on the capsid surface since crystal morphology and diffraction were unaffected by the drugs. As a final check, radioactive drug was soaked into the crystal and shown to bind in a stoichiometry of about 60 per capsid (this stoichiometry was later confirmed with binding studies using HRV 14 in solution) (11).

It is important to discuss here the validity of the structure of the virion-drug complex if one soaks the drug into crystals rather than crystallizing the drug-virion complex. As will be shown later, the conformational changes imposed by the drug are distal to the virion packing contacts, and it is therefore unlikely that protein movement is restricted by crystal packing. It should also be noted that such studies with virus crystals are unique in that because the virions are large, the relative percentage of the capsid involved in virion packing is negligible. Finally, if one exposes rhinovirus crystals to conditions that are known to affect capsid structure, the crystals quickly disintegrate, suggesting that such conformational changes are probably stronger than packing forces.

1.   Data Collection and Analysis

Data were collected at the Cornell Synchrotron, and the films were processed with the Cyber 205 Supercomputer at Purdue. Using the native structure factors and native phases, a difference map was calculated. This map was difficult to interpret, since it was a complex mixture of positive and negative peaks, because regions of viral protein had moved into and out of several areas.

To generate a more interpretable map, a method of making "synthetic" maps was devised. When the crystals are soaked with drugs, it is unlikely that 100% of the binding sites will contain drug. Because of this, the new structure factors (F_{obs}) are actually a composite of new and native structure factors. This can be represented mathematically by:

$$F_{\text{new structure}} = |f_{\text{observed}} - (1 - k)F_{\text{native}}|$$

The value of k was determined empirically by subtracting two maps until an interpretable map resulted. One of these maps was calculated with the f_{obs} and the native phases, and the other map was calculated with f_{native} and native phases. The native map was multiplied by a fraction then subtracted from the new, f_{obs}, map, and the resultant map was examined. This process was continued until the fraction $(1 - k)$ yielded a map where peptides were contiguous and, wherever there had been obvious peptide movement, the old structure had been completely subtracted away. In this final map, the amplitude of the drug's electron density was of the same magnitude as the surrounding protein density, and nowhere in the peptide density that had been moved by the drug was the amplitude significantly lower than the unaltered protein.

2.   Examination of Capsid/Drug Interactions

The next step was to interpret the new structure. As shown in Figure 6, this new map was not difficult to interpret, and it was not difficult to reposition the amino acids that had been moved by the drug.

There was a new section of density that was not connected to any of the viral proteins and was presumed to be the electron density of the drug. This density was found in the middle of the β-barrel of VP$_1$ (Fig. 7) and corresponded to the structure of the WIN 52,084 compound. The density showed two planar bulges where the phenoxy and oxazoline rings were positioned, and the aliphatic chain assumed a slightly bent conformation as it skirted around tyrosine 128 on its way to the planar isoxazole ring. The rings were positioned into the center of the planar bulges in the density, and the aliphatic chain was placed into the density with a slow dihedral twist, since it was assumed that this orientation represented a lower energy state than one with cis bonds.

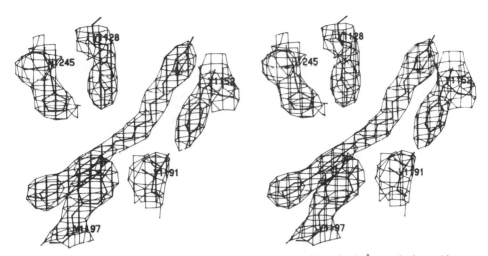

Figure 6 WIN 52,084 electron density at approximately 3-Å resolution. Also shown are portions of the surrounding viral electron density and the side chains fitted to it.

After the drug was oriented into its density, the protein surrounding the drug was examined for specific interactions (Fig. 8). With this particular compound, there may be a hydrogen bond between the nitrogen of the oxazoline ring and asparagine 1219 of VP_1, and there is a strong stacking interaction between the phenyl ring of tyrosine 1197 of VP_1 and the phenoxy group of the drug (the first number represents the viral protein; the next three represent the residue number—e.g., 1219 is residue 219 in VP_1). Although these are examples of positive binding interactions, tyrosine 1128 seems to point toward the aliphatic chain, making it bend around the tyrosine hydroxyl. The rest of the interactions are less specific, in that the deepest portion of the drug-binding pocket at the isoxazole end of the drug binds in a region of very hydrophobic residues.

There are many large conformational changes in the region of VP_1 (Fig. 9) called the FMDV loop (so named because of its sequence homology with an antigenic portion of the foot-and-mouth disease virus). The FMDV loop is found on the floor of the canyon approximately at the VP_1, VP_2, and VP_3 interface. When the drug binds, this portion of VP_1 is twisted about Gly 1214 and Gly 1222, which act as hinges for the conformational movement. One of the side chains on this FMDV loop that has the most dramatic movements is Met 1221. In the native structure, the sulfur of Met 1221 is located precisely where the phenoxy ring of WIN 52,084 is found in the structure of the virus/drug complex. When the drugs bind to the capsid, the sulfur is moved

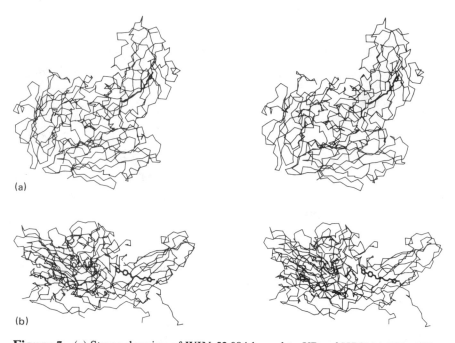

Figure 7 (a) Stereo drawing of WIN 52,084 bound to VP_1 of HRV 14. VP_1, VP_2, VP_3 are displayed as c-alpha tracings with the top β-barrel representing VP_1, the bottom β-barrel representing VP_2, and the left β-barrel representing VP_3. The orientation in this diagram is such that the icosahedral fivefold axis is pointing out of the paper at the top right portion (the top of the VP_1 β-barrel), and the reader is looking toward the RNA interior. (b) Another view of WIN 52,084 binding to the asymmetric unit of rhinovirus 14. In this view, the icosahedral fivefold axis is at the right, running up and down the paper; the RNA is at the bottom, and the solvent is at the top. In this view, the canyon is clearly visible at the top right portion of the diagram.

away from the RNA interior as the entire FMDV loop is displaced toward the floor of the canyon. His 1220 is moved the largest distance, and since it forms the lining of the solvent-exposed canyon region, it may contribute to the pI change.

Smaller changes occur elsewhere in VP_1 as well. Structural changes occur in residues 1151–1155 (Fig. 10), and even smaller changes occur between residues 1100 and 1109. Together, these changes represent concerted movement in the β-barrel such that the hydrogen-bonding patterns that support the β-barrel are maintained (33).

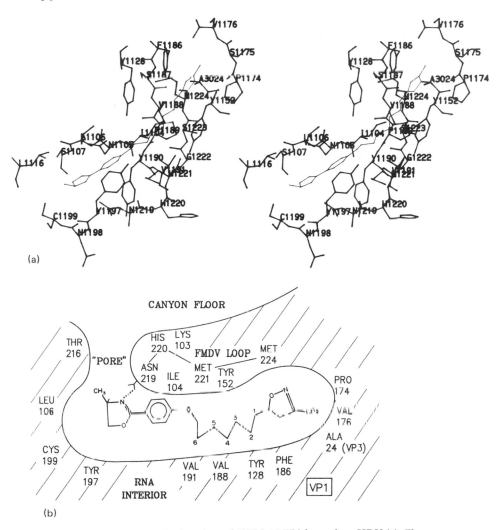

Figure 8 (a) Stereoscopic drawing of WIN 52,084 bound to HRV 14. Shown are residues within 3.6 Å of the drug. In this numbering system the first number designates the viral protein type ($VP_1 = 1$, $VP_2 = 2$, $VP_3 = 3$, and $VP_4 = 4$), and the last three numbers represent the amino acid number. The orientation here is the same as in Figure 7a, with the drug being the finer lines. (b) Schematic drawing of the WIN 52,084 environment.

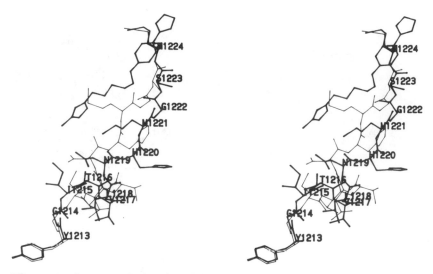

Figure 9 Stereoscopic drawing of the conformational changes in the FMDV loop. The fine lines represent the native structure, and the thick lines represent the new drug-bond structure. Shown here is WIN 52,035 bound with its orientation opposite to WIN 52,084. The diagram orientation is the same as in Figure 7a.

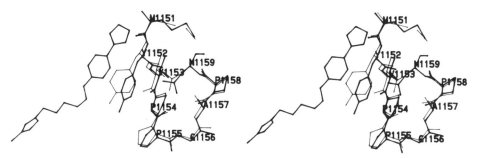

Figure 10 Stereoscopic drawing of the conformational changes in residues 1151–1159 when the drugs bind. Shown here is WIN 52,035 bound. The orientation for the diagram is the same as in Figure 7a. The native structure is represented by thin lines, and the new structure is represented by dark lines.

C. Mechanism of Action

Now that the antiviral compound/capsid structure has been described in atomic detail, can we use it both to understand the mechanism of capsid stabilization and to optimize drug efficacy? The first step to optimize drug efficacy is to develop postulates that can explain the drug's effects.

Two mechanisms have been developed to explain drug-mediated capsid stabilization (11). The first utilizes the observation that the drugs cover the entrance to channels in the capsid that lead to the RNA interior. It has been postulated that the heavy-atom derivative $Au(CN)_2^-$, used to solve the native HRV 14 structure, traveled down these channels in order to reach the final reaction sites (1). The flux of ions into the RNA interior has been shown to have a pivotal role in the swelling and disassembly of some plant viruses, and it was thought that a similar phenomenon might be part of the disassembly pathway of HRV 14 (28–30). In this first mechanism it was suggested that the drugs cover those ion channels that are necessary for capsid swelling and disassembly. As will be shown with other compounds and computer graphics, this model does not explain all of the drug properties.

The second model for drug action is based on the thermodynamics of drug binding. This model simply suggests that the drug bound in the pocket stabilizes the β-barrel, the collapse of which may be essential for disassembly. One way to understand how this might work is by comparing drug binding with micelle formation. When phospholipids are in aqueous solutions, they have a low entropy term, because they order water molecules around their nonpolar tails in order to stay in solution. To decrease their Gibbs free energy, they shed their water molecules to form what appears to be a more ordered structure — micelles or phospholipid bilayers. In the same way, these drugs bind to the capsid in a high-affinity, energetically favorable way, since they are able to become less ordered in the hydrophobic environment of the drug-binding pocket by shedding their ordered water molecules.

The mechanism of the drug stabilization can now be understood using general concepts of protein structure/function. It is thought that structural proteins do not and should not undergo conformational changes, because they are near their Gibbs free-energy minima of folding. To move the structure out of the bottom of this energy well requires a large energy input from the environment. Allosteric enzymes, on the other hand, need to be structurally dynamic and are therefore not at their lowest packing energy. Because of this, it takes much less energy to move the peptide chains. In the case of the drug binding to the VP_1 β-barrel, the large entropy input of drug binding may decrease the overall energy of the capsid. This may move the capsid farther down its energy well and therefore may increase the energy required to make the conformational changes necessary for disassembly.

One prediction that can be made from this model is that drug binding is proportional to biological efficacy (barring large differences in pharmacological effects such as cytotoxicity, membrane permeability, interactions with serum proteins, etc. between different compounds). This is an important step in drug design in that one can assume that to increase binding efficacy is to increase biological efficacy. This assumption allows one to ignore the possibility of strange secondary conformational effects upon drug binding, which might be difficult to understand or to model. This approximation has been shown to be valid in preliminary binding studies (11,31).

Further evidence supporting this latter hypothesis comes from work on bacteriophage T_4 lysozyme (34). In these studies, point mutations were made in the lysozyme sequence in areas where an increase in the bulk of a side chain could be accommodated without a significant change in structure—for instance, a gly→ala mutation. Such mutations did not alter enzymatic activity or the crystallographic structure, but they did increase the stability of the enzyme as measured by heat denaturation experiments. Since there were not significant changes in the structure, they argued that the enhanced stability came from the fact that in order to unfold the structure, the larger hydrophobic groups (e.g., gly→ala) must be placed into water, and this process is unfavorable because of the decrease in the entropy of unfolding. In the same way, the drugs can be thought to stabilize the capsid, since in order to unfold, they must now expose their hydrophobic residues in the drug-binding pocket and expel the hydrophobic drug into water. Because of this, hydrophilic compounds are not expected to work as well as the current compounds, since there would not be as large a decrease of entropy of unfolding.

D. Mathematical Examination of Drug/Virus Interactions

One interesting result from the work on WIN 52,084 was that even though a racemic mixture was soaked into the rhinovirus 14 crystals, only the S form (which is 10-fold more biologically active than the R form) was visible in crystal structure. It was suggested that the enhanced binding of the S form might be due to hydrophobic interactions between the methyl group and a pocket formed by Leu 1106 and Ser 1107. The R form cannot be oriented properly and should bind like the desmethyl compound 51,711.

To further examine this effect of chirality on drug efficacy, energy calculations have been performed in the region of the oxazoline methyl (32). For these calculations, the position of the drug and the surrounding protein was held fixed as the oxazoline ring was allowed to rotate about the phenoxy bond. For each 10° step in the 360° rotation, the Van der Waals forces were calculated (Fig. 11). When these calculations were performed on WIN 52,084, a minimum was found roughly at 10–30°, which agreed with the crystallographic results. At this angle, the oxazoline ring is held in an orientation favoring hydrogen bonding with asparagine 1219. When these calculations were repeated with the R form of WIN 52,084 and the desmethyl compound, there was a very broad minimum, with very little evidence of a preferred orientation.

Interestingly, gem dimethyl has the same biological activity as the racemic mixture of WIN 52,084 and has a potential minimum at the biologically relevant 10–30°. The gem dimethyl shows several other minima as well, but none quite as low as the 10–30° well. In the case of the ethyl substituent, the well is better defined with the S isomer than the R isomer, with the R-isomer having only a shallow minimum at 10°, and showed lower minima at other angles.

The importance of this work is that it presents a mathematical way to show a phenomenon observed with biological and crystallographic studies. These studies were performed by looking at only a portion of the binding phenomenon, but this abbreviated approach led to some tentative conclusions with conventional computers. This shows that one can perform drug modeling using energy calculations without having to use a supercomputer. Even so, the conclusions from these calculations might explain one aspect of the drug efficacy, and they can lead to the development of better compounds.

E. Studies with Other Members of This Family of Compounds

Another way to understand which drug/virus interactions are important to drug binding is by determining the x-ray structures of several modified drugs and trying to correlate the new binding modes with their respective efficacies. The group at Purdue has examined nine compounds to date (11,33) (Fig. 12). The first generalization that can be made about these compounds is that all cause nearly identical conformational changes upon binding to the virion even though they have very different structures.

One important finding, upon reexamination of the Win 51,711 data, was that the desmethyl compound may actually be able to bind with either the isoxazole or the oxazoline group in the deepest region of the pocket (33). The reason this is suspected is that even though the data for the difference Fourier is of good quality and yields an excellent map in the protein regions, it shows ambiguous density around the drug itself. It is therefore possible that WIN 51,711 can bind in both directions so that the density of the drug is the average of these two binding modes. This is further supported by studies with some of the other compounds where there were fewer data used for the

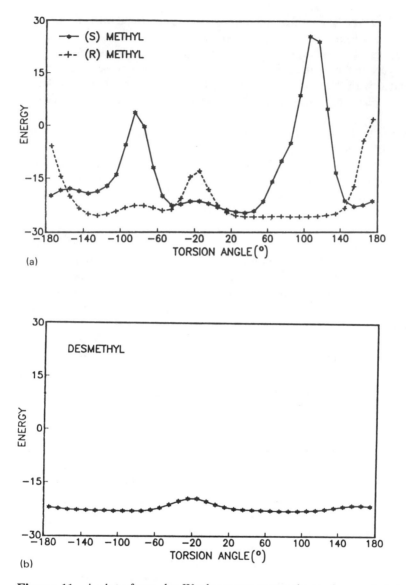

(a)

(b)

Figure 11　A plot of van der Waals energy versus the torsion angle between the oxazoline and phenyl rings for compounds 1–4, bound in the HRV 14 virus pocket. The pocket consists of all residues within 8 Å of any atom of the appropriate compound. All calculations were performed on a VAX 11785 using Chem-x. The intramolecular van der Waals energy was calculated using a 6–12 function.

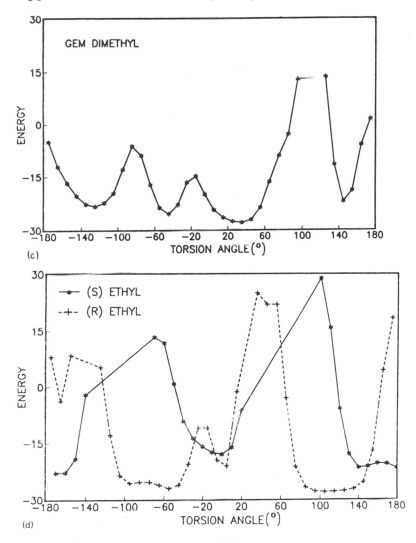

(c)

(d)

Fourier calculations yet the orientation and density of the compounds were obvious.

It was then postulated that the methylation of the $n = 7$ compound (WIN 51,711) may predispose the isoxazole to bind first. To test for this, the R methyl form of WIN 52,084 (33) was examined. The R form of WIN 52,084 is 10-fold less effective than the S form and is of equal efficacy to WIN 51,711, but it binds in the same orientation as the R form of WIN 52,084. It can therefore be concluded that although the methylation may determine the orientation, the orientation does not necessarily dictate the efficacy.

Compound Bound		MIC (μM)

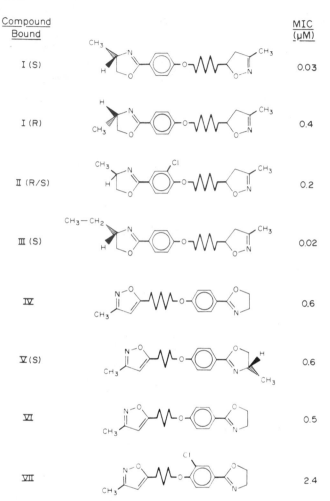

I (S)	0.03
I (R)	0.4
II (R/S)	0.2
III (S)	0.02
IV	0.6
V (S)	0.6
VI	0.5
VII	2.4

Figure 12 Structures of the compounds examined crystallographically to date with their respective efficacies. The compounds are drawn in the orientation as bound to HRV 14 using WIN 52,084 as the standard. MIC is the concentration of drug necessary to inhibit the number of plaques on a monolayer of HeLa cells by 50%.

To see if the stereochemistry of this chiral center holds true with larger substituents, an ethylated compound was examined. The x-ray structure of the ethyl compound also showed the S form bound, even though the crystals were soaked in a mixture of R and S enantiomers. Indeed, as was found in the case of WIN 52,084, the S form was 10 times more active. So it does seem that if there is a small substituent in the oxazoline ring, the drug will bind with the isoxazole end first, but the stereochemistry of this chiral center itself determines efficacy. This concurs with the results from mathematical calculations.

From the examination of other compounds, it may actually be that the methyl and ethyl forms of WIN 51,711 are the odd compounds. With the compounds studied thus far, when the compound has an aliphatic chain of $n = 5$ instead of $n = 7$, it binds with the oxazoline end inserted first (Fig. 13). These shorter compounds bind to the deepest recesses of the pocket. This was expected, since that portion of the pocket is the most hydrophobic and could therefore better accommodate the drug.

Since the methylation of WIN 51,711 (WIN 52,084) seems to cause the drug to bind with the isoxazole end inserted first, it was wondered whether the same would happen if the aliphatic chain was 5 carbons long instead of 7. This turns out not to be the case. In fact, even if the compound is mono- or dichlorinated at the phenoxy ring, the orientation is still the same. Interestingly in either orientation, asparagine 1219 is positioned so that it can hydrogen-bond to the drug.

The chlorination of the phenoxy ring makes the compounds more hydrophobic, and the chlorine in the monochloric seems to stack with tyrosine 1128 in the pocket (Figs. 13,14), yet these compounds are less efficacious in HRV 14. This could possibly be explained by the fact that the tyrosine 1128 side chain is very slightly moved (about 3–4 Å) by the chlorine,

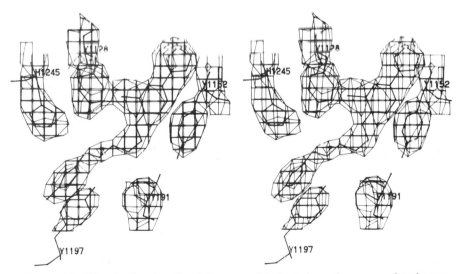

Figure 13   The election density of the monochlorinated $n = 5$ compound and some of the surrounding viral protein.

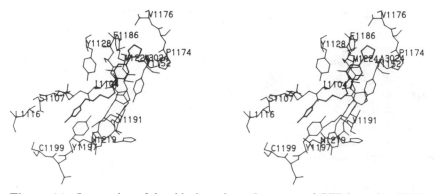

Figure 14 Interaction of the chlorinated $n = 5$ compound (VII) bound to HRV 14. The orientation in this stereo drawing is the same as in Figure 7a. The drug is represented by thick lines.

and this movement may increase the overall energy of binding and therefore diminish the binding efficacy.

Full understanding of the subtle differences between the efficacy of these various compounds awaits full mathematical calculations of the various binding modes. With these nine compounds, there is a large data base to test the results of such calculations.

F.   Comparisons of the Efficacies of These Compounds Against the Different Serotypes of Rhinovirus

Another way to utilize the virus/drug complex structure is by comparing the sequences of different viruses and, assuming that the structure will be homologous about homologous sequences, trying to understand their respective antiviral sensitivities (Table 1). It should first be noted that although comparisons between the different serotypes can be valuable and informative, it may be impossible to completely understand all of the differences in antiviral sensitivity, since drug efficacy may also be affected by those distal residues affecting capsid stability.

One residue that is conserved among all rhinoviruses and polioviruses is asparagine 1219. As previously mentioned, Asn 1219 may be hydrogen-bonded to all of the compounds studied thus far. Interestingly, this residue is serine in Mengo and glycine in FMDV (35), and the drugs are ineffective against both viruses. The loss of hydrogen bonding with residue 1219 may lead to the loss of drug efficacy, but other amino acid changes in the entrance to the drug pocket may prevent pocket accessibility. Indeed, after the initial drug studies were

Table 1 List of Residues Within 3.6 Å of the Bound WIN Compounds, and Comparisons with Aligned Sequences of Other Picornaviruses

Viral protein	Residue number	HRV 14 amino acid type	Interaction	HRV 2, HRV 39, HRV 49	PV 1 Mahoney	PV 1 Sabin	PV 2 Lansing	PV 3 Leon	Mengo	FMDV (A10)
1	134	Ile	Phenolic oxygen	Ile	Ile	Ile	Ile	Ile	Leu	Leu
1	106	Leu	Phenyl	Leu	Tyr	Tyr	Tyr	Tyr	Leu	Leu
1	107	Ser	Methyl on oxazoline	Gln	Lys	Lys	Lys	Lys	Ser	Ala
1	115	Leu	Oxazoline	Phe	Leu	Leu	Leu	Leu		
1	123	Tyr	Phenolic oxygen, C-3 in aliphatic chain	Ile	Leu	Phe	Phe	Phe	Val	Ile
1	152	Tyr	C-4, C-2, C-1 of aliphatic chain	Tyr	Tyr	Tyr	Tyr	Tyr	Cys	Val
1	174	Pro	Isoxazole	Ala	Pro	Pro	Pro	Pro	Pro	Pro
1	176	Val	Methyl of isoxazole	Val	Ile	Ile	Val	Ile	Val	Ala
1	186	Phe	Isoxazole	Phe	Ile	Ile	Ile	Ile	Phe	Leu
1	188	Val	C-2 and C-3 of aliphatic chain	Leu	Val	Val	Val	Val	Val	Leu
1	191	Val	C-6 of aliphatic chain	Leu	Val	Val	Val	Val	Asn	Thr
1	197	Tyr	Phenol C-7 and C-5 of aliphatic chain	Tyr	Tyr	Tyr	Tyr	Tyr	Leu	Leu
1	199	Cys	Oxazoline	Met	His	His	His	His	Ala	Thr
1	219	Asn	Phenyl; N of oxazoline	Asn	Asn	Asn	Asn	Asp	Ser	Gly
1	221	Met	Phenyl	Met	Phe	Phe	Phe	Phe	Phe	Met
1	224	Met	C-1 of aliphatic chain	Leu	Leu	Leu	Leu	Leu	Leu	Ala
3	24	Ala	Isoxazole	Ala	Ala	Ala	Ala	Ala	Ile	Val

MIC (μM)

Compound	HRV 14	HRV 2	HRV 39	HRV 49	PV 1 Mahoney	PV 1 Sabin	PV 2 Lansing	PV 3 Leon	Mengo	FMDV (A10)
WIN 51711	0.4	3.8	9.3	4.7	8.7	1.1	0.8	1.1	Inactive	Inactive
WIN 52084	0.06	0.1	2.2	0.8	>9.3	6.9	5.7	1.2	Inactive	No data

Abbreviations for viruses: HRV, human rhinovirus; PV, poliovirus; FMDV(A10), foot-and-mouth disease virus strain A10 (32).

performed, the structure of Mengo virus was solved and showed an extensive insertion in the VP_1 protein which filled in that region corresponding to the canyon in rhinovirus between VP_1 and VP_2 (3). This insertion should block the entrance of the drug into the β-barrel of VP_1. To test for this, drug-binding studies were performed on Mengo virus in solution with radioactive drug, and it was found that the drug was unable to bind (unpublished results).

There are large differences in drug efficacy between some of the rhinovirus serotypes, with WIN 51,711 and WIN 52,084 being generally less effective against rhino 2, 39, and 49 than against rhino 14. This might be explained by the fact that Val 188 and Val 191 in rhino 14 are both leucine in rhino 2, 39, and 49. These changes could cause steric hindrance in drug binding. That these effects are less pronounced with WIN 52,084 might be due to the fact that the positive effects of the additional methyl may overcome some of the deleterious effects of the valine to isoleucine changes.

G.   Studies with Drug-Resistant Mutants

When rhinovirus is propagated in the presence of these antiviral compounds, three different types of drug resistant mutants arise: (1) mutants resistant to low concentrations of drug; (2) mutants resistant to high concentrations of drug; and (3) mutants that require the drug for growth. By examining these changes, we might better understand the virus-drug interactions important for drug binding and the virus-virus interactions necessary to confer the drug's stabilization, and we might be able to see what mutant virions will occur in the future if the drug becomes marketable and how to counteract them.

Approximately 30 mutants, which can grow in the presence of high concentrations of WIN 52,084 ($n = 7$), have been sequenced. Interestingly, all of these mutations map to only one of two sites: cysteine 1199 or valine 1188. Valine 1188 was found to mutate to methionine or leucine, and cysteine 1199 is mutated to tryptophan, arginine, or tyrosine (Table 2).

The valine 1188 to leucine mutation was first modeled graphically and then later confirmed crystallographically (Fig. 15). In both the predicted and actual structures it was obvious that the new residue would sterically interfere with the binding of the drug compounds. Importantly, it was possible to correctly model a single mutational change in the pocket. This result may give more credence to the drug activity comparisons between the various serotypes that depend heavily on such structural comparisons.

When cysteine 1188 is mutated to the larger side chains such as tyrosine and tryptophan, simple modeling predicts that side chains will cause severe steric hinderence to drug binding. The actual x-ray structure determination of this class of mutants is under way at Purdue.

Table 2 The Effect of Mutations on MIC (μM) Values[a]

Virus		WIN 52,084	WIN 51,711	WIN 52,035 ($n = 5$)	WIN 54,563 ($n = 5$)
HRV 14 WT		0.06	0.4	0.2	0.75
HRV 14 mutant	1199 Cys→Trp	2.7	5.3	1.2	1.4
HRV 14 mutant	1199 Cys→Arg				
HRV 14 mutant	1199 Cys→Tyr				
HRV 14 WT					
HRV 14 mutant	1188 Val→Leu	1.0	6.1	1.2	>8
HRV 14 mutant	1188 Val→Met				
HRV 2	1188 is Leu	0.1	3.8		
HRV 39	1188 is Leu	2.2	9.3		
HRV 49	1188 is Leu	0.8	4.7		

[a]Listed are the MIC values—the concentration of drug necessary to inhibit infection (as measured by plaque assays) 50%.

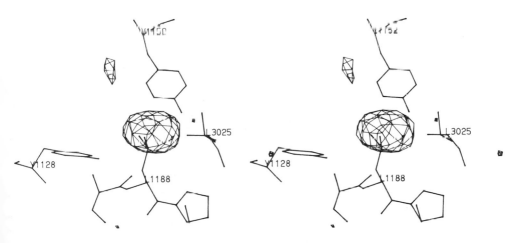

Figure 15 Drug-resistant mutant structure when valine 1188 is mutated to isoleucine. The density shown is the difference map of $F_{\text{mutant}} - F_{\text{native}}$, applying native phases. This positive peak arises from the extension of the side chain as valine is mutated to isoleucine.

Examination of this mutant has led to one of the most exciting results of the use of graphics to design drugs in this system (Fig. 16). According to the structure of the shorter $n = 5$ compound bound to HRV 14, it was predicted that the shorter compounds could still bind to this mutant in its normal position in the deepest portion of the pocket. These compounds were then tested against this mutant and, indeed, were found to be effective. This result is also exciting because half of the mutations expected to occur when the $n = 7$ compound is used can be overcome by simply using the $n = 5$ compound.

It should be noted, though, that all mutations may not simply be a change in side chain. In some cases they may also cause a conformational change. This same cautionary note must be applied to studies where the structure of other rhinovirus serotypes are extrapolated from the HRV 14 structure.

Studies are under way to further examine the low resistant and dependent mutants. Perhaps the most interesting studies will be on the drug-dependent mutants. Clearly, with these mutants, the drug is able to bind, but somehow it is no longer able to exert its effect. The easiest way to explain how this might occur is by invoking the thermodynamic mechanism of action. The overall stability of a virus capsid is a tenuous state; it must be stable enough to bind to the cell and infect but must be unstable enough to unfold once inside the cell. In the native virions the drugs may tip the scale and make the capsids too stable to unfold. In the case of the drug-dependent mutants, a mutation(s)

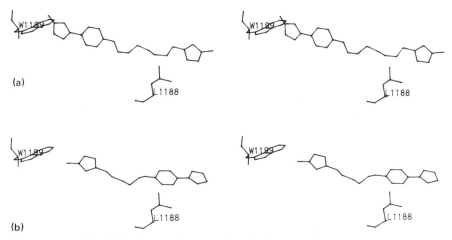

Figure 16 Modeled drug-resistant mutant when cysteine 1199 is mutated to tryptophan concomitantly with WIN 52,084 bound (a), or with the shorter $n = 5$ compound bound (b). Also shown is the valine 1188 to isoleucine mutation.

may have occurred that made the capsid so unstable that it cannot survive very well outside the cell. Now, in the presence of the drug, the capsid has enough stability to survive outside the cell but is not so stable that it cannot unfold inside the endosomal vesicle. It will be very interesting to see where mutations have occurred that have made the capsids so unstable.

H. Future Studies and Drug Design

Even though we have determined the structures of several complexes, we are at a very early stage in our understanding of drug binding and action. One of the most important areas of future work will be the computational analysis of the various compounds. This work is perhaps the most important because of the unique nature of this antiviral project. Most drugs have an enzymological target, and the synthetic chemists can capitalize on the chemical mechanism of the catalyzed reaction to optimize efficacy. With these compounds, all that can be done is to optimize drug binding, since there is not a reaction involved. We need to be able to understand, mathematically, how much each portion of the compound contributes to the binding efficacy so that sensible modifications can be made. For instance, the chlorination of the phenoxy ring results in a less effective compound even though the structure of the complex suggests a stacking arrangement with a neighboring tyrosine. We need to be able to mathematically understand our results to date and to be able to correctly predict the changes in binding of the compounds we have already studied.

A potential strategy is to make the compounds irreversible by putting a covalent modification on them such as an azido group. This is probably not a good idea because of toxicity problems. Since serum albumins are important carriers in the bloodstream, putting such an active group on them will increase their affinity to nonspecific binding sites, thereby potentially increasing their toxic side effects. One of the unique properties of these compounds as they are currently designed has been that they have such an uncanny specificity for viral capsids. In the bloodstream they bind tenuously to the albumins and wait until they can "latch onto" a passing virion with a high affinity.

Another strategy is to try to make the compounds more hydrophilic so that higher serum doses can be attained. The problem here is that the binding pocket is almost entirely hydrophobic, and to change polarity is predicted to, and indeed does, diminish activity greatly. Another problem is that increasing the polarity at one end while keeping the other end nonpolar to maintain activity may turn the compounds into detergents, which will obviously be deleterious to cell membranes.

Perhaps the most important information to be gained to date from the present knowledge is not only what new compounds can be designed but also what compounds simply will not work. Currently, the structures of some of the antibodies that neutralize HRV 14 are being studied (T. Smith, M. Rossmann, and R. Reuckert, unpublished data). Antibody binding and subsequent neutralization may be associated with pI changes in the capsid and, in the case of poliovirus, may require divalent attachment. By studying the structures of these antibodies (and hopefully the examination of the complex of Fab with peptides representing the antigenic sites), one might be able to model or "dock" the Fab to the rhinovirus surface. By doing so, it might be possible to understand the conformational changes associated with neutralization. For instance, it may be possible that antibodies to NIM Ia bind divalently across the icosahedral twofold axis, and subsequent conformational changes disrupt the virion. Future drug studies might someday examine compounds to mimic such neutralization, although this type of antiviral will be difficult to develop.

IV. CONCLUSIONS

Although much is now understood as to how and where currently available antirhinovirus compounds bind, we are still at a very early stage in our understanding of some of the details of both drug action and binding. X-ray crystallography has been essential in defining both the virus (receptor) structure and its interaction with drugs. It would have been impossible to predict that the compounds would bind to the site that they do, because the pocket is so constricted in the native structure. It would have also been impossible to predict that binding to this site would confer such capsid stability.

It is important to note that all of these studies have been made practical and efficient because of the great technological advances in x-ray sources and computational power. Future studies will continue to rely heavily on these advances for the rapid examination of new compounds, new mutants, and mathematical modeling of drug binding.

These compounds will be an important proving ground for thermodynamic calculations, as the energy of binding of the various components will be compared to their K_d's and biological efficacies. This is a nearly perfect system for such calculations, since the conformational changes are identical among all of the compounds, and the interactions are nearly all simple hydrophobic/Van der Waals contacts.

Eventually, these studies will lead to much better compounds, which can be used to treat viral infection. Along the way, they are elucidating an important aspect of viral infection that has been very poorly understood— viral uncoating.

ACKNOWLEDGMENTS

I would like to thank Michael Rossmann's group at Purdue, Roland Reuckert's group at the University of Wisconsin, and the antiviral group at Sterling-Winthrop Research Institute for all of the work that this chapter reviews. The work described here was truly a collaborative effort of many excellent scientists rather than any one person, and this collaboration has been a fruitful one. Special thanks go to John Badger at Purdue for Figures 12–16, Audi Treasurywala for Figure 11, E. Wimmer for Figure 2, and Michael Rossmann for his support in all aspects of the work. The work described here was supported by NIH, NSF, Sterling-Winthrop grant to Michael Rossmann, and a Jane Coffin Childs grant to myself.

REFERENCES

1. Rossmann, M. G., E. Arnold, J. W. Erickson, E. A. Frankenberger, J. P. Griffith, H. J. Hecht, J. R. Johnson, G. Kamer, M. Luo, A. G. Mosser, R. R. Rueckert, B. Sherry, and G. Vriend, Structure of a human common cold virus and functional relationship to other picornaviruses. *Nature 317*:145–153 (1985).

2. Hogle, J. M., M. Chow, and D. J. Filman, Three-dimensional structure of poliovirus at 2.9 Å resolution. *Science 229*:1358–1365 (1985).

3. Luo, M., G. Vriend, G. Kamer, I. Minor, E. Arnold, M. G. Rossmann, U. Boege, D. G. Scraba, G. M. Duke, and A. C. Palmenberg, The structure of Mengo virus at atomic resolution. *Science 235*:182–191 (1987).

4. Stauffacher, C. V., R. Usha, M. Harrington, T. Schmidt, M. V. Hosur, and M. V. Johnson, The structure of cowpea mosaic virus at 3.5 Å resolution. In *Crystallography in Molecular Biology*, D. Moras, J. Drenth, B. Strandberg, D. Suck, and K. Wilson, eds., pp. 293–308 (1987).

5. Harrison, S. C., A. J. Olson, C. E. Schutt, F. K. Winkler, and G. Bricogne, Tomato bushy stunt virus at 2.9 Å resolution. *Nature 276*:368–373 (1978).

6. Abad-Zapatero, C., S. S. Abdel-Meguid, J. E. Johnson, A. G. W. Leslie, I. Rayment, M. G. Rossmann, D. Suck, and T. Tsukihara, Structure of southern bean mosaic virus at 2.8 Å resolution. *Nature 286*:33–39 (1980).

7. Lijas, L., T. Unge, T. A. Jones, K. Fridborg, S. Lovgren, U. Skoglund, and B. Strandberg, Structure of satellite tobacco necrosis virus at 3.0 Å resolution. *J. Mol. Biol. 159*:93–108 (1982).

8. Hogle, J. M., A. Maeda, S. C. Harrison, The structure and assembly of turnip crinkle virus. I: X-ray crystallographic structure analysis at 3.2 Å. *J. Mol. Biol. 191*:625–638 (1986).

9. Hosur, M. V., T. Schmidt, R. C. Tucker, J. E. Johnson, T. M. Gallagher, B. H. Selling, and R. R. Reuckert, The structure of an insect virus at 3.0 Å resolution. *Proteins Struct. Function Genet. 2*:167–176 (1987).

10. Vriend, G., and M. G. Rossmann, Determination of the orientation of a randomly placed crystal from a single oscillation photograph. *Acta Crystallogr.* (in press).

11. Smith, T. J., M. J. Kremer, M. Luo, G. Vriend, E. Arnold, G. Kamer, M. G. Rossmann, M. A. McKinlay, G. D. Diana, and M. J. Otto, The site of attachment in human rhinovirus 14 for antiviral agents that inhibit uncoating. *Science 233*: 1286–1293 (1986).

12. Rueckert, R. R., *Comprehensive Virology*, Vol. 6. H. Fraenkel-Conrat and R. R. Wagner, eds. Plenum, New York, pp. 131–213 (1976).

13. Abraham, G., and R. J. Colonno, Many rhinovirus serotypes share the same cellular receptor. *J. Virol. 51*:340–345 (1984).

14. Koch, F., and G. Koch, *The Molecular Biology of Poliovirus*. Springer-Verlag, New York (1985).

15. Palmenberg, A. C., In vitro synthesis and assembly of picornaviral capsid intermediate structures. *J. Virol. 44*:900–906 (1982).

16. Jacobson, M. F., J. Asso, and D. Baltimore, Further evidence on the formation of poliovirus proteins. *J. Mol. Biol. 49*:657–669 (1970).

17. Toyoda, H., M. J. H. Niclin, M. V. Murray, C. W. Anderson, J. J. Dunn, F. W. Studier, and E. Wimmer, A second virus-encoded proteinase involved in proteolytic processing of polio virus polyprotein. *Cell 45*:761–770 (1986).

18. Rueckert, R. R., Picornaviruses and their replication. In *Fundamental Virology*, B. Fields and D. K. Knipe, eds. Raven Press, New York, pp. 357–390 (1986).

19. Arnold, E., M. Luo, G. Vriend, M. G. Rossmann, A. C. Palmenberg, G. D. Parks, M. J. H. Nicklin, and E. Wimmer, Implications of the picornavirus capsid structure for polyprotein processing. *Proc. Nat. Acad. Sci. USA 84*:21–25 (1987).

20. Diana, G. D., M. A. McKinlay, M. J. Otto, J. Akullian, and C. Oglesby, {[(4,5-Dihydro-2-oxazolyl)phenoxy]alkyl}isoxazoles. Inhibitors of picornavirus uncoating. *J. Med. Chem. 28*:1906 (1985).

21. McKinlay, M. A., and B. A. Steinberg, Oral efficacy of WIN 51,711 in mice infected with human poliovirus. *Antimicrob. Agents Chemother. 29*:30 (1985).

22. Otto, M. J., M. P. Fox, M. J. Fancher, M. F. Kuhrt, G. D. Diana, and M. A. McKinlay, In vitro activity of WIN 51,711, a new broad-spectrum antipicornavirus drug. *Antimicrob. Agents Chemother. 27*:883–886 (1985).

23. Fox, M. P., M. J. Otto, and M. A. McKinlay, Prevention of rhinovirus and poliovirus uncoating by WIN 51711, a new antiviral drug. *Antimicrob. Agents Chemother. 30*: 110 (1986).

24. Caliguiri, L. A., J. J. McSharry, and G. W. Lawrence, Effect of arildone on modifications of poliovirus in vitro. *Virology 105*:86 (1980).

25. McSharry, J. J., L. A. Caliguiri, and H. J. Eggers, Inhibition of uncoating of poliovirus by arildone, a new antiviral drug. *Virology 97*:307 (1979).

26. Diana, G. D., U. J. Salvador, E. S. Zalay, R. E. Johnson, J. C. Collins, D. Johnson, W. B. Hinshaw, R. R. Lorenz, W. H. Thielking, and F. Pancic, Antiviral activity of some β-diketones. 1. Aryl alkyl diketones. In vitro activity against both RNA and DNA viruses. *J. Med. Chem. 6*:750–756 (1977).

27. Diana, G. D., J. Salvador, E. S. Zalay, P. M. Carabateas, G. L. Williams, J. C. Collins, and F. Pancic, Antiviral activity of some β-diketones. 2. Aryloxy alkyl diketones. In vitro activity against both RNA and DNA viruses. *J. Med. Chem. 6*:757–761 (1977).

28. Incardona, N. L., and P. Kaesberg, A pH-induced structural change in bromegrass mosaic virus. *Biophys. J. 4*:11 (1974).
29. Robinson, I. K., and S. C. Harrison, Structure of the expanded state of tomato bushy stunt virus. *Nature 297*:563–568 (1982).
30. Kruse, J., K. M. Kruse, J. Witz, C. Chauvin, B. Jacrot, and A. Tardieu, Divalent ion-dependent reversible swelling of tomato bushy stunt virus and organization of the expanded virion. *J. Mol. Biol. 162*:393–417 (1982).
31. Fox, P., F. Dutco, and M. A. McKinlay (unpublished results).
32. Diana, G. D., M. J. Otto, M. A. McKinlay, R. C. Oglesby, A. Treasurywala, E. G. Maliski, M. G. Rossmann, and T. J. Smith, Enantiomeric effects of homologues of disoxaril on the inhibitory activity against human rhinovirus 14. *J. Med. Chem. 31*: 540–544 (1988).
33. Badger, J., I. Minor, M. J. Kremer, M. A. Oliveira, M. Luo, M. G. Rossmann, M. A. McKinlay, G. D. Diana, F. J. Dutto, R. R. Reuckert, B. Heinz, T. J. Smith, J. P. Griffith, D. M. A. Guerin, and S. Krishnaswamy, Structural analysis of a series of antiviral agents complexed with human rhinovirus 14. *Proc. Natl. Acad. Sci. USA 85*: 3304–3308 (1988).
34. Matthews, B. W., H. Nicholson, and W. J. Becktel, Enhanced protein thermostability from site directed mutations that decrease entropy of unfolding. *Proc. Natl. Acad. Sci. USA 84*:6663–6667 (1987).
35. Palmenberg, A. C. (unpublished results).

11

Conformation Biological Activity Relationships for Receptor-Selective, Conformationally Constrained Opioid Peptides

Victor J. Hruby
University of Arizona, Tucson, Arizona

B. Montgomery Pettitt
University of Houston, Houston, Texas

405

I. INTRODUCTION

There has been a revolution in our ability to undertake the rational design of peptide hormones and neurotransmitters. Unparalleled experimental and theoretical developments in peptide chemistry and biophysics methodology and rapid developments of new biological assay methods and molecular biological approaches have provided new tools for the design, synthesis, and analysis of peptides with extraordinary biological properties including (1) superpotency; (2) in vivo stability against degradative enzymes; (3) antagonist biological activities; (4) high receptor selectivity; (5) ability to cross membrane barriers; and (6) highly prolonged in vitro and in vivo biological responses. In some cases, it has been possible to design peptides with all of these desirable activities.

Although a good deal of fundamental science is still needed to establish general approaches, it is now clear that, although most peptide hormones and neurotransmitters are short-lived and easily biodegradable in the biological system (they are designed by nature to be so), this is not an intrinsic property of peptides. Indeed, in several cases, peptide hormone or neurotransmitter analogs have been designed that possess extraordinary potency, prolonged biological activity, and even oral activity (for examples see Refs. 1–6). In some cases stability to enzyme degradation has been demonstrated (e.g., 7,8), but clearly prolonged biological activity need not be related to the enzymatic stability. In any case, there now is ample precedent for suggesting that the rational design of peptide ligands for the endocrine and central nervous system (CNS) is possible.

In many successful cases of designed peptide ligands for receptors, conformational constraint has been a central theme (7,9–12). Although numerous approaches are possible within this context (12), perhaps the most successful have involved cyclization or transannular stabilization of secondary or tertiary structure. Often these peptide analogs are sufficiently constrained that they can only assume a relatively limited number of conformations. Thus study of their conformational and dynamic properties becomes accessible using modern one- and two-dimensional nuclear magnetic resonance (NMR) and other spectroscopic methods in conjunction with modern molecular mechanics methods to examine possible low-energy conformations and molecular dynamics methods to explore the thermally accessible conformational space (13). When coupled to modern molecular graphics, these tools provide working conformational models that serve as reasonable starting points for the further design of analogs to test developing ideas of conformation–biological activity relationships.

Equally important has been the explosive development of new quantitative assay methods both in vitro and in vivo. Peptide hormone and neurotransmitter receptors serve as extraordinarily sensitive and precise monitors of the stereoelectronic, structural, and conformational requirements for a particular hormone or neurotransmitter. Hence, careful quantitative evaluation of biological activities of analogs provides essential data for the design of further analogs. Careful integration of chemical, physical, and biological methodologies is essential for successful rational design of potent and specific peptide hormone and neurotransmitter analogs.

In this chapter we will review studies utilizing the above approach that have led to the design of conformationally constrained cyclic enkephalin analogs with extraordinary δ opioid receptor selectivities and the use of the results from these studies to begin δ opioid receptor mapping studies. In addition, we will examine a designed series of somatostatin-like peptide analogs with little or no somatostatin-like biological activity but with extraordinary potency and specificity for μ opioid receptors. These latter studies represent a new approach to peptide receptor ligand design that is referred to as the "molecular template" approach.

II. GENERAL CONSIDERATIONS

A. Multiple Opioid Receptors

In general, peptide hormones and neurotransmitters have several receptor systems with which they interact under various physiological conditions. For example, the classical peptide hormone oxytocin has been known for many years to interact with both uterine and mammary gland receptors (14,15). In addition, it has avian vasodepression activity (the classical assay for the hormone), pressor effects in mammals, and antidiuretic and natriuretic effects (14). More recently it has been shown to have a variety of CNS effects (15–18). From the results from many laboratories, we postulated some time ago that, in general, different receptors utilized different structural *and* conformational features of the native hormone for interaction at the various receptors (19–21). Furthermore, it was postulated that agonist and competitive antagonist analogs would utilize *different* structural and conformational features for interacting with a specific receptor (11,19–22) for the hormone—that is, that the binding "message" was different from the structural and conformational features required for transduction (agonist activity). Much evidence now exists to support these suggestions for a number of peptide hormone and neurotransmitter systems.

In this regard, the opioid receptor systems provide a very fruitful area for the application of these ideas. It was suggested some time ago (23–25) that there exists at least three different opioid receptor systems—δ (delta), μ (mu), and κ (kappa)—and perhaps others as well. In the meantime, much evidence has appeared to fully support these suggestions (e.g., see reviews 26–28). Moreover, from the work presented here and from other studies, there is now overwhelming evidence that all of these receptors have different structural requirements for peptide-receptor interaction. Thus, the pharmacophore for each receptor type is different, which has often been ignored in previous efforts to understand "the biologically active conformation" for the opioids. Investigators have often used a single assay to evaluate "opioid activity" and thus have obtained results derived from interaction of a given ligand with several different opioid receptors, further confusing the issue.

B. Structure–Function Analysis of Opioid Peptides—A Brief Overview

Several thousand opioid peptide analogs have been reported, and undoubtedly many more are known, since there has been much activity by pharmaceutical companies in this area. Several reviews of opioid peptide structure-function analysis have appeared (e.g., 29–31), and each year *Peptides* publishes a comprehensive review of the extensive literature appearing the previous year on the multiple biological activities of the opioid peptides (see Ref. 33 for a recent example). It is not the purpose of this section to review comprehensively the literature that exists, but rather to examine a few key issues regarding structure and function that have emerged from classical structure-function analysis.

In any effort to examine the natural endogenous opioid peptides, especially the enkephalins [Met[5]]enkephalin, H–Tyr–Gly–Gly–Phe–Met–OH, and [Leu[5]]enkephalin, H–Tyr–Gly–Gly–Phe–Leu–OH, and the more recently discovered dynorphins, e.g., dynorphin A, H–Tyr–Gly–Gly–Phe–Leu–Arg–Arg–Ile–Arg–Pro–Lys–Leu–Lys–Trp–Asn–Asn–Gln–OH, one is immediately faced with discussing structure-function analysis at multiple opioid receptors. In retrospect, it would appear that many previous structure-function studies made no distinction. Nonetheless, though questions still remain, there is general agreement that dynorphin peptides have κ receptor selectivity, whereas the enkephalins have selectivity for δ and μ receptors with slight preference for δ receptors. Most structure-activity studies have concentrated on the enkephalins. Several general structural features have emerged from these studies as apparently critical for strong peptide opioid receptor agonist interaction. (1) An L-tyrosine or substituted L-tyrosine residue with an amino terminus is needed; N-acylated analogues have very low potency. (2) Glycine-2 can be substituted with most D amino acids with maintenance of high potency, but analogs containing L amino acids generally have low potency. The exception is that an L-Pro residue can be used in the morphiceptin peptides. (3) The glycine residue in position 3 generally cannot be readily substituted for either D or L amino acids, but it can simply be left out in many analogs and still retain high potency. (4) The phenylalanine in position 4 can be substituted with many other amino acids with the maintenance of moderate potency, but the most potent analogs are generally N-methyl-substituted phenylalanine or ring-substituted phenylalanine analogs. (5) Finally, the leucine (or methionine) in the 5 position can simply be eliminated and replaced by an amide group, or a variety of D or L amino acids, α-amino acid amides, or α-amino alcohols with the maintenance of high potency.

These studies have provided a few potent, highly receptor-selective analogs. Although one may argue the relative merits of the various ligands for specific applications, it would appear that the following peptide analogs are examples of linear peptides with reasonable receptor selectivities which we will define as $\geqslant$ 100-fold: (1) μ receptor agonists—H–Tyr–D–Ala–Gly–N–MePhe–Gly-ol (DAGO) (34) and H–Tyr–Pro–N–MePhe–D–Pro–NH$_2$, (PLO17) (35), μ receptor antagonists—no linear peptide analogues (see later); δ receptor agonists—linear peptide analogues, H–Tyr–D–Thr–Gly–Phe–Leu–Thr–OH (36); δ receptor antagonists—none known, though N,N–diallyl–Tyr–Aib–Aib–Phe–Leu–OH (37) is close to 100; κ receptor agonists and antagonists—none are known, though dynorphin A (1–9), H–Tyr–Gly–Gly–Phe–Leu–Arg–Arg–Ile–Arg–OH, is at least 15-fold selective.

Many physical studies have been made on a variety of linear enkephalins and enkephalin analogs (for recent reviews see Refs. 38,39). It is perhaps not surprising, therefore, that there are about as many models for the "biologically active" conformation as there are proposers. The multiple conformations possible for the enkephalins, the difficulties of unambiguous interpretation of biophysical data in terms of conformation and topology in such cases, and the lack of consideration of the multiple opioid receptor problem have made it difficult to interpret most previous results in terms of conformation–biological activity relationships at a specific receptor.

C. Why Use Conformational Constraints in Peptide Neurotransmitter Research?

From the above considerations, it seems reasonable to suggest that further conformational constraints would be required to more precisely define conformation–biological activity relationships at specific opioid receptors. Conformational constraints provide many potential advantages (12) in the exploration of peptide neurotransmitter conformational structure–biological activity relationships. This is particularly the case if one can arrive at constrained peptide analogs that possess high receptor binding potency and have a single or relatively restricted number of possible conformations. Under these circumstances a variety of structural changes would be possible without significantly affecting the overall conformational properties, and hence specific structural changes can be made to explore specific structural, topographical, conformational, and dynamic properties of a particular "site" in the peptide ligand that are compatible with high receptor-ligand potency, selectivity, etc. (receptor mapping). Using this approach, several opportunities for rational chemical design directly related to biology are likely to present themselves, including the following: (1) increased potency at the receptor(s); (2) increased receptor selectivity (each receptor has different conformational requirements); (3) development of a receptor antagonist (conformational constraint is consistent with receptor recognition but not transduction); (4) receptor-related prolonged biological activity (ligand remains in the "receptor compartment" much longer); (5) increased stability to biological degradation (e.g., enzymes, both specific and nonspecific); (6) more predictive insights into the "biologically active" conformation; (7) constrained analogs can serve as templates for further analysis of conformation–biological activity relationships.

The use of conformational constraints has been successfully applied to a number of neurotransmitter peptides (for recent reviews see 12,38–40). In the area of the opioid peptides, pioneering work was done by Schiller and co-workers, who placed dibasic D amino acids in position 2 and then prepared a series of cyclic lactam structures by cyclization of the ε amino group on this amino acid with the C-terminal backbone carboxylate in [Leu^5]enkephalin analogs (41–43). In this series, the cyclic analog H–Tyr–D–Lys–Glu–Phe–Leu⌐ appears to be the most selective, with about a 40-fold selectivity for the μ vs. the δ receptor. In a somewhat different approach, amino acid side chain to amino acid side chain lactam ring formation was accomplished in both pentapeptide and des-Gly^3 tetrapeptide cyclic analogs (44,45). To date the most selective analog appears to be H–Tyr–D–Orn–Phe–Asp–NH$_2$, which has about a 210-fold selectivity for the μ vs. the δ receptor. In the meantime, we have developed δ and μ receptor ligands more highly selective which are also conformationally constrained, via the rational design features discussed in Sections III and IV of this chapter.

D. Approaches to Peptide Conformations in Solution

In this section we give a brief, selective review of theoretical and experimental methods useful in conformational studies and concentrate on techniques where the interplay between theory and experiment is the greatest. The experimental tools with perhaps the widest applicability are the one- and two-dimensional NMR spectroscopies. The 2-D experiments, especially correlation spectroscopy (COSY) and nuclear Overhauser enhancement spectroscopy (NOESY), are particularly sensitive to conformational structure for examination of solution conformation.

Vibrational spectroscopies, such as infrared (IR) and Raman, most clearly in the N–H and carbonyl stretching regions, are sensitive to hydrogen-bonding environment. Consequently these spectroscopies provide a complementary experimental tool to NMR. In other selected cases, energy transfer measurements (fluorescence techniques) and circular dichroism (CD) spectroscopy can provide additional valuable information.

Although these experiments can be used to construct physical models of the compounds, such static models may be somewhat misleading in detail. Using the available force fields for peptides and related compounds, it is possible to refine a given structure via geometry optimization or energy minimization (46,47). Even this coarse approach will already reveal that a number of low-energy structures may be able to satisfy the experimental data. The number of possible structures found by energy minimization demonstrates the intrinsic complexity of the problem, namely, that one must deal with a thermal distribution of conformations in solution. Such a realistic view of the conformational problem is immediately apparent from molecular dynamics and non-Boltzmann simulation techniques (46,47). These approaches allow one to pass from the underlying energy surface to the intramolecular free-energy surface. A number of approximate theories of the effective solvent modified intramolecular potential also yield similar insights (at a fraction of the computer time) into the distribution of conformers sampled in solution (47,48).

Given such a free-energy surface, the height of the barriers then determines, in part, the rates of transitions. Experiments then will be sensitive to conformational changes within their own time scale. This is especially important in making the connection between a molecular dynamics simulation of a peptide in solution which may last for 10's to 100's of picoseconds versus the time resolution for NMR of nanoseconds and longer.

1. Spectroscopic Methods

Various NMR spectroscopic methods are currently the most widely used experimental methods and in principle are capable of providing direct conformational information about peptides in solution. Whereas the earliest studies primarily concentrated on rather simple, short peptides, the increased usage of Fourier transform methods and two-dimensional techniques has led to the structural elucidation of ever more complex peptides. A number of reviews have recently appeared on a range of applications (49–51).

Proton and ^{13}C NMR of peptides in the solid state (crystalline or matrix) is a method capable of yielding very high resolution spectra (49). Samples for this technique do not have to be of the same crystalline quality needed for diffraction techniques, which is a practical advantage.

It is, of course, in the liquid state that most peptides are biologically active. For the NMR time scales, different conformations can be distinguished for single-bond dihedral rotational barriers of 4 or 5 kcal/mol or higher. Although spectrometers and experimental design techniques have greatly increased in sophistication, some of the greatest progress has involved the additional advantage gained by designed synthetic conformational restrictions, especially cyclizations to reduce the number of conformers accessible in solution.

The techniques of fluorescence spectroscopy have been used to study the conformational and dynamical aspects of peptides in solution for at least two decades (52). The information obtained in such experiments is somewhat indirect. However, these data can be used to test various hypotheses about suggested conformations related to side chain spatial arrangements. Experimental advances in this area, such as the use of synchroton sources (53), have allowed the measurement of rotational correlation times well below a nanosecond and thus hold a great deal of promise in the future for such relaxation time measurements.

Infrared and Raman vibrational spectroscopies have long been used for studying the conformations of peptides in various solvents (54–57). In most cases the evidence from these experiments is in the form of N–H stretching frequencies. These spectra have frequently been taken in dilute CCl_4 or mixtures of CCl_4 and $CHCl_3$. Some studies have been performed in H_2O and D_2O. Such studies have given a wealth of indirect data on the molecular conformations. This is indirect information, because the geometric parameters that specify a conformation are not measured from the spectrum but are given by a model (with force field) that is fit to reproduce some features of the spectrum (58). These techniques, however, are useful for discerning whether multiple conformations exist. It is in this capacity that many valuable studies have been performed. Although in relatively nonpolar solvents few (two or three) conformations for dipeptides are predicted, the case in aqueous solution is not as clear (47,57).

Circular dichroism spectroscopy can also be a very valuable method for examining overall conformational properties of peptides and certain specific conformational parameters as well (59). In particular, CD can readily be used to examine α-helical and β sheet structures, and more recently it has been developed for the examination of various reverse turn conformations. Perhaps the most useful application for specific conformational information with peptides is the use of the quadrant rule to examine the helicity (right-handed or left-handed) of the disulfide bond in peptides.

2. Uses of Molecular Modeling

In even its simplest form, the molecular model can provide a useful tool in the conception of a compound's activity. By using either a set of physical models or a graphics program, one is given an immediate intuitive view of the molecular structure. This usefulness is related to the explicit chemical constraints that such model building incorporates.

If we imagine a limiting procedure by which the bonds and angles are made essentially rigid at their equilibrium positions, then only the torsions are left free to deform. The only constraint then applicable to the dihedral degrees of freedom are those imposed by the Van der Waals size of the atoms in question. Such nonbonded interactions generally take place at a distance of three or more chemical bonds.

The hard sphere approach to modeling steric contacts is a very valuable "zeroth-order" approximation to the allowed conformational space. Such models, although long used in the chemical physics literature to model a variety of systems, including scattering of small molecules and simple molecular fluids, were first used by Ramachandran and co-workers (60) in the prediction of peptide conformations. These crude representations are immediately useful in a cursory examination of what is or is not reasonable, such as ring closure or interpreting information from 2-D NMR experiments.

Although the rigid bonding structures–hard sphere models are quite primitive in terms of predicting what is allowed, they are certainly most instructive in terms of what is not allowed. Even in this sense the extreme nature of the interaction leads to disallowing conformations that more sophisticated approaches show are eminently reasonable, such as a C_{7ax} conformer for the blocked alanine residue.

The main differences between the rigid models and more realistic force fields, even in vacuo, are due to the fact that small deviations in bond angles and to a lesser extent bond lengths costing 1 or 2 kcal/M can relieve hundreds of kcal/M in Van der Waals strain. Also electrostatics, especially in the form of hydrogen-bonding interactions, can give considerable stabilization to certain conformations. Thus the techniques of molecular mechanics can take modeling efforts far beyond the simplest considerations with only a small price to pay in complexity.

3. Molecular Mechanics

The use of empirical force fields combined with the techniques of minimization and constrained minimization for exploring energy surfaces is generally referred to as molecular mechanics. This approach to conformational problems has been widely used to study the smallest polyatomic systems to proteins. A number of reviews (46,47,61) and a monograph (62) have given quite thorough presentations of the material in this field.

In most conformational studies molecular mechanics is the next step in conceptual complexity used to refine the ideas from the model-building stage. In general practice, one starts with a number of possible guesses to the likely conformations and then refines the geometry of such estimates by searching for "nearby" minima on a potential energy surface. Even a vacuum potential energy surface for a short polypeptide will have so many local minima that even slight alterations in the minimization procedure or algorithm may find more than one minimum near a given starting structure.

One of the simplest procedures adopted is to directly minimize the guess conformers without the aid of any restraints. If a conservative minimization technique such as a steepest-descent method is used, then one will proceed to a minimum that in some sense is nearest to the starting structure. On the other hand, more robust algorithms, such as conjugate gradient or adopted basis Newton-Rhaphson, will frequently bypass a shallow local minimum in search of a deeper extremum.

It is not uncommon to impose a constraint on the search as a method of guiding the search toward a supposed minimum energy structure. Such constraints can either by rigid constraints, such as fixing bond lengths or angles, or flexible constraints. In the latter case, the restraint usually takes the form of an energy penalty—an extra term added to the empirical energy surface that keeps various degrees of freedom from wandering too far from a preset geometry without paying a substantial energy penalty.

A useful approach for probing the surface for selected degrees of freedom that uses the method of constrained minimization is called "mapping." In such a procedure one uses energy penalties to constrain certain degrees of freedom and then minimizes the system. The geometry specifying n constraints is then slightly changed, and the system is reminimized. This is continued until an n-dimensional energy subsurface is completely mapped out. This is most frequently used for $n \leq 3$ for obvious graphical (visualization) reasons. Such a procedure is really nothing more than the logical extension of the Ramachandran technique to systems with more realistic energy surfaces (i.e., flexible, soft sphere models). However, as only a few interesting degrees of freedom at a time can be conveniently viewed in this fashion, such a technique, in even the best cases, is limited. In larger systems great care must be exercised, or such mapping procedures may not even yield meaningful results. An example might be when a cyclic coordinate such as a torsion angle is mapped, and upon completion of the cycle the energy does not come back to its original value. This sort of problem occurs when in the course of repeated straining and minimizing, the system is induced to undergo an "essentially irreversible" conformational transition in an unconstrained part of the molecule. Such is the price of using sophisticated potential model, as this sort of problem cannot arise in a rigid, hard sphere model. Another difficulty related to this is the multiple minimum problem. How does one know that all the conformers that may potentially satisfy our criteria have been found? This is a question that is better addressed by statistical mechanics. In terms of computer simulations both stochastic (Monte Carlo) and deterministic (molecular dynamics) methods as well as a variety of methods in between these extremes may be used to further examine the conformation populations (46,47). In addition, these techniques and other, more analytical methods allow for the inclusion of solvent (48). Solvent effects on conformational populations can be profound (47,68).

4. Molecular Dynamics

Molecular dynamics simulations are capable of sampling configuration space and are thus useful in calculating the averages needed for evaluation of thermodynamic quantities. Given a potential energy function for the system of interest, one only needs a starting configuration to begin. From this point one need only solve the equations of motion for the system which usually includes the surrounding solvent. Most applications use Newton's equations of motion, although Hamilton's equations are also occasionally used. For the most detailed calculations, the solute molecule(s) of interest and the surrounding solvent molecules are explicitly included in the computed phase space trajectory. Although this technique is computationally demanding, it may be used to discern information about the thermal fluctuations in the system and provide the average quantities necessary to compute changes in thermodynamic properties with respect to either conformation or chemical composition.

One common computer simulation technique in conformational searches is the use of high-temperature quenched dynamics (63). In this method one runs a trajectory, either in vacuum or on a solvent modified potential, at very high temperature, several hundred to a few thousand degrees Kelvin. Next, one takes a number of the coordinates separated in time from the trajectory and subjects each to an exhaustive minimization. The use of nonphysiological temperatures allows barriers that would only infrequently be crossed at room temperature to be traversed readily. Thus, one can wander quite far from the starting structure and sample a wide range of possible conformers.

In most cases a large number of the quenched high-temperature configurations minimize to very strained high-energy structures, but a reasonable percentage of the selected configurations minimize to low-energy and therefore probable conformations. We have used this technique to complete a search for the low-energy structures of enkephalin analogs after an extensive search by model-building techniques. As the high-temperature dynamics has no bias about what the structure should be, it is a handy companion method, even for relatively small molecules. For large molecules, such as enzymes, it is nearly indispensable as a search technique (63).

Another major use of computer simulations is to compute relative free energies including the effects of solvent. By using non-Boltzmann sampling techniques, the free energy map for 1 (or in some cases 2) degrees of freedom can be computed. The probability ratio is then easily related to the free-energy difference. Although such techniques easily give the most reliable measure of free-energy differences theoretically feasible, they are quite computer-intensive (46,47).

5.   New Techniques

To understand the behavior of solutes in an aqueous environment, it is essential to have methods for determining both inter- and intramolecular solvent-mediated interactions which are both reliable as well as relatively inexpensive. It is clear that a liquid solvent medium can have a profound influence on reaction rates (46). It is now widely accepted that conformational equilibria are also strongly affected by the presence of solvents (47). The simplest effects are demonstrated by the changes in equilibrium bond lengths and bond angles on going from gas to liquid phase as measured by diffraction experiments on few-atom molecules. However, for solutes that possesses less rigid degrees of freedom than covalent bonds and angles, such as torsions, the effects on the equilibrium populations can be striking (47,64). It is the single-bond torsions about dihedral angles that are the most important for governing conformational changes in biomolecules.

A simple example to demonstrate this is a system that contains four heavy (nonhydrogenic) atoms connected by a dihedral angle such as 1,2-dichloroethane (64). In the gas phase this molecule is nearly entirely in the trans conformation. The two chlorines are as far apart as possible. But in aqueous solution the equilibrium is changed until essentially no trans population remains. This shift from trans to gauche has to do with stabilizing dipolar interactions. For polypeptides, hydrogen-bonding competition also comes into play. N-methylalanyl acetamide and its glycine analog have been the subject of a number of theoretical solvation studies (47,65–69). Although such molecules are stable only in the C_7 conformations at room temperature without solvent, several studies both experimental and theoretical have indicated a marked increase in flexibility about the two central single bond dihedrals, $\varphi(C_\alpha-N-C'-C_\alpha)$ and $\psi(N-C'-C_\alpha-N)$ in aqueous solution. The theoretical studies performed with integral equation methods (67,69) and field theoretical techniques (47) offer a substantial (several orders of magnitude) savings in computer time required for their evaluation. However, work continues on validating the details of the predictions made by such approximate methods.

III. DESIGN OF CONFORMATIONALLY CONSTRAINED DELTA OPIOID RECEPTOR-SELECTIVE PEPTIDES

A. Considerations and Studies Leading to [*D*-Pen², *D*-Pen⁵]Enkephalin

The above considerations, especially IIA, IIB, and IIC, served as the primary impetus for the development, starting in 1981, of the δ receptor-specific enkephalin analogs. One additional observation was also important to our design considerations. As previously discussed, Schiller and co-workers had demonstrated the potential usefulness of side chain to backbone cyclization as a way to constrain the conformational freedom in enkephalins with lactam analogs such as H–Tyr–*D*–A₂bu–Gly–Phe–Leu⌐, which are selective for μ (vs. δ) opioid receptors. We thought it might be interesting to apply the concept of pseudoisosteric cyclization which had been successfully developed for our cyclic superpotent α-melanotropin analogs (3). From this perspective, the Gly² and Met⁵ residues in enkephalin were reminiscent of the Met¹ and Gly¹⁰ residues in α melanotropin. Hence substitution of the Gly² residue by a *D*–Cys² and the Met⁵ residue by a *D* (or *L*)–Cys⁵ to give a 14-membered cyclic structure seemed a good starting point.

On examining the literature, we found that Sarantakis (70) had reported in a patent the preparation of [*D*–Cys², *L*–Cys⁵]enkephalin and that the compound had analgesic activity, although no data on receptor specificity were reported. However, we wished to further constrain the proposed cyclic analog, and decided to do this by utilizing geminal dimethyl groups for restricting the conformation of the planned 14-membered ring system, an approach that we had demonstrated leads to conformational restriction in oxytocin antagonists (11,19,20,22,71–73). Thus, we first prepared the enkephalinamide (EA) analogs [*D*–Pen², Cys⁵]EA (1) and [*D*–Pen², *D*–Cys⁵]EA (2) (Table 1) (74) and utilized the mouse vas deference (MVD) and guinea pig ileum (GPI) for selectivity and potencies, and found them to be quite δ opioid receptor selective. At about the same time, Schiller et al. (75) reported that [*D*–Cys², *D*–Cys⁵]EA (3) and [*D*–Cys², *D*–Cys⁵]EA (4) had high potency but very little receptor selectivity (Table 1) in the same assay systems. These results indicated that the much higher delta opioid receptor selectivity of the D–Pen^2 analogs 1 and 2 was primarily due to the much *decreased* potency of 1 and 2 in the GPI (principally μ receptor) relative to 3 and 4, whereas relatively high potency is retained in the MVD assay (primarily δ receptor) system. Thus, the more highly constrained and sterically demanding D–Pen^2–containing analogs bring greater receptor selectivity. Preliminary NMR spectroscopic studies (76) indicated that indeed D–Pen^2–containing analogs are the more conformationally constrained but that the origins of the biological differences between them and the D–Cys^2 containing analogs 3 and 4 must be due to conformational effects in the C-terminal portion of the cyclic peptides 1 and 2. We interpret this as due to the transannular effect(s) of the geminal dimethyl groups of D–Pen^2 in the 14-membered ring system.

Earlier structure-function studies (77–79) with linear enkephalin analogs had indicated that carboxylate terminal enkephalins were relatively more potent in the MVD (δ receptor) assay whereas carboxamide terminal analogs were relatively more potent in the GPI (μ receptor) assay. We therefore decided to examine the properties of the carboxylate terminal analogs of 1 and 2 (82). As shown in Table 1, both carboxylate terminal peptides 5 and 6 became slightly less potent in the GPI (μ receptor) assay relative to the corresponding carboxamide analogs 1 and 2, respectively, but both 5 and 6 showed increased potency relative to 1 and 2 in the MVD (δ receptor) assay. Thus compound 5, DPLCE, was found to be at the time the most δ opioid receptor-selective compound as measured by these in vitro assays.

The receptor-binding affinities to opioid receptors in rat brain membrane preparations using [^{3}H]naloxone (a mildly selective μ opioid antagonist) and [^{3}H]DADLE (a nonselective δ opioid agonist) were examined (74,80,81), and though qualitatively similar results were obtained, the specificities observed for these compounds for δ vs. μ opioid receptor were quantitatively lower. Several important factors may account for these differences: (1) species differences; (2) differences in tissue—i.e., peripheral vs. central tissue; (3) heterogeneity of binding parameters, populations, and other properties of the receptor subtypes; and (4) lack of discrimination of the receptor subtypes by the competing tritiated ligands.

Despite these problems we were highly encouraged by our results and sought to further increase δ selectivity in this cyclic series. Studies in which D–Cys was placed in position 2 and either D- or L-penicillamine was substituted in position 5 gave potent and highly selective analogs (80,81), but none were better than DPLCE (5).

This led us to examine the possible conformations for DPLCE and DPDCE and the corresponding D–Cys^2 and D (or L)–Pen^5 analogs. Classical reverse-turn conformations such as β turns, C$_7$ turns (γ turns), etc. were

Table 1 Biological Activities of Cyclic Enkephalin Analogs in GPI and MVD Assays

Compound[a]	IC_{50} (nM)[b] GPI	MVD	$\dfrac{IC_{50}\,(GPI)}{IC_{50}\,(MVD)}$
1. [D–Pen², Cys⁵]EA	118.	3.6	33.
2. [D–Pen², D–Cys⁵]EA	117.	16.8	7.
3. [D–Cys², Cys⁵]EA	1.51	0.76	2.
4. [D–Cys², D–Cys⁵]EA	0.78	0.30	2.6
5. [D–Pen², Cys⁵]E	213.	0.32	666.
6. [D–Pen², D–Cys⁵]E	1,350.	6.27	215.
7. [D–Pen², Pen⁵]E	2,720.	2.5	1,088.
8. [D–Pen², D–Pen⁵]E	6,930.	2.19	3,164.
9. [D–Pen², D–Phe⁴, Cys⁵]E	40,000.	84.	476.
10. [D–Pen², N–MePhe⁴, D–Pen⁵]E	180,000.	596.	300.
11. [D–Pen², Tic⁴, D–Pen⁵]E	⩾300,000.	1,500.	⩾200.
12. [D–Pen², β–MePhe(E), D–Pen⁵]E	42,700.	23.4	1,820.

examined. Interestingly we noted in many of these models for the D–Pen^2 as well as for the D (or L)–Pen^5 analogs that the β-hydrogens on the half-cysteine residues whether D–Cys^2 or D (or L)–Cys^5, respectively, were not especially sterically hindered by the side-chain groups on positions 1, 4, and 2 (or 5). It thus seemed possible that despite the conformational constraints imposed by the geminal β,β-dimethyl groups already on the D (or L)–Pen residue in the 14-membered ring system, a second pair of geminal dimethyl substitutions might be placed in the 14-membered ring system. We therefore decided to prepare the peptides H–Tyr–D–Pen–Gly–Phe–Pen–OH (7) and H–Tyr–D–Pen–Gly–Phe–D–Pen–OH (8). Indeed, the synthesis of these compounds proceeded well, the monomers were obtained in high yield (83), and purification could be readily accomplished by partition chromatography followed by gel filtration (83). The biological activities of 7 and 8 in the in vitro bioassays using the GPI and MVD assays are shown in Table 1. The results are indeed satisfying, with DPDPE 8 being the most selective δ opioid receptor ligand reported to date using these assay systems, and DPLPE being nearly as good. Receptor-binding studies using rat brain membrane preparations were made on these compounds using [^{3}H]naloxone and [^{3}H]DADLE (the results are shown in Table 2) and compared with a few other selective delta opioid ligands. Clearly DPDPE and DPLPE are highly δ opioid receptor-selective ligands.

Recently we (84) and others (85–87) have made more extensive binding

Table 2 Receptor-Binding Affinities of Selected Cyclic Enkephalin Analogs with δ Opioid Receptor Selectivity in Rat Brain Membrane Preparations

Compound[a]	IC$_{50}$ (nM)[b]		$\dfrac{IC_{50}\,(NAL)}{IC_{50}\,(DADLE)}$
	[^{3}H]NAL	[^{3}H]DADLE ([^{3}H]DPDPE)	
8. [D–Pen^2, D–Pen^5]E	3710	10. (2.3)	371. (1613)
7. [D–Pen^2, Pen^5]E	2840	16.2 (2.8)	175. (1014)
5. [D–Pen^2, Cys^5]E	178	11.7 (0.9)	15.2 (198)
6. [D–Pen^2, D–Cys^5]E	157	26.	6.0
Morphine	23.3	27.2	0.86
[D–Thr^2, Leu^5, Thr^6]E	36.3	6.4	5.7
[D–Ser^2, Leu^5, Thr^6]E	88.	5.7	15.4

[a]E = enkephalin.
[b]Values of the mean ($\pm$ SEM—not shown) of three to six determinations, each done in triplicate.

studies with DPDPE and DPLPE and other opioid peptide ligands using the tritiated analog [³H]DPDPE as the δ opioid ligand. From both equilibrium binding studies and saturation binding studies it was found that DPDPE has a K_D of ~1.24 nM at neuroblastoma × glioma hybrid NG 108-15 cells (a pure δ receptor), 1.61 nM in the guinea pig brain, and 3.3–5.2 nM in the rat brain depending on location in the brain. Where direct comparisons are possible, very similar results were obtained by Cotton et al. (85). In a somewhat different approach, James and Goldstein (87,88) have demonstrated that DPDPE and DPLPE are the most delta receptor-selective compounds known. More recently Clark et al. (89) have shown that DPDPE is the first peptide found with a low affinity for the μ_1 opiate binding site, and Gulya et al. (90) have utilized this highly selective tritiated ligand to examine the localization of δ opioid receptor in the rat brain using light microscopic autoradiography. In addition, numerous in vivo studies using DPDPE and DPLPE have demonstrated that indeed δ opioid receptors have distinct biological effects which differ from those of μ and κ opioid receptors, and much more work along these lines can be anticipated in the future. Space does not allow discussion of these interesting and important studies.

B. Solution Conformation of [D–Pen², D–Pen⁵] Enkephalin from NMR Studies

The cyclic 14-membered ring structure of DPDPE coupled with the presence of two geminal dimethyl carbon atoms in the 14-membered ring would suggest that this highly δ opioid receptor-selective peptide should have a relatively limited number of available conformations. In this section we will briefly outline the NMR parameters for DPDPE with special emphasis on those parameters related to conformational properties. We have examined the proton NMR of DPDPE both in aqueous solution and in dimethylsulfoxide. DPDPE appears to have similar proton NMR spectra in both solvents. However, we have done more extensive studies in aqueous solution, and thus our discussion will concentrate on studies in this solvent.

Despite its relatively simple structure, the complete proton assignment for DPDPE presented some difficulties. First, several of the αCH protons were near the water peak, making it difficult to examine NH–αCH coupling constants and connectivities. A method that did not require solvent saturation methods was developed (91) and could be used for both 1-D and 2-D COSY and NOESY experiments. Two-dimensional COSY experiments were done in D_2O and in H_2O/D_2O (90:10) and were coupled with delayed COSY experiments and pH titration experiments to distinguish the D–Pen² residues from the D–Pen⁵ residue and the Tyr¹ and Phe⁴ residues (92). The delayed COSY experiments were needed to distinguish the D–Pen² from D–Pen⁵ β-

methyl groups which required examination of the long-range couplings of $C\alpha H$ to the $C\gamma H_3$ protons in the D-penicillamine residues.

The unambiguous assignments of the pro-R and pro-S methyl groups in the D–Pen residues and of the pro-R and pro-S hydrogens of the β-methylene groups in Tyr[1] and Phe[4] could not be made by these studies. However, subsequent studies have indicated that for D–Pen[2] the most upfield β-methyl protons were the pro-S, and the downfield β-methyl protons were the pro-R. Resonances for the strongly coupled alpha and β-proton for Tyr[1] and Phe[4] had to be simulated, since they were non-first-order. The simulated spectra are shown in Figure 1 along with the spectra for DPDPE in this region. The best-fit chemical shifts and coupling constants for all of the protons in DPDPE are given in Table 3 (93).

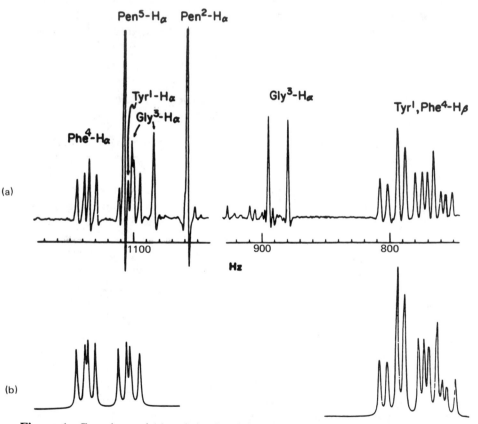

Figure 1 Experimental (a) and simulated (b) NMR spectra for the α and β proton regions of $[D$–Pen^2, D–Pen$^5]$enkephalin in aqueous solution

Table 3 ¹H NMR Chemical Shifts (in ppm) and Coupling Constants (in Hz) for $[D\text{-Pen}^2, D\text{-Pen}^5]$Enkephalin

Residue	δCH_3	$\delta_\alpha H$	$\delta_\beta H$	δ Aromatic	δNH	$^3J_{NH-\alpha CH}$	$^3J_{\alpha\beta}$	$^2J_{\beta\beta}$	$^2J_{\alpha\alpha'}$
Tyr¹		3.19 3.07	4.35	6.73 7.04			6.2 9.2	−13.9	
D-Pen²	0.85 1.49		4.25		8.09	8.1			−15
Gly³			3.42 4.20		8.41	4.2 8.5			
Phe⁴		3.19 3.05	4.45	7.20 (m)	8.32	6.8	5.5 9.0	−14.4	
D-Pen⁵	1.33 1.38		4.43		7.38	8.4			

The temperature dependence of the four peptide amide protons was determined. There was some difficulty in obtaining the D–Pen[5] amide NH proton temperature-dependent chemical shift, because this proton was "buried" in the same region of the spectrum as the Phe[4] aromatic protons. However, use of 2-D NMR spectral methods made it possible to determine its temperature dependence as well. At pH 3.1 the temperature dependencies were as follows: (1) D–Pen[2], -3.7×10^{-3} ppm/°C; (2) Gly[3], -4.3×10^{-3} ppm/°C; (3) Phe[4], -4.7×10^{-3} ppm/°C; and (4) D–Pen[5], -2.5×10^{-3} ppm/°C. Thus it would appear that there are no strong intramolecular amide hydrogen bonds in DPDPE.

A most interesting feature of the ^{1}H NMR of DPDPE is the very large nonequivalence of the Gly[3] αCH_2 protons (Table 3). Generally for most peptides there is a very small chemical-shift difference ($\Delta \delta = 0.0$–0.10 ppm) for these diastereotopic hydrogens, in part because of the general conformation flexibility around a Gly residue. However, in DPDPE the chemical-shift difference is 0.80 ppm, and these and even larger chemical shift differences are seen for other penicillamine-containing cyclic enkephalin analogs (Table 4). In the case of DPDPE, it might be suggested that this large chemical shift difference is due to a preferential interaction of the aromatic group, especially of Phe[4] with one of the Gly[3] α-hydrogens. However, as shown in Table 4, when the aromatic amino acid Phe[4] is replaced by an aliphatic amino acid, Acc (α-aminocyclohexane carboxylate), an analog is obtained that displays an almost identical chemical shift for these protons (Table 4). Additionally, when a tetrahydroisoquinoline carboxylate residue is placed in this position (91,94), a residue in which the aromatic ring is maintained in a conformation compatible with more certain interaction with

Table 4 Chemical Shift Nonequivalence of Gly[3] α-Hydrogens in Cyclic Enkephalin Analogs and Other Peptides

Peptide[a]	δ Gly[3] αCH_s	$\Delta \delta$	Ref.
H–Tyr–D–Pen–Gly–Phe–D–Pen–OH	3.42, 4.22	0.80	92
H–Tyr–D–Pen–Gly–Acc–D–Pen–OH	3.67, 4.51	0.84	94
H–Tyr–D–Pen–Gly–Tic–D–Pen–OH	3.68, 5.04	1.36	94
H–Tyr–D–Pen–Gly–Phe–D–Cys–OH	3.53, 3.98	0.45	76
H–Pen–Leu–Ile–Gln–Asn–Cys–Pro–Leu–Gly–NH$_2$	3.87, 3.96	0.09	72
Met–Gly–Met	b	0.00	95
Phe–Gly–Phe–Gly	b	0.10	95

[a]Acc = α-aminocyclohexane carboxylate; Tic = tetrahydroisoquinoline carboxylate.
[b]Not given in reference.

the Gly[3] α-protons, the chemical shift difference increases to 1.36 ppm for these hydrogens (Table 4). The results for DPDPE are consistent with the rotamer analysis for DPDPE (vide infra) in which the most populated χ^1 conformation places the Phe[4] aromatic ring more than 4 Å away from the Gly[3] α-CH$_2$ protons—that is, outside of the shielding or deshielding region of the aromatic ring.

The likely explanation for the large chemical-shift difference for these two Gly α-CH$_2$ protons is related to the quite rigid conformation of the peptide backbone in the 14-membered ring. The bulky disulfide bond and geminal dimethyl groups of the D–Pen[2] and D–Pen[5] residues tend to limit backbone flexibility and force peptide carboxyl groups away from the interior of the 14-membered ring. As a consequence of this, one of the Gly α-CH$_2$ protons is fixed in the shielding zone and the other in the deshielding zone of the peptide carbonyl of the peptide bonds adjacent to the α-CH$_2$ protons, especially the Gly[3] CO–Phe[4] NH, the carbonyl group of which is directly adjacent to the Gly[3] α-CH$_2$ protons. These results are consistent with the observation that the Gly[3] α-CH$_2$ protons are both shielded and deshielded relative to their "normal" position in most peptides. In this regard, it should be pointed out that the small nonequivalence of Gly α-CH$_2$ protons in most peptides previously has been explained (72,95,96) by suggesting that one of the protons (pro-R) was shielded more than the other (pro-S) as a result of the slight difference in orientation of these hydrogens with respect to the carbonyl group of the peptide bond. With a more rigid peptide backbone, this effect can apparently be greatly amplified.

As pointed out above, the temperature dependence of the peptide amide protons indicates that although these NH protons are somewhat solvent-shielded for such a small peptide, there are likely no significant amide hydrogen bonds for DPDPE in aqueous solution. Rather, as would be suggested from studies of solvent effects on peptides, it seems reasonable that the hydration of the peptide backbone in aqueous solution would tend to weaken the intramolecular hydrogen bonds and promote hydrophobic clustering of the nonpolar side-chain groups. The NMR results suggest, therefore, that all of the amide protons found in the 14-membered ring system are partially shielded from the solvent by their relative proximity to the hydrophobic side chain groups of D–Pen[2], Phe[4], and Tyr[1] (and possibly D–Pen[5]). With regard to the hydrophobic clustering of side-chain groups, we have consistently observed NOEs on the Bruker AM 250 spectrometer between the protons on the two β-methyl groups of D Pen[2] and the Tyr[1] *and* Phe[4] aromatic protons in DPDPE (Fig. 2).

Much less clear are the occasional observations of NOEs between the protons on the β-methyl groups of D–Pen[5] and the aromatic protons. In such 2-D NOE studies it is critical that all J coupling effects be eliminated so that

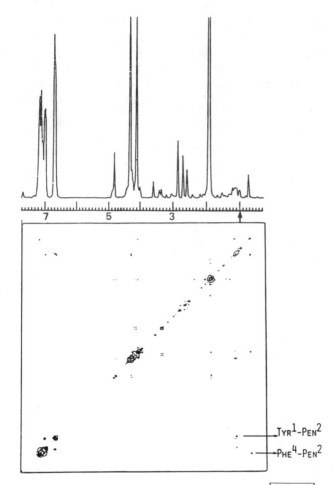

Figure 2 NMR NOESY experiments for [D–Pen^2, D–Pen^5]enkephalin in aqueous solution at 250 MHz.

only the NOEs are seen. We believe that this is the case for the NOEs seen between the D–Pen^2 β-methyl protons and the Tyr^1 and Phe^4 aromatic protons shown in Figure 2. These results therefore suggest that DPDPE possesses a rather compact conformation in aqueous solution in which the hydrophobic aromatic side chains of Tyr^1 and Phe^4 and the D–Pen^2 β-methyl groups are in close proximity to form a lipophilic topological arrangement. A number of conformations are possible within this context. Model building was begun, and a starting conformation was obtained (Fig. 3A). These model-building exercises indicated that C$_7$ and type I, II, and III β

turns can be built, but the lack of a strong intramolecular hydrogen bond suggested a more skewed reverse turn—i.e., a type IV β turn with the Gly[3] and Phe[4] residues serving as the i + 1 and i + 2 residues. A more precise definition of the likely conformation requires careful evaluation of low-energy conformations using molecular mechanics calculations (see below). However, there is one more conformational feature that can be examined from the NMR parameters which can help in this process, namely the side-chain conformations for Tyr[1] and Phe[4].

Table 3 summarizes the αCH–βCH coupling constants for Tyr[1] and Phe[4]. Calculation of the side-chain rotamer populations using the parameters of De Leeuw and Altona (97) indicate that the gauche (+) ($+60°$) conformer is largely excluded for both Tyr[1] and Phe[4] χ^1 values, while both the gauche($-$) ($-60°$) and trans ($\pm180°$) conformers are allowed. The rotamer populars are as follows: (1) for Tyr[1]—gauche($-$) 27%, and trans 73%; (2) for Phe[4]—gauche($-$) 30%, and trans 70%, though the reverse is possible in both cases because the diastereoisotopic β hydrogens are not stereochemically assigned. Excellent models for DPDPE could be built with either of these side-chain conformations for Tyr[1] and Phe[4]. However, to more clearly define low-energy conformations consistent with all the NMR, we turned to molecular mechanics calculations in an effort to find one (or more) low-energy conformations for DPDPE that would be consistent with all of the NMR data. The details of the approach and some of the results are outlined below.

C. Conformational Analysis of [D–Pen^2, D–Pen^5]-Enkephalin Using Molecular Mechanics Calculations

We have recently performed an extensive conformational analysis on [D–Pen^2, D–Pen^5]enkephalin (DPDPE) (92). As discussed earlier, in an effort to overcome the conformational complexity in small linear peptides such as the enkephalins, we have synthetically incorporated conformational constraints including amino acid side-chain to side-chain cyclization and geminal dimethyl substitution in medium-size rings (11,12,19–21) in an effort to obtain analogs constrained in a desired active conformation for a specific receptor.

For our theoretical modeling studies we modified the CHARMM protein parameters set to accommodate both D and L penicillamine. The empirical energy function used to obtain the energy-minimized structures included potential energy terms for bond lengths, bond angles, bond dihedral angles, improper dihedral angles, Van der Waals and electrostatic terms for nonbonded interactions, and a hydrogen-bonding potential. For these initial computations solvent molecules were not explicitly included in the calculations, but the effect of bulk solvent H_2O was approximated by employing a dielectric constant of 80, which is appropriate for a small molecule such as DPDPE (67). The neutral zwitterionic structure of DPDPE was used.

The structural starting points for conformational energy minimization calculations were obtained by utilizing several strategies which included structural models built having minimal constraints or with structural "constraints" that were imposed on the basis of interpreted NMR spectra. Each starting structure was then thoroughly minimized in energy (structure optimization), and the results were categorized according to energy. In all cases, any structural constraints initially imposed on the three-dimensional structure of DPDPE were relaxed during the calculation, and the energy minimization was allowed to finish without any conformational constraints. Our starting structure is shown in Figure 3A and a variety of other possible C_5, C_7, and various β-turn conformations with intramolecular hydrogen bonds were examined, given that all structures had to satisfy the obvious ring closure constraints.

None of the C_7 conformations or the β-turn conformations that resulted from the geometry optimization studies using these initial conformations led to conformations consistent with the NMR data, in that many φ angles so obtained were outside the range ($\pm 25°$) consistent with ^3J NMR parameters, though some of the C_7 conformations (e.g., structure in Fig. 3a) and β-turn conformations (e.g., Fig. 3b) were interesting. The overall energies found were lowest when experimentally derived data was used in the model building prior to energy minimization. From these sorts of studies, one of the lowest energy conformations obtained was about 10.1 kcal/mole and had no intramolecular hydrogen bond (Fig. 3c). In this search, the most stable intramolecular hydrogen bond-containing conformations involved a β-turn conformation with the D–Pen^5–NH to D–Pen^5–CO intramolecular hydrogen bond and an imbedded C_7-like conformation and an overall energy equal to -10.6 kcal/mole (Fig. 3d). However, its conformation was inconsistent

---

Figure 3 Stereostructures of [D–Pen^2, D–Pen^5]enkephalin representing the following structures: (a) a low-energy starting conformation with two C_7 turns with $\varepsilon = 1$ (note the near salt bridge); (b) a β-turn structure—this and all subsequent runs done with $\varepsilon = 80$ (note the H bond from Tyr OH to –COO$^-$; (c) β-turn structure with rings outside NOE distance; (d) β-turn (3_{10}) structure with embedded C_7 (weak H bonds), rings still outside NOE distance; (e) β-turn structure, no intramolecular H bonds, rings within NOE distance; (f) structure extended, no β-turn structure. See text for discussion.

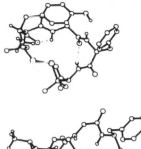
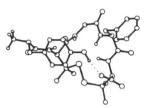
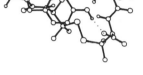
(a)

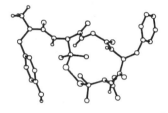
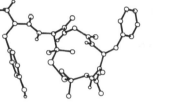
(b)

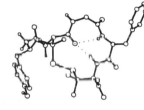
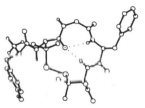
(c)

(d)

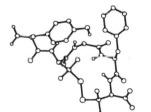
(e)

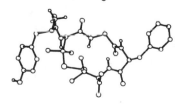
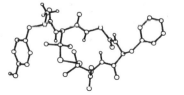
(f)

with some of the conformational features implied by the NMR experiments, such as the aromatic rings relative to the rest of the molecule.

By using the NMR-derived coupling constant parameters, anisotropy effects, especially on the Gly[3] diastereotopic α-hydrogens, and the proximity of the Tyr[1] *and* Phe[4] aromatic rings to the Pen[2] β-methyl group(s) as determined by NOESY experiments, a number of lower-energy candidates were obtained. In the process, a careful examination of side-chain dihedral angles was necessary. These studies led to a number of low energy conformations with overall energies ranging from -6 kcal/mole to -11 kcal/mole. None contained strong intramolecular hydrogen bonds but some contained weak ones; most had type IV β-turn conformations as defined by Lewis et al. (98). None of this group, after energy minimization, satisfied all of the NMR criteria.

This led us to further model building in which constraints consistent with the $J_{NH-\alpha CH}$ values were included and, in addition, conformations consistent with large chemical shift nonequivalence of the Gly[3] diastereotopic α-hydrogens. The anisotropic effects that led to this extraordinarily large nonequivalence was not due to the aromatic rings in DPDPE (vide supra). We postulated that this was the result of a somewhat "constrained" glycine residue with one of the α protons in the shielding cone of a peptide bond and the other in a deshielding region. An additional conformational consideration was the observation from the NOESY NMR studies that the Tyr[1] *and* Phe[4] aromatic ring protons were within a distance ($\leqslant 4.5$ Å) which allowed interaction with the D–Pen[2] β-methyl groups (Tyr[1] interacts with both β-methyl groups) but not extensively with the D–Pen[5] β-methyl groups. This led us to examine conformations consistent with these observations. Both right-handed and left-handed disulfide conformations were examined.

Interestingly, we found that often the low-energy conformations come in pairs, which primarily differed in conformation by the differences in their disulfide helicity [right-handed ($+$) or left-handed ($-$)] but otherwise with only minor perturbations in the rest of the structure. Energy minimization of a number of possible conformations led to the four low-energy conformations shown in Table 5 as the only conformations that satisfied the NMR criteria. [In fact, conformer 1′ (Fig. 3e; Table 5) does not satisfy the criteria for the Phe[4] φ angle, but is left in because of its close conformational similarity to conformer 1.] It is interesting that for both the Phe[4] and Tyr[1] side chains the gauche($+$) ($+60°$) conformation appears to be excluded. We have investigated this question by building models of 2′ and 1 (Table 5) with either or both χ_1 values changed from the ± 180 to $-60°$ or vice versa and then performing a geometry optimization. These changes had virtually no effect on the backbone conformations and only minor effects (± 1 kcal) on the overall energy. Overall, we found for the particular empirical force field we used that

Table 5 Low-Energy Backbone Conformations of DPDPE Satisfying All NMR Constraints

Residue	Angle	1	1'	2	2'
Tyr[1]	ψ	139	157	162	164
	ω	-176	-173	-173	-173
	χ_1	-171	-164	-164	-163
	χ_2	58	51	50	51
D–Pen[2]	φ	94	116	114	111
	ψ	83	53	27	14
	ω	-179	169	175	173
	χ_1	-167	-166	179	-180
	χ_2	-97	-137	87	143
Gly[3]	φ	-75	-108	-109	-98
	ψ	-41	12	-17	-18
	ω	-177	-176	177	177
Phe[4]	φ	-94	-128	-74	-72
	ψ	-50	-70	-63	-46
	ω	-177	-174	176	-175
	χ_1	-60	-56	180	179
	χ_2	102	103	62	68
D–Pen[5]	φ	87	69	83	83
	χ_1	-56	68	45	-70
	χ_2	74	-51	-140	119
	$\leqslant$CSSC	106°	-99°	102	-110
	F (kcal)	-12.4	-10.0	11.2	13.7

some distortion of bond angles and some dihedral angle strain is apparently compatible with low-energy conformations as a result of the significant stabilization provided by the intramolecular Van der Waals forces. The electrostatic effect was small because of the assumed solvent shielding.

Examining the conformational properties of the energy-minimized structures of the conformers in Table 5 indicated that the carbonyl groups of the amide bonds in the 14-membered ring (D–Pen[2] to Gly[3], Gly[3] to Phe[4], and Phe[4] to D–Pen[5] amide bonds) were all pointing out away from the 14-membered ring on the side opposite the two lipophilic aromatic rings and the β,β-dimethyl groups of D–Pen[2], to give an amphiphilic-like structure. A three-dimensional stereostructure for the low-energy conformation 2' in Table 4 is given in Figure 4. We did examine the effect of coordinated φ, ψ flips of the peptide amide bonds (the kind, for example, that convert a type 1 to a type 2β turn) and found that all such conformations were of much higher energy. An example of one of these conformations is given in Figure 3f.

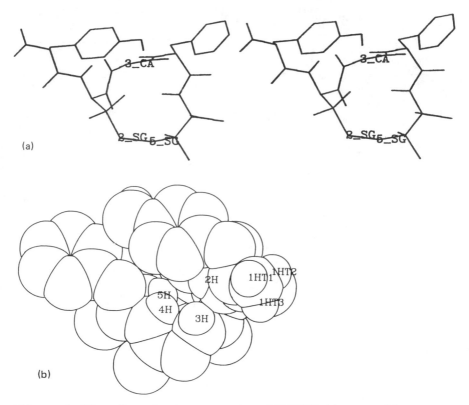

(a)

(b)

Figure 4 Three-dimensional representation of DPDPE: (a) stereo stick structure (color plate); (b) space-filling structure.

D. Molecular Dynamics Investigations of [D–Pen², D–Pen⁵]Enkephalin

In the previous section a series of molecular mechanics calculations were described. In any such search, whether or not one has truly covered all the possible, relevant conformations is always a concern. Since the number of configurations (only considering dihedral rotations) goes as the number of rotamers sampled per dihedral (times the number of dihedrals), it is possible that one has missed an important or relevant conformer, even in a molecule with only five amino acid residues and an internal macrocyclic constraint such as DPDPE. Several recent studies have shown how time-consuming a truly detailed search of polypeptide conformational space can be (92,99–102).

Thus, it is important to have a method that establishes the confidence level of a less than complete search.

We have employed a search technique based on annealing high-temperature molecular dynamics snapshots (63). A number of individual configurations from the trajectory are selected and then thoroughly mini-mized. A similar technique has also proved quite useful in the study of glasslike configurations obtained from a liquid-state simulation (103). In our technique a molecular simulation was run for the $[D\text{–}\overline{Pen^2, D\text{–}Pen^5}]$-enkephalin in a continuum aqueous solvent. The temperature chosen was about 1000°K. This elevated temperature allowed the molecule to explore a number of configurations that are separated by barriers that would be very infrequently crossed at room temperature as previously discussed. Thus the dynamics is used essentially to perform a search for other conformers that were not found in the model-building work already done. After an extensive heating and equilibration period, a 20-psec trajectory was obtained for the same model potential surface used earlier. From the resulting trajectory, 20 configurations were taken separated by 1-psec intervals. Each of these sets of coordinates was then subjected to an extensive energy refinement. A number of the configurations minimized to relatively high-energy conformations and may therefore be rejected as improbable in solution.

In the course of examining the remaining conformers, within 5 kcal/mol of the minimum, no configurations were found that differed significantly from the previous search. In several cases the resulting structures found in the quenched molecular dynamics search were related to previously described structures by symmetry-related rotations about side-chain dihedrals. Most common in such cases were 120° ring flips of the phenylalanine and tyrosine side chains.

During the process of heating the molecule to 1000°K, several inter-mediate equilibrations were used. An extensive equilibration run near 300°K was employed. During that run a highly correlated motion of the Phe and Tyr side chains was noticed. In the lowest energy minimum previously reported, the two aromatic rings were placed such that they were situated "on top" or roughly parallel to the macrocycle. During the dynamics the thermal energy of the molecule of course displaced it from its minimum-energy conformer. In the process the rings were found to move together in a positively correlated fashion, thus always exposing a similar orientation of the rings to the solvent. Associated with these side-chain motions we also noted at a higher temperature a hindered crank shaft motion about the disulfide dihedrals. This motion was hindered by the presence of the pair of geminal dimethyl groups from the two penicillamine residues and therefore only went from $+120°$ to $-120°$ via $\pm180°$.

Further conformationally restricted analogs of DPDPE have been synthesized and characterized pharmacologically. In particular the highly restricted tetrahydroisoquinoline carboxylate analog $[D–\overline{\text{Pen}}^2, \text{Tic}^4, D–\overline{\text{Pen}}^5]$enkephalin (DPTDPE) has been shown to have good specificity but less potency than $[D–\overline{\text{Pen}}^2, D–\overline{\text{Pen}}^5]$enkephalin (94).

DPTDPE was also examined by traditional molecular mechanics for energy minima. The low-energy conformer was found to be very similar in overall shape to that found for the DPDPE with the isoquinoline ring and the tyrosine ring in a similar position to that found in $[D–\overline{\text{Pen}}^2, D–\overline{\text{Pen}}^5]$-enkephalin. Thus from such a static calculation one might have predicted that the two compounds would have similar pharmacological profiles.

During a 10-psec dynamical simulation, a similar disulfide crank shaft motion was noted in the DPTDPE compound. Interestingly, this motion was found to disturb the mutual orientation of the Tic aromatic ring and the tyrosine ring, which was found in the other bis-penicillamine compound. This result is certainly suggestive of a dynamical difference in the two compounds being partly responsible for the difference in activity between the compounds. Although this dynamic hypothesis is attractive, more work remains to be performed to substantiate its validity. In our previous energy minimization studies we found that the lowest-energy conformers often came in pairs that differed only in their helicity about the disulfide bridge. Thus, even in the preliminary static calculations, we can see in retrospect that the disulfide crank shaft conformations were prominent in the $[D–\overline{\text{Pen}}^2, D–\overline{\text{Pen}}^5]$ compounds. However, it would not have been possible to even postulate such a "dynamic" conformational disruption from the simple molecular mechanics calculations.

Currently, dynamics calculations are in progress with the explicit inclusion of water. These studies will reveal the time scales for various small internal motions and will also serve as the starting materials for conformational free-energy profiles in solution.

E. Design of DPDPE Analogs for Delta Opioid Receptor Mapping and Investigation of the "Biologically Active" Conformation

The development of a conformational model for the conformationally constrained, cyclic, highly delta opioid receptor-specific peptide DPDPE provides us with an opportunity to utilize this conformational structure as a "template" for exploring the "biologically active" conformational structural and dynamic requirements of the δ opioid receptor (receptor mapping). Exploring the topochemical requirements for a specific receptor relative to other closely related receptors by rational design principles involves a number of underlying assumptions and requires the utilization and availability of a number of physical, chemical, and biological tools. It is perhaps worthwhile to briefly outline some of these assumptions and requirements.

Table 6 lists some of the basic assumptions utilized in efforts for receptor mapping of ligand requirements for a particular receptor. With respect to these assumptions, we would make the following comments (the numbers used here correspond to the numbers of Table 6) regarding our efforts using DPDPE.

1. The high δ receptor selectivity of DPDPE in several assay systems is compatible with the identity of a specific δ receptor and justifies the use of DPDPE as a template for it.

2. We will explore the validity of this assumption in our design of new analogs of DPDPE. Different assays must be used to assess this.

3. From the standpoint of peptide neurotransmitters, this can probably be true only if the ligand has a greatly reduced number of conformations available. From the standpoint of the receptor, it must be emphasized that bioassays often (generally) measure effects somewhat downstream from the ligand-receptor interaction, often making interpretation difficult.

Table 6 Some Assumptions in the Rational Design of Ligands in Peptide Neurotransmitter Receptor Mapping

1. The receptor has specific structural, conformational, and dynamic requirements for its ligands which clearly distinguish it from other receptors.
2. Different receptors will utilize different topochemical features of the same ligand for receptor interaction.
3. The bioassay methods used to examine particular receptor-ligand interactions faithfully reflect the specific ligand-receptor interactions.
4. The overall conformational and dynamic properties of the ligands in solution are in some consistent way related to conformational properties at the receptor.
5. Appropriate structural modifications of the side-chain (and perhaps other) groups can be made while maintaining most of the overall topographical properties of the neurotransmitter ligand.
6. Biophysical methods are available to assess the effects of structural perturbation of the ligand on its conformation and dynamics.
7. All aspects of any conformational model should be testable by specific structural changes which can be examined for biological effects in the standard assays.
8. Agonist and competitive antagonist analogs need not (and generally will not) interact with a receptor utilizing the same topochemical structural features.

4. How they are related to each other is subject to modification in the course of study as more information becomes available.

5. We have some specific suggestions about this (see below).

6. We will generally utilize NMR, CD, and Raman spectroscopic methods and molecular mechanics and molecular dynamics studies to assess these effects.

7. It is essential that any model be testable.

8. There is a good deal of evidence for this at a number of peptide hormone and neurotransmitter receptors. However, there are so few δ receptor-specific antagonists known that it is not possible to assess the situation at the δ receptor at this time.

Most of our investigations of δ receptor mapping involve structural modifications that will not drastically affect the peptide backbone conformation. Therefore, structural modifications will primarily involve changes in the side-chain moieties (β carbon or further removed). We also will make some structural modifications aimed at specifically testing our conformational model for DPDPE and its possible relationship to biological potency and specificity. Specific changes in configuration at the α carbon, substitutions at α carbons, and substitutions at the peptide amide NH protons will be examined. One change in configuration that does not have very important consequences in terms of selectivity or potency at the δ receptor is replacement of D–Pen^5 with a L–Pen^5 residue (DPLPE) (Table 1), where we saw virtually no difference in potency at δ receptors and only a slight difference at μ receptor.

We have performed both NMR studies and energy calculations on DPLPE, and the two studies show virtually the same overall topological properties particularly with regard to the relationships of the aromatic rings of Tyr^1 and Phe^4 and the D–Pen^2 side chain. The major difference appears to be the relationship of the carboxylate group to the rest of the molecule (a single configurational effect), and apparently this is acceptable to the δ receptor, which, as may be recalled, prefers a charged C-terminal group. It might be interesting to determine if this would hold in the carboxamide series, which generally has less specificity for the δ receptor and greater μ selectivity. We also have investigated configurational requirements at the Phe^4 position.

Our model building indicates that use of a D–Phe^4 residue would disturb the topochemical relationships of the side-chain groups in position 4 relative to positions 1 and 2, although some conformational compensation is possible so as to maintain the overall topological structure. Since the $[D$–Pen^2, L–Cys$^5]$E analog had the highest potency in the δ receptor MVD assay (Table 1), we made the D–Phe^4 substitution in this compound (9, Table 1).

Interestingly, as shown in Table 1, [D–Pen², D–Phe⁴, Cys⁵]E (9) loses about 250-fold in potency in the MVD (δ) assay. It nonetheless retains high δ selectivity (∼ 500-fold) because of a concomitant drop in potency in the GPI (μ) assay (Hurst et al., unpublished results). Thus, it would appear both the δ and μ receptor systems can accommodate this configurational change but at some expenditure in binding energy due to the unfavorable energy needed to obtain the desired topological arrangement of this Phe⁴ side-chain moiety in the D–Phe⁴ analog. Additional studies in the DPDPE series should provide detailed insight into the reasons for loss of binding at both receptor types. Other studies regarding configurational requirements are in progress.

We next decided to explore changes that would be expected, based on our conformational model, to greatly disrupt the DPDPE conformation. Our first effort along these lines involved substitution of the Phe⁴ NH proton with a methyl group. As discussed previously, the NMR results and conformation calculations indicate that this NH is somewhat buried in a lipophilic pocket involving the aromatic side-chain groups. Placement of a methyl group in this pocket is not possible sterically and thus should lead to a disruption of the conformation of DPDPE. Indeed, this analog [D–Pen², N–MePhe⁴, D–Pen⁵]E (10, Table 1) showed greatly reduced potency in the MVD assay (Table 1) and reduced selectivity as well, although it still favored the delta receptor. Interestingly, in this analog the chemical shift difference between the diastereotopic αCH protons of Gly³ is eliminated, perhaps because, as our NMR suggests, a cis peptide bond is now possible at the Gly³–N–MePhe⁴ bond, and possibly cis-trans isomerism reduces the anisotropic effect of the carbonyl group to virtually zero. This would be consistent with our suggestion (vide supra) that the large chemical shift differences in these protons in most D penicillamine-containing cyclic enkephalin analogs is due to the anisotropic effect of this carbonyl group in the constrained 14-membered ring system.

Tetrahydroisoquinoline carboxylate (Tic), as mentioned in Section IIID, is an interesting amino acid residue (A, Fig. 5) in this context. By appropriate disconnection, it can be viewed either as a constrained analog of 2′-methylphenylalanine (B, Fig. 5) or of N-methylphenylalanine (C, Fig. 5). More interesting is an examination of the conformations allowed for the Tic residue (Fig. 6). Note that in the Tic residue one can readily distinguish the gauche(−) from gauche(+) conformation by NMR. We have placed Tic into the 4 position of DPDPE. NMR analysis indicated that the Tic⁴ residue is in the gauche(+) conformation (94). Other conformational features are currently under investigation. As shown in Table 1, [D–Pen², Tic⁴, D–Pen⁵]-enkephalin (11) has greatly reduced potency in the MVD (δ receptor) but does retain considerable receptor specificity. It may be that a gauche(+) conformation in position 4 is not compatible with a strong interaction with

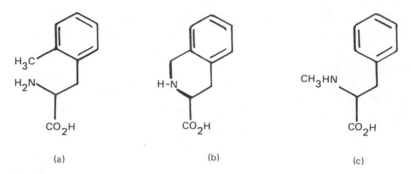

Figure 5 Structure of tetrahydroisoquinoline carboxylate (Tic; a), 2′-methyl-phenylalanine (b), and N-methylphenylalanine (c).

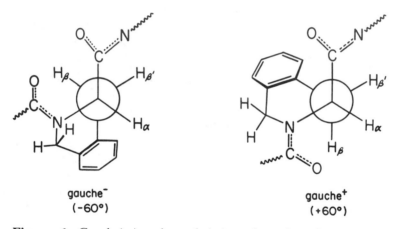

Figure 6 Gauche(−) and gauche(+) conformation of tetrahydroisoquinoline carboxylate.

the δ opioid receptor (low potency), but it does appear to be compatible with transduction, since the analog is a full agonist.

A very promising, but to this time largely unexplored, approach to rational design of peptide receptor, acceptor, and enzyme ligands is the utilization of side-chain conformation bias of amino acid residue to control side-chain topological relationships. Aromatic residues (Phe, Tyr, His, Trp, etc.) are particularly promising in this regard because of their inherent conformational properties and because of their central importance in many peptide hormones and neurotransmitters. The importance of Tyr[1] in all opioid receptors is well documented, and the possible relative importance of

Phe[4] in controlling δ vs. μ vs. κ ligand-receptor interactions needs further evaluation by rational design.

The classical low-energy conformations for β-substituted amino acids such as phenylalanine in a peptide are given in Figure 7. Examination of these models using standard steric and structural electronic considerations suggests that the gauche(+) conformation is the least stable (highest energy) conformation and that the gauche(−) and trans conformations are more nearly equivalent. This simple analysis is consistent with the conformational populations found for side-chain groups of aromatic amino acids in proteins by x-ray analysis. Further examination of these structures indicates that the two β hydrogens are diastereotopic. Therefore, in the asymmetric environment of a receptor, they may interact differently and have vastly different structural requirements at the receptor. Further examination of these conformers indicated that substitution of *one* of these hydrogens (pro-R or Pro-S) will have different consequences on the conformational bias of the side-chain group. For example, in the *L* amino acid shown in Figure 7 (R = phenyl), it might be predicted that generally if the pro-S hydrogen is replaced with a methyl group, the gauche(−) conformer becomes greatly favored, but if the pro-R hydrogen is replaced with a methyl group, the trans conformation will be favored. These conformational biases should provide critical insights into the topological relationships important to activity and specificity at a particular receptor. Note also that NMR can be used to distinguish the gauche(−) and trans conformers in, say, the pro(S)-substituted analog if the appropriate bias predicted is actually obtained.

Thus we have been preparing all of the possible isomers (threo and erythro) of β-methylphenylalanine (β-McPhe) and of other β methyl amino acids to examine their use in rational design (104). In Table 1 the results with what is probably the L-erythro-β-McPhe[4] analog are most interesting.

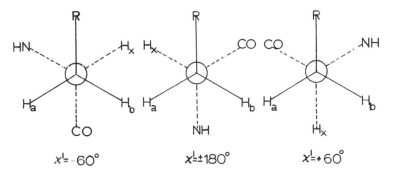

Figure 7. Classical gauche(−), trans, and gauche(+) conformations for β-substituted α amino acids.

Although the analog <u>12</u> (Table 1) loses some potency at the δ receptor, the loss is minimal, and high receptor selectivity is retained. These results suggest that the gauche($-$) conformation is probably that preferred by the δ receptor, but that the conformation at the 4 position is not highly critical for determining receptor selectivity. In this regard, however, it is interesting to note that the β,β-dimethylphenylalanine (β,β-Me$_2$Phe) analog has also been made and has greatly reduced potency ($>$1000-fold less potent than DPDPE) but also less selectivity. Molecular dynamics simulations (Kao and Hruby, unpublished) indicate that in this analog the aromatic side chain of β,β-dimethylphenylalanine becomes "frozen" in the trans conformation. Obviously this is not compatible with interaction of the analog with the δ opioid receptor. Interestingly, however, [D–$\overline{\text{Pen}}^2$, $\beta\beta$-Me$_2$Phe, D–$\overline{\text{Pen}}^5$]-enkephalin and [D–$\overline{\text{Pen}}^2$, β-MePhe^4, D–$\overline{\text{Pen}}^5$]enkephalin have nearly identical, albeit weak, interactions at the μ receptor, suggesting that the trans side-chain conformation at position 4 may be compatible with the initial binding recognition at this receptor. Much more work clearly remains to be done to determine the precise conformational properties and topological arrangements in these compounds and the effect of these properties on bioactivity in vitro and in vivo. However, the results we have obtained suggest that this kind of conformational and topological modeling can provide an important new approach to peptide ligand design.

F. Future Perspectives

There are several directions suggested by the research to date that could provide further insights into the conformational, structural, and dynamic requirements of the δ opioid receptor and to the rational design of even more potent agonist analogs and the development of antagonists. A few will be briefly outlined below.

   1.   Further examine the effects of β-subsituted erythro vs. threo L (and D) aromatic amino acids in position 4 on receptor potency and selectivity in DPDPE. These should also be examined in the context of Pen-containing analogs that have a D–Cys^2 or a $L(D)$–Cys^5 substitution.

   2.   Further examine the effect of 2'(6'), 3'(5'), 4' substitutions in the Phe^4 residue on δ receptor potency and selectivity and on the conformational properties of DPDPE.

   3.   Examine the effects of β-substituted erythro and threo L (and D) analogs of tyrosine on δ receptor selectivity and potency and on conformational properties in the DPDPE series.

   4.   The role of the Gly^3 residue in DPDPE is not clear, and in view of the

results of Schiller et al. with the cyclic amides (44,45), it would be interesting to delete this amino acid and/or substitute it with alanine, D-alanine, α-aminoisobutyric acid, etc.

    5. The β,β-dimethyl groups of D–Pen^2 and $D(L)$–Pen^5 are diastereoisotopic. It would be interesting to explore the effect of large β substituents on opioid receptor potency and selectivity and on DPDPE conformation and dynamics. Also β-substituted erythro and threo cysteine derivatives would be very interesting.

    6. Further examine the conformational space available to DPDPE and analogs using quenched molecular dynamics and non-Boltzmann sampling calculations to fully determine all possibilities consistent with the data. The use of these methods in conjunction with analog design will be of great interest.

    7. Much more effort is needed to examine the conformational, structural, and dynamic features that differentiate the δ and μ receptors (and eventually the κ receptor as well). Again, molecular graphics, molecular mechanics, and molecular dynamics methods will be invaluable.

    8. Receptors, pure and in quantity, are needed.

Exciting new results and directions can be expected to emerge from these studies.

IV. DESIGN OF CONFORMATIONALLY CONSTRAINED μ OPIOID RECEPTOR-SELECTIVE PEPTIDES

A. Considerations and Studies Leading to D–Phe–C̄ys–Tyr–D-Trp–Orn–Thr–P̄en–Thr–NH$_2$ (CTOP), a Highly μ Opioid Receptor-Selective Antagonist

Somatostatin-14 is a regulatory peptide of structure H–Ala–Gly–C̄ys–Lys–Asn–Phe–Phe–Trp–Lys–Thr–Phe–Thr–Ser–C̄ys–OH, which has high potency at receptors that control the release of growth hormone, glucagon, and insulin (105). It was also observed, though these observations have been largely ignored, that at a much higher concentration, somatostatin can interact weakly with the opioid receptor system (106,107). These observations led us to consider the possibility of developing a somatostatin analog with high potency and selectivity at the opioid receptor system and little or no "somatostatinlike" activities. Although this thinking is contrary to most approaches to ligand design in that activities that are 100- or 1000-fold less for a peptide neurotransmitter are considered to be "nonphysiological" and/or "of no importance," it has been our contention that in fact such activities are of great potential physiologically, since the activities are still in the micromolar to millimolar range. Thus design for the low-affinity ("nonphysiological") receptors at the expense of the high-affinity ("physiological") receptors is in fact a reasonable approach and an important new method for rational drug design.

About this time a most interesting study appeared (108), in which it was reported that the somatostatin analog D–Phe–Cys–Phe–D–Trp–Lys–Thr–Cys–Thr(ol) had superagonist activity in terms of inhibition of growth hormone release, a classical physiological receptor for somatostatin, and also had high binding potency at opioid receptors. From this observation, we decided to investigate the possibility of designing a somatostatin-related peptide in conjunction with conformational constraints (12) that would have high opioid receptor potency and selectivity but greatly reduced or no somatostatinlike activities. We have had considerable success in doing this.

Since somatostatin and many of its potent analogs are disulfide-containing peptides, we began by investigating the effect of further constraining such cyclic peptides by penicillamine (Pen). The advantages of this residue have already been discussed in other contexts (see above; 11, 12, 15, 19–22). Our starting peptides were H–D–Phe–Cys–Phe–D–Trp–Lys–Thr–Cys–Thr-OH (1, Table 7) and related peptides containing Pen at position 2 (2) or position 7 (3) or both positions 2 and 7 (4, Table 7). Using rat brain binding assays to evaluate μ vs. δ receptor selectivity and binding at the somatostatin receptor, very interesting results were obtained. The initial results showed (109) that whereas the cysteine-containing analog 1 had no μ vs. δ opioid receptor selectivity, it was slightly more potent than somatostatin in binding to opioid receptors. Most importantly, 1 was 50 times less potent than somatostatin in binding to somatostatin receptors. When Pen was placed in position 2 in 1 to give the analog 2, a significant decrease in binding at both μ and δ receptors occurred, and the analog had a very slight δ receptor selectivity. Conversely, when a Pen residue was placed in position 7 in 1, the analog obtained, 3, showed greatly *increased* binding at the μ receptor relative to 1 but little change from 1 in binding to the δ receptor (Table 7). Interestingly, the bis-penicillamine analog 4 showed intermediate potency at both receptors and, like 1, no selectivity at the μ vs. δ receptor. It should also be pointed out that all of these compounds were quite a bit less potent (30–150 times) than somatostatin in binding to somatostatin receptors. Nonetheless, all of these analogs had higher binding potency at somatostatin than at opioid receptors.

Our next major objective was to modify the basic lead structure 2 in such a

Table 7 Binding Potencies and Receptor Selectivities of Penicillamine-Substituted Cyclic Somatostatinlike Octapeptides in Binding Assays with Rat Brain Homogenates

Compound	[³H]NAL IC$_{50}$ (nM)	[³H]DADLE IC$_{50}$ (nM)	[¹²⁵I]CGP23996 IC$_{50}$ (nM)	[³H]DADLE / [³H]NAL	[¹²⁵I]GGP / [³H]NAL
Somatostatin	27,400	16,400	6	0.60	0.0002
1. D–Phe–Cys–Phe–D–Trp–Lys–Thr–Cys–Thr–OH	4,500	5,000	300	0.90	0.067
2. D–Phe–Pen–Phe–D–Trp–Lys–Thr–Cys–Thr–OH	61,000	38,000	800	0.65	0.013
3. D–Phe–Cys–Phe–D–Trp–Lys–Thr–Pen–Thr–OH	931	5,400	170	5.8	0.18
4. D–Phe–Pen–Phe–D–Trp–Lys–Thr–Pen–Thr–OH	10,000	9,300	1,000	0.93	0.10
5. D–Phe–Cys–Tyr–D–Trp–Lys–Thr–Pen–Thr–OH	290	3,800	1,600	13.	5.5
6. D–Phe–Cys–Tyr–D–Trp–Lys–Thr–Pen–Thr–NH$_2$	3.5	950	690	271.	197.

manner as to obtain increased potency and selectivity at opioid receptors while diminishing interaction at somatostatinlike receptors. To this end, we replaced the Phe^3 residue with a Tyr residue. This analog ($\underline{5}$, Table 7) showed increased potency at μ receptors and specificity for μ vs. δ receptors. In addition, for the first time, an analog was obtained with greater binding at the μ receptor than at the somatostatin receptor (Table 7). Preparation of an analog of $\underline{5}$ with a carboxamide terminal led to analog H–D–Phe–Cys–Tyr–D–Trp–Lys–Thr–Pen–Thr–NH$_2$ (CTP, $\underline{6}$, Table 7) with higher μ vs. δ receptor selectivity. This analog, which we refer to as CTP, has μ vs. δ opioid receptor selectivity > 270-fold, and μ opioid vs. somatostatin receptor selectivity > 190-fold (110).

Although analog $\underline{6}$ binds with considerably greater potency at μ opioid vs. somatostatin receptors in the brain, competitive binding studies (Table 7) with the somatostatin analog [^{125}I]CGP 23996 shows that $\underline{6}$ still binds with an EC$_{50}$ that is submicromolar at somatostatin receptors. Thus we examined structural modifications compatible with the same conformational features as CTP but with decreased somatostatinlike binding activity. Previous studies by Nutt et al. (111) had demonstrated that somatostatin analogs in which substitutions were made for the basic residue in position 5 (as defined in our analogs) could possess greatly reduced somatostatinlike potency. We therefore replaced the Lys^5 residue with the basic amino acid residues Arg and Orn and with the neutral amino acid residue norleucine (Nle) (112,113). The results with analogs $\underline{7}$, $\underline{8}$, and $\underline{9}$ (Table 8) are very gratifying. Substitution of the Lys^5 residue with Arg^5 gave an analog CTAP ($\underline{7}$, Table 8) with similar binding potencies at μ and δ opioid binding sites CTP but greatly reduced binding (about 20-fold) at somatostatin receptors. Please note that in these binding studies we are now utilizing the highly δ receptor-selective radiolabeled ligand [^{3}H]DPDPE (84) rather than the relatively nonselective δ opioid peptide analog [^{3}H]DADLE, so that much higher selectivity at μ vs. δ receptor binding sites is now observed. In any case, CTAP ($\underline{7}$) is an analog with very little somatostatinlike binding activity. Even more selective is the Orn^5 analog $\underline{8}$ (Table 8), which has slightly increased binding at the μ receptor, slightly decreased binding at the δ opioid receptor, and greatly *decreased* ($\geqslant 30$-fold) binding at the somatostatin receptor. This analog is a very potent and μ opioid receptor-selective compound (112,113) with a 4800-fold selectivity for the μ vs. δ opioid receptor and an 8100-fold selectivity for the μ opioid vs. somatostatin brain receptor. Interestingly, the Nle^5 analog, in which the Nle residue is isosteric to the Orn residue but neutral rather than basic, is less potent and μ opioid receptor-selective ($\underline{9}$, Table 8).

Our discussion to this point has concentrated on the in vitro binding properties of the peptide analog. What we will briefly do now is outline their in vitro and in vivo biological activities. Though this is not the major theme

Table 8 Binding Potencies and Receptor Selectivities of Penicillamine-7-Substituted Somatostatinlike Octapeptides in Opioid and Somatostatin Binding Assays with Rat Brain Homogenates

Compound	[³H]NAL IC₅₀ (nM)	[³H]DPDPE IC₅₀ (nM)	[¹²⁵I]CGP23996 IC₅₀ (nM)	$\dfrac{[³H]DADLE}{[³H]NAL}$	$\dfrac{[¹²⁵I]CGP}{[³H]NAL}$
Somatostatin	27,400	16,400[a]	6.0	0.60	0.0002
5. D-Phe-Cys-Tyr-D-Trp-Lys-Thr-Pen-Thr-NH₂ (CTF)	3.73	8,400	690	2,270	185
7. D-Phe-Cys-Tyr-D-Trp-Arg-Thr-Pen-Thr-NH₂ (CTAP)	3.50	4,490	13,200	1,280	3,770
8. D-Phe-Cys-Tyr-D-Trp-Orn-Thr-Pen-Thr-NH₂ (CTOF)	2.80	13,520	22,700	4,800	8,100
9. D-Phe-Cys-Tyr-D-Trp-Nle-Thr-Pen-Thr-NH₂ (CTNP)	9.64	5,570	ND	578	—

[a]Versus [³H]DADLE.

of this paper, a few words about these activities provide insight into the biological impetus for these studies. Details can be found elsewhere (114–118).

Basically these peptides have been found to be opioid μ receptor antagonists. Most of the compounds reported here have been tested in several assays for opioid activity including the guinea pig ileum (GPI) (μ primarily, and κ receptors), the mouse vas deferens (MVD) (δ primarily, and μ and κ receptors), the hot-plate test in mice (μ and δ receptor-mediated analgesia), etc. The most comprehensive studies thus far have been done with CTP (6, Tables 7 and 8). CTP itself had no agonist actions in the GPI assay, and in the MVD it did produce agonist activities but at very high ($> 10,000$ nM) concentrations that were inhibited by naloxone and the delta antagonist ICI 174,864, indicating very weak delta agonist activity (these agonist activities have never been observed in vivo). At much lower concentrations (10–1000 nM), CTP produced dose-related inhibition of the highly μ receptor-selective peptide agonist PLO17 in the MVD but did not antagonize the agonist activity of the highly delta opioid selective agonist DPDPE. CTP is therefore a highly potent and selective μ opioid receptor antagonist. Similarly in the GPI, CTP produced a potent inhibitory effect on the μ agonist ligand PLO17.

When tested in vivo, CTP was also found to have no agonist (analgesic) effects itself. However, at very low concentrations, and in a dose-related fashion, CTP could antagonize the analgesic effect caused by the μ receptor agonist PLO17 with a pA$_2$ value of about 10.5. Furthermore, this compound showed very prolonged in vivo activity with a $t_{\frac{1}{2}}$ of inhibition of over 270 min. This is to be contrasted with naloxone, which under the same conditions has a $t_{\frac{1}{2}}$ of inhibition of about 21 min. Clearly, these peptides show extraordinary promise as opioid receptor antagonists to probe the physiological and pharmacological roles of μ opioid receptors.

B.   Solution Conformation of D–Phe–Cys–Tyr–D–Trp–Lys–Thr–Pen–Thr–NH$_2$ (CTP) from NMR Studies

A major working hypothesis in this research has been the idea that the major conformational features related to the reverse-turn conformation (β turn) involving residues 3, 4, 5, and 6 of these cyclic octapeptide analogs (e.g., 119) has been retained. Stabilization of this reverse-turn structure has been suggested to involve an intramolecular hydrogen bond between the Thr^6 NH proton and the Tyr^3 carbonyl oxygen (in some cases and under some conditions, a C$_7$ reverse turn also is possible). The major intention in our design was that although this secondary structural feature would be maintained, the conformationally constraining penicillamine residue could alter conformational properties of side-chain groups (e.g., Tyr^3, Cys^2, Thr^8, etc.) by its transannular effects, stabilize the disulfide helicity to right-handed (or left-handed), and otherwise modulate topological relationships at the "wings" (residues 1, 2, 3, 7, and 8) of the peptide in ways that would be critical to interaction with opioid receptors while at the same time disfavoring interactions with somatostatin receptors. Thus, from the beginning, careful NMR investigations have been ongoing to establish that in fact the basic "template" conformation has been maintained and to determine the changes in conformation and topology that accompany structural perturbation, especially those leading to large changes in bioactivity. Although a very considerable amount of work has been done in this regard (120–122), we will report here primarily on the results from our NMR studies on CTP in aqueous solution (120).

To obtain the proton NMR chemical shifts, coupling constants, and other pertinent NMR parameters, we have utilized extensive 1-D NMR, 2-D COSY (DQF), and NOESY experiments; temperature dependence and pH dependence studies; delayed COSY experiments for determination of long-range connectivities; and computer simulations. We also have performed heteronuclear COSY experiments and J-resolved spectroscopy. The complete ·chemical shift assignments and coupling constants for CTP in aqueous solution are given in Table 9. Careful evaluation of the results of these experiments led to the conclusion that indeed CTP does possess a type II′ β-turn in the critical central tetrapeptide sequence $-Tyr^3-D-Trp^4-Lys^5-Thr^6$ with an intramolecular H bond between the Thr^6 NH proton and the Tyr^3 carbonyl oxygen. In addition, NQF measurement indicates that the disulfide helicity is left-handed for this and other related analogs that have high potency and selectivity for the μ opioid receptor. Studies of several other analogs suggest that the basic conformational features seen for CTP (particularly in the critical region involving the 3, 4, 5, and 6 positions) are retained but that conformational and topological changes about the other residues best correlate with substantial changes in biological potency and receptor selectivity.

C. Conformation Model for CTP and Relation to Biological Activity

The results above have led us to construct a conformation model for the solution conformation of CTP. A picture of the three-dimensional structural model for CTP is shown in Figure 8. The type II′ β turn is evident, and one should also note the disulfide region of the structure. Although we believe the overall conformational features for CTP correspond to those illustrated here,

Table 9 ¹H 300-MHz NMR Parameters for D–Phe–Cys–Tyr–D–Trp–Lys–Thr–Pen–Thr–NH$_2$ in Aqueous Solution

Amino Acid	δ_{NH}	$^3J_{NH-C\alpha H}$	δ_α	δ_β	δ_γ	δ_δ	δ_ε	$^3J_{\alpha\beta}$	$^3J_{\beta\beta}$
D-Phe[1]			4.35	3.34, 3.25				6.0, 8.2	−13.9
Cys[2]	8.64	7.16	5.07	2.73, 2.85				5.4, 8.8	−14.1
Tyr[3]	8.56	8.33	4.68	2.95				6.4, 7.8	
D-Trp[4]	8.49	7.82	4.41	3.09, 2.95				3.9, 11.3	−13.9
Lys[5]	8.24	7.26	3.95	1.14, 1.52	0.28, 0.51	1.25	2.66	3.7, 10.5	
Thr[6]	8.72	5.18	4.38	4.26	1.16			6.4	
Pen[7]	8.02	7.97	4.78						
Thr[8]	8.15	7.84	4.42	4.26	1.23			4.4	
Amide	7.60								

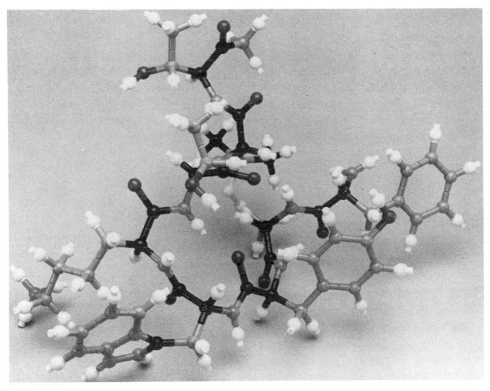

Figure 8 Three-dimensional structure of CTP.

careful energy minimization studies and conformational searches have not been performed but are in progress. The results obtained thus far, however, support the concept that the strong preference we have induced for the μ vs. somatostatin receptors is primarily the result of structural and conformational properties associated with the C-terminal and N-terminal portions of these molecules. Furthermore, the results seem to demonstrate that the reverse-turn structure in the "central" sequence of these somatostatinlike analogs can serve as a template for the design of μ opioid receptor specific analogs with little or no somatostatinlike activity in vitro or in vivo. Thus, "receptor mapping" of the μ opioid receptor to determine the μ receptor pharmacophore for antagonists is possible.

D.   Conclusions and Future Perspectives

We have developed a concept that we believe to be a new general approach in the design of receptor-specific ligands for peptide neurotransmitters (and hormone receptors). This approach utilizes "nonphysiological" actions of endogenous peptides as starting points for the design of agonist or antagonist ligands for that receptor at the expense of the putative "physiological" activities of the neurotransmitter peptide. Essentially we are suggesting that all ligand-receptor interactions of a particular endogenous peptide, even those that cover as much as a 1000–10,000 concentration range, *are* or *can be* "physiologically" important or can be made so by design of ligands for these "low-affinity" receptors. Physiological relevance comes not from some arbitrary definition of an appropriately potent biological response of an endogenous peptide but rather from the successful design of a potent and selective ligand for the receptor in question.

From the standpoint of the progress already made with the somatostatin-like μ antagonist analogs, we are most excited about future prospects. We have designed analogs that are the most μ receptor-selective opioid ligands reported thus far. Receptor mapping by further exploring the specific topological requirements of the μ receptor by analog design involving the C-terminal and N-terminal portions of the CTP, CTOP, and related peptides is in progress. Clearly, manipulations of the topological properties of the aromatic residues in positions 1, 3, and 4 should provide critical new insights. These can now be planned with help from computer-aided molecular modeling, and such studies are in progress. Use of constrained aromatic amino residues should be particularly helpful here. Also further manipulation of the Pen[7] residue with larger R groups at the β-carbon atom could be most interesting. We are optimistic that even greater specificities for the μ antagonist receptor will be possible and that the pharmacophore for this receptor can be determined in detail. The extent to which this pharmacophore can interact and overlap with the μ receptor agonist pharmacophore should be quite interesting to investigate with these peptides.

V.   PROBLEMS AND PERSPECTIVES FOR RATIONAL DESIGN OF RECEPTOR-SELECTIVE PEPTIDES

We are optimistic about the prospects for continued developments in the rational design of receptor-selective peptides. The availability of modern computer-assisted graphics systems for structural model building and design, especially when coupled with the powerful techniques being developed in molecular mechanics and molecular dynamics which can be utilized quite readily with computers already available and especially those that will become generally available in the very near future, provides important new tools that are crucial for success. A major problem at this point is the lack of understanding and appreciation of the specific properties of peptides and proteins by the synthetic, organic, and medicinal chemists who are best equipped to design and synthesize specific structural features into peptide ligands. The concept of "peptide mimetics" is appealing to many scientists currently examining the problem of rational design of peptide ligands. However, it seems apparent to us that many of the ideas in the area appear to be more wishful thinking than a careful analysis of the conformational, dynamic, and topological features that peptides generally have or can assume in the course of a ligand-receptor interactions.

In particular, dynamic conformational changes seem to be of critical importance for receptor-ligand recognition, transduction, and reversal. Clearly, a much better understanding of this aspect of this problem, generally referred to, depending on the perspective of the scientist involved, as the "folding problem," the "docking problem," the "transduction process," etc., is needed. The uses of conformational constraints, structurally based conformational bias, and template-based design discussed in this paper are perhaps useful approaches, but clearly much more development is needed. Despite the difficulties of the problems remaining, we are optimistic. Receptors are exquisitely sensitive "hosts" for examination of rational design of ligands. This is particularly true at this time, as biologists continue to develop ever more sensitive and specific assays, both in vitro and in vivo, that can relate structural, conformational, and dynamic properties to the biological response. The simultaneous use of a large variety of assays by the scientist interested in rational drug design is a prerequisite to success, and such systems are increasingly available. Obviously the availability of large quantities of receptors in a bioactive form would greatly accelerate progress. Clearly a multidisciplinary approach is needed, and the general recognition of this will produce increasingly sophisticated and successful approaches to rational design.

ACKNOWLEDGMENTS

We are particularly grateful to our many chemical and biological collaborators whose creativity, hard work, and enthusiasm have made this report possible. Thanks are especially due Henry I. Mosberg, Robin Hurst, Lung-Fa Kao, John T. Pelton, Wieslaw Kazmierski, Elizabeth Sugg, Professor Henry I. Yamamura and his colleagues, Professor Thomas F. Burks and his colleagues, Professor Frank Porreca, and Professor Georges Van Binst. V. J. H. especially thanks Professor Martin Karplus for a stimulating year in his laboratory at Harvard during a sabbatical, and a Guggenheim Fellowship for support. The work in our laboratories was supported by grants from the National Science Foundation (V.J.H.), the U.S. Public Health Service (V.J.H. and B.M.P.), and the Robert A. Welch Foundation (B.M.P.).

REFERENCES

1. Veber, D. F., F. W. Holly, R. F. Nutt, S. J. Bergstrand, S. F. Brady, R. Hirschmann, M. S. Glitzer, and R. Saperstein, Highly active cyclic and bicyclic somatostatin analogues of reduced ring size. *Nature* 289:512–514 (1979).

2. Sawyer, T. K., P. J. Sanfilippo, V. J. Hruby, M. H. Engle, C. B. Heward, J. B. Burnett, and M. E. Hadley, [Nle^4, D-Phe^7]-α-melanocyte stimulating hormone: A highly potent α-melanotropin with ultralong biological activity. *Proc. Natl. Acad. Sci. USA 77*: 5754–5758 (1980).

3. Sawyer, T. K., V. J. Hruby, P. S. Darman, and M. E. Hadley, [4-Half-cystine, 10-half-cystine]-α-melanocyte stimulating hormone: A cyclic α-melanotropin exhibiting superagonist biological activity. *Proc. Natl. Acad. Sci. USA 79*:1751–1755 (1982).

4. Manning, M., A. Misicka, S. Stoev, E. Nawrocka, W. A. Klis, A. Olma, K. Bankowski, B. Lammek, and W. H. Sawyer, Studies leading to orally active antagonists of the antidiuretic (V$_2$) and basopresson (V$_1$) responses to arginine vasopressin (AVP). In *Peptides: Structure and Function*, C. M. Deber, V. J. Hruby, and K. D. Kopple, eds. Pierce Chemical Co., Rockford, Ill., pp. 599–602 (1985).

5. Chan, W. Y., V. J. Hruby, T. W. Rockway, and J. Hlavacek, Design of oxytocin antagonists with prolonged action: Potential tocolytic agents for the treatment of preterm labor. *J. Pharmacol. Exp. Ther.* 239:84–87 (1986).

6. Nestor, J. Jr., R. Tahilramani, T. L. Ho, G. I. McRae, B. H. Vickery, and W. J. Bremner, New luteinizing hormone-releasing factor antagonists. In *Peptides: Structure and Function*, V. J. Hruby and D. H. Rich, eds. Pierce Chemical Co., Rockford, Ill., pp. 861–864 (1983).

7. Veber, D., Conformational considerations in the design of somatastatin analogs showing increased metabolic stability. In *Peptides: Structure and Biological Function*, E. Gross and J. Meienhofer, eds. Pierce Chemical Co., Rockford, Ill., pp. 409–419 (1979).

8. Castrucci, A. M. L., M. E. Hadley, T. K. Sawyer, and V. J. Hruby, Enzymological studies of melanotropins. *Comp. Biochem. Physiol. 78B*:519–524 (1984).

9. Marshall, G. R., F. A. Gorin, and M. L. Moore, Peptide conformation and biological activity. *Annu. Rep. Med. Chem. 13*:277–238 (1978).

10. Hruby, V. J., J. L. Krstenansky, and W. L. Cody, Recent progress in the rational design of peptide hormones and neurotransmitters. *Annu. Rep. Med. Chem. 19*:303–312 (1984).

11. Meraldi, J. P., V. J. Hruby, and A. I. R. Brewster, Relative conformational rigidity in oxytocin and [1-penicillamine]oxytocin: A proposal for the relationship of conformational flexibility to peptide hormone agonism and antagonism. *Proc. Natl. Acad. Sci. USA 74*:1373–1377 (1977).

12. Hruby, V. J., Conformational restrictions of biologically active peptides via amino acid side chain groups. *Life Sci. 31*:189–199 (1982).

13. Vida, J. A., and M. Gordon, eds., *Conformationally Directed Drug Design*, ACS Symposium Series 251, American Chemical Society, Washington, DC, 1984; Hruby, V. J., ed., *The Peptides: Analysis, Synthesis, Biology, Vol 7: Conformation in Biology and Drug Design*. Academic Press, New York (1985).

14. Hruby, V. J., and C. W. Smith, Structure-activity relationships of neurohypophyseal peptides. In *The Peptides: Analysis, Synthesis, Biology, Vol. 8: Chemistry, Biology and Medicine of Neurophypophyseal Hormones and Their Analogs*, C. W. Smith, ed. Academic Press, New York, pp. 77–207 (1987).

15. Hruby, V. J., Structure activity of the neurohypophyseal hormones and analogues, and implications for hormone-receptor interactions. *Biochem. Actions Hormones 13*:191–241 (1986).

16. Amico, J. A., and A. G. Robinson, eds., *Oxytocin: Clinical and Laboratory Studies*, Elsevier/North Holland, New York (1985).

17. Jost, K., M. Lebl, and F. Brtnik, eds., *Handbook of Neurohypophyseal Analogs*, Vol. 2, CRC Press, Boca Raton, Fla. (1987).

18. Hoffman, P. L., Central nervous effects of neurohypophyseal peptides. In *The Peptides: Analysis, Synthesis, Biology*, Vol. 8: *Chemistry, Biology and Medicine of Neurohypophyseal Hormones and Their Analogs*, C. W. Smith, ed. Academic Press, New York, pp. 239–295 (1987).

19. Hruby, V. J., Structure and conformation related to the activity of peptide hormones. In *Perspectives in Peptide Chemistry*, A. Eberle, R. Geiger, and T. Wieland, eds. S. Karger, Basel, pp. 207–220 (1981).

20. Hruby, V. J., Relation of conformation to biological activity in oxytocin, vasopressin and their analogues. In *Topics in Molecular Pharmacology*, A. S. V. Burgen and G. C. K. Roberts, eds. Elsevier/North Holland, Amsterdam, pp. 99–126 (1981).

21. Hruby, V. J., and M. E. Hadley, Binding and information transfer in conformationally restricted peptides. In *Design and Synthesis of Organic Molecules Based on Molecular Recognition*, G. van Binst, ed. Springer-Verlag, Berlin, pp. 269–289 (1984).

22. Hruby, V. J., and H. I. Mosberg, Structural, conformational and dynamic considerations in the development of peptide hormone antagonists. In *Hormone Antagonists*, M. K. Agarwal, ed. W. de Gruyter, Berlin, pp. 433–474 (1982).

23. Martin, W. R., C. G. Eades, J. A. Thompson, R. E. Hupper, and P. E. Gilbert, The effects of morphine and nalorphine-like drugs in the non-dependent and morphine-dependent chronic spiral dog. *J. Pharmacol. Exp. Ther. 97*:517–523 (1976).

24. Lord, J. A. H., A. A. Waterfield, J. Hughes, and H. W. Kosterlitz, Endogenous opioid peptides: Multiple agonists and receptors. *Nature 267*:495–499 (1977).

25. Chang, K. J., B. R. Copper, E. Hazum, and P. Cuatrecasas, Multiple opiate receptors: Different regional distribution in the brain and differential binding of opiates and opioid peptides. *Mol. Pharmacol. 16*:91–104 (1979).

26. Iwamoto, E. T., and W. R. Martin, Multiple opioid receptors. *Med. Res. Rev. 1*:411–440 (1981).

27. Goldstein, A., and I. F. James, Multiple opioid receptors: Criteria for identifi-
     cation and classification. *Trends Pharmacol. Sci.* 5:503–505 (1984).

28. Paterson, S. J., L. E. Robson, and H. W. Kosterlitz, Opioid receptors. In *The
     Peptides: Analysis, Synthesis, Biology*, Vol 6: *Opioid Peptides: Biology, Chemis-
     try, and Genetics*, S. Udenfriend and J. Meienhofer, eds. Academic Press, New
     York, pp. 147–189 (1984).

29. Rapaka, R. S., G. Barnett, and R. L. Hawks, eds., *Opioid Peptides, Medicinal
     Chemistry*. NIDA monograph 69, Washington, D.C.: U.S. Government Print-
     ing Office (1986).

30. Hansen, P. E., and B. A. Morgan, Structure-activity relationships in enkephalin
     peptides. In *The Peptides: Analysis, Synthesis, Biology*, Vol. 6: *Opioid Peptides:
     Biology, Chemistry, and Genetics*, S. Udenfriend and J. Meienhofer, eds.
     Academic Press, New York, pp. 269–321 (1984).

31. Miller, R. J., and P. Cuatrecasas, Enkephalins and endorphins. *Vitam. Horm.*
     36:297–382 (1978).

32. Morley, J. S., Structure-activity relationships of enkephalin-like peptides. *Annu.
     Rev. Pharmacol. Toxicol.* 20:81–110 (1980).

33. Olson, G. A., R. D. Olson, and A. J. Kastin, Endogenous opiates: 1985. *Peptides*
     7:907–933 (1986).

34. Handa, B. K., A. C. Lane, J. A. H. Lord, B. A. Morgon, M. J. Rance, and G. F.
     C. Smith, Analogues of β-LPH[61–64] possessing selective agonist activities at
     mu-opiate receptors. *Eur. J. Pharmacol.* 70:531–540 (1981).

35. Chang, K. J., E. T. Wei, A. Killian, and J. K. Chang, Potent morphiceptin
     analogs: Structure activity relationships and morphine-like activities. *J. Phar-
     macol. Exp. Ther.* 227:403–408 (1983).

36. Zajac, J. M., G. Gacel, F. Petit, P. Dodey, P. Rossignol, and B. P. Roques,
     Deltakephalin, Tyr–D–Thr–Gly–Phe–Leu–Thr: A new highly potent and fully
     specific angonist for opiate δ-receptors. *Biochem. Biophys. Res. Commun.*
     111:390–397 (1983).

37. Cotton, R., M. B. Giles, L. Miller, J. S. Shaw, and T. Timms, ICI 174,864: A
     highly selective antagonist for the opioid-delta receptor. *Eur. J. Pharmacol.*
     97:331–332 (1984).

38. Rapaka, R. S., Research topics in the medicinal chemistry and molecular
     pharmacology of opioid peptides—present and future. *Life Sci.* 39:1825–1843
     (1986).

39. Schiller, P. W., Conformational analysis of enkephalin and conformation-
     activity relationships. In *Peptides: Analysis, Synthesis, Biology*, Vol. 6: *Opioid
     Peptides: Biology, Chemistry, and Genetics*, S. Udenfriend and J. Meienhofer,
     eds. Academic Press, New York, pp. 219–268 (1984).

40. Hruby, V. J., Design of peptide hormone and neurotransmitter analogues.
     Trend Pharmacol. Sci. 6:259–262 (1985).

41. DiMaio, J., and P. W. Shiller, A cyclic enkephalin analog with high in vitro
     opiate activity. *Proc. Natl. Acad. Sci. USA* 77:7162–7166 (1980).

42. Schiller, P. W., and J. DiMaio, Opiate receptor subclasses differ in their
     conformational requirements. *Nature* 297:74–76 (1982).

43. DiMaio, J., T. M.-D. Nguyen, C. Lemieux, and P. W. Schiller, Synthesis and pharmacological characterization in vitro of cyclic enkephalin analogues: Effect of conformational constraint on opiate receptor selectivity. *J. Med. Chem.* 25:1432-1438 (1982).

44. Schiller, P. W., T. M.-D. Nguyen, and J. Miller, Synthesis of side chain to side chain cyclized peptide analogues on solid supports. *Int. J. Peptide Protein Res.* 25:171-177 (1985).

45. Schiller, P. W., T. M.-D. Nguyen, C. Lemieux, and L. A. Maziak, Synthesis and activity profiles of novel cyclic opioid peptide monomers and dimers. *J. Med. Chem.* 28:1766-1771 (1985).

46. McCammon, J. A., and S. C. Harvey, *Dynamics of Proteins and Nucleic Acids*, Cambridge University Press, New York (1987).

47. Pettitt, B. M., and M. Karplus, Interaction energies. In *Topics in Molecular Pharmacology*, Vol. 3, R. S. V. Burgen, G. C. K. Roberts, M. S. Tute, eds. Elsevier, Amsterdam, pp. 75–113 (1986).

48. Pettitt, B. M., and P. J. Rossky, New approaches to solvent mediated interactions. *Isr. J. Chem.* 27:156-160 (1986).

49. Opella, S. J., and L. M. Gierasch, Solid-state nuclear magnetic resonance of peptides. In *The Peptides: Analysis, Synthesis, Biology*, Vol. 7, V. J. Hruby, ed. Academic Press, New York, pp. 405-436 (1986).

50. Kessler, H., and W. Bermel, Conformational analysis of peptides by two-dimensional NMR spectroscopy. In *Applications of NMR Spectroscopy to Problems in Stereochemistry and Conformational Analysis*, A. P. March and Y. Takeuchi, eds. VCH Publishers, New York (1986).

51. Kessler, H., W. Bermel, A. Müller, and K. H. Pook, Modern nuclear magnetic resonance spectroscopy of peptides. In *The Peptides: Analysis, Synthesis, Biology*, Vol. 7: *Conformation in Biology and Drug Design*, V. J. Hruby, ed. Academic Press, New York, pp. 437-473 (1985).

52. Weber, G., What we have learned about proteins from the study of their excited states. In *Excited States of Biological Molecules*, J. B. Birks, ed. Wiley, New York, pp. 363-374 (1976).

53. Munro, J., I. Pecht, and L. Stryer, A subnanosecond motion of tryptophan residues in proteins. *Proc. Natl. Acad. Sci. USA* 76:56-60 (1979).

54. Avignon, M., P. V. Huong, L. Lascombe, M. Marraud, and J. Neel, Etude par spectroscopie infra-rouge, de la conformation de quelques composés peptidiques modèles. *Biopolymers* 8:69-89 (1969).

55. Avignon, M., C. Garrigou-Lagrange, and P. Bothorel, Conformational analysis of dipeptides in aqueous solution. 2. Molecular structure of glycine and alanine dipeptides by depolarized Rayleigh scattering and laser Raman spectroscopy. *Biopolymers* 12:1651-1669 (1973).

56. Oboodi, R. M., C. Alva, and M. Diem, Solution-phase Raman studies of alanyl dipeptides and various isotopomers: A reevaluation of the amide III vibrational assignment. *J. Phys. Chem.* 88:501-505 (1984).

57. Rao, C. P., P. Balaram, and C. N. R. Rao, Infrared spectroscopic study of C_7 intramolecular hydrogen bonds in peptides. *Biopolymers* 22:2091-2104 (1983).

58. Wilson, E. B., C. C. Decius, and P. C. Cross, *Molecular Vibrations*. McGraw-Hill, New York (1955).

59. Woody, R. W., Circular dichroism of peptides. In *The Peptides: Analysis, Synthesis, Biology*, Vol. 7: *Conformation in Biology and Drug Design*, V. J. Hruby, ed. Academic Press, New York, pp. 16–144 (1985).

60. Ramachandran, G. N., C. Ramakrishnan, and V. Sasisakharan, Stereochemistry of polypeptide chain configurations. *J. Mol. Biol. 7*:95–99 (1963).

61. Zimmerman, S. S., Theoretical methods in the analysis of peptide conformation. In *The Peptides: Analysis, Synthesis, Biology*, Vol. 7: *Conformation in Biology and Drug Design*, V. J. Hruby, ed. Academic Press, New York, pp. 165–212 (1985).

62. Burkart, U., and N. L. Allinger, *Molecular Mechanics*. ACS, Washington, D.C. (1982).

63. Elber, R., and M. Karplus, Multiple conformational states of proteins: A molecular dynamics analysis of myoglobin. *Science 235*:318–321 (1987) and references therein.

64. Zichi, D. A., and P. J. Rossky, Molecular conformational equilibria in liquids. *J. Chem. Phys. 84*:1712–1723 (1986).

65. Rossky, P. J., M. Karplus, and A. Rahman, A model for the simulation of an aqueous dipeptide solution. *Biopolymers 18*:825–854 (1979).

66. Rossky, P. J., and M. Karplus, Solvation. A molecular dynamics study of a dipeptide in water. *J. Am. Chem. Soc. 101*:1913–1937 (1979).

67. Pettitt, B. M., and M. Karplus, The potential of mean force surface for the alanine dipeptide: A theoretical approach. *Chem. Phys. Lett. 121*:194–201 (1985).

68. Mezei, M., P. K. Mehrotra, and D. L. Beveridge, Monte-Carlo determination of the free energy and internal energy of hydration for the Ala dipeptide at 25°C. *J. Am. Chem. Soc. 107*:2239–2245 (1985).

69. Pettitt, B. M., M. Karplus, and P. J. Rossky, Integral equation model for aqueous solvation of polyatomic solutes: Application to the determination of the free energy surface for the internal motion of biomolecules. *J. Phys. Chem. 90*:6335–6345 (1986).

70. Sarantakis, D., Peptides with morphine-like activity. U.S. Patent 4098781 (1979).

71. Hruby, V. J., K. K. Deb, J. Fox, J. Bjarnason, and A. T. Tu, Conformational studies of peptide hormones using laser Raman and circular dichroism: A comparative study of oxytocin agonists and antagonists. *J. Biol. Chem. 253*:6060–6067 (1978).

72. Mosberg, H. I., V. J. Hruby, and J.-P. Meraldi, Conformational study of the potent peptide hormone antagonist [1-penicillamine, 2-leucine]-oxytocin in aqueous solution. *Biochemistry 20*:2822–2828 (1981).

73. Hruby, V. J., H. I. Mosberg, J. W. Fox, and A. T. Tu, Conformational comparisons of oxytocin agonists, partial agonists and antagonists using laser Raman and circular dichrosim spectroscopy. Examination of 1-pencillamine and diastereoisomeric analogues. *J. Biol. Chem. 257*:4916–4924 (1982).

74. Mosberg, H. I., R. Hurst, V. J. Hruby, J. J. Galligan, T. F. Burks, K. Gee, and H. I. Yamamura, [D-Pen², L-Cys⁵]enkephalinamide and [D-Pen², D-Cys⁵]-enkephalinamide, conformationally constrained cyclic enkephalinamide analogues with delta receptor specificity. *Biochem. Biophys. Res. Commun. 106*:506–512 (1982).

75. Schiller, P. W., and J. DiMaio, Aspects of conformational restriction in biologically active peptides. In *Peptides: Structure and Function*, V. J. Hruby and D. H. Rich, eds. Pierce Chemical Co., Rockford, Ill., pp. 269–278 (1983).

76. Mosberg, H. I., and P. W. Schiller, ¹H n.m.r. investigation of conformational features of cyclic enkephalin amide analogs. *Int. J. Peptide Protein Res. 23*:462–466 (1984).

77. Morley, J. S., Structure-activity relationships of enkephalin-like peptides. *Am. Rev. Pharmacol. Toxicol. 20*:81–110 (1980).

78. Kosterlitz, H. W., J. A. H. Lord, S. J. Paterson, and A. A. Waterfield, Effect of the changes in the structure of enkephalins and of narcotic analgesic drugs on their interactions with μ- and δ-receptors. *Br. J. Pharmacol. 68*:333–342 (1980).

79. Ronai, A. Z., I. P. Berzétei, J. I. Székeley, E. Miglécz, J. Kurgyis, and S. Bajusz, Enkephalin-like character and analgesia. *Eur. J. Pharmacol. 69*:263–271 (1981).

80. Mosberg, H. I., R. Hurst, V. J. Hruby, J. J. Galligan, T. F. Burks, K. Gee, and H. I. Yamamura, Conformationally constrained cyclic enkephalin analogs with pronounced delta opioid receptor agonist selectivity. *Life Sci. 32*:2565–2569 (1983).

81. Mosberg, H. I., R. Hurst, V. J. Hruby, K. Gee, K. Akiyama, H. I. Yamamura, J. J. Galligan, and T. F. Burks, Cyclic penicillamine containing enkephalin analogs display profound delta receptor selectivities. *Life Sci. 33* (Suppl. I):447–450 (1983).

82. Mosberg, H. I., R. Hurst, V. J. Hruby, K. Gee, H. I. Yamamura, J. J. Galligan, and T. F. Burks, Bis-penicillamine enkephalins possess highly improved specificity toward delta opioid receptors. *Proc. Natl. Acad. Sci. USA 80*:5071–5874 (1983).

83. Hurst, R., Receptor specific enkephalin analogs. Master's thesis, University of Arizona, Tucson (1984).

84. Akiyama, K., K. Gee, H. I. Mosberg, V. J. Hruby, and H. I. Yamamura, Characterization of [³H][2-D-penicillamine, 5-D-penicillamine]-enkephalin binding to delta opiate receptor in the rat brain and neuroblastoma-glioma hybrid cell line (NG 108-15). *Proc. Natl. Acad. Sci. USA 82*:2543–2547 (1985).

85. Cotton, R., H. W. Kosterlitz, S. J. Paterson, M. J. Rance, and J. R. Traynor, The use of [³H][D-Pen², D-Pen⁵]enkephalin as a highly selective ligand for the delta binding site. *Br. J. Pharmacol. 84*:927–932 (1985).

86. Corbett, A. D., M. G. C. Gillan, H. W. Kosterlitz, H. T. McKnight, S. J. Paterson, and L. E. Robson, Selectivities of opioid peptide analogues as agonists and antagonists at the delta receptor. *Br. J. Pharmacol. 83*:271–279 (1984).

87. James, I. F., and A. Goldstein, Site-directed alkylation of multiple opioid receptors. 1. Binding selectivity. *Mol. Pharmacol. 25*:337–342 (1984).

88. Goldstein, A., and I. F. James, Multiple opioid receptors criteria for identification and classification. *Trend Pharmacol. Sci. 5*:503–505 (1984).

89. Clark, J. A., Y. Itzhak, V. J. Hruby, H. I. Yamamura, and G. W. Pasternak, [*D*-Pen^2, *D*-Pen^5]enkephalin (DPDPE): An α-selective enkephalin with low affinity for μ opiate binding sites. *Eur. J. Pharmacol. 128*:303–304 (1986).

90. Gulya, K., D. R. Gehlert, J. K. Wamsley, H. Mosberg, V. J. Hruby, and H. I. Yamamura, Light microscopic autoradiographic localization of delta opioid receptors in the rat brain using a highly selective bis-penicillamine cyclic enkephalin analogue. *J. Pharmacol. Exp. Ther. 238*:720–726 (1986).

91. Kao, L.-F., and V. J. Hruby, Suppression or differentiation of solvent resonance by a combination of DEFT with a two-dimensional sequence. *J. Magn. Reson. 70*:394–407 (1986).

92. Hruby, V. J., L.-F. Kao, B. M. Pettitt, and M. Karplus, The conformational properties of the delta opioid peptide [*D*-Pen^2, *D*-Pen^5]enkephalin in aqueous solution determined by NMR and energy minimization calculations. *J. Am. Chem. Soc. 110*:3351–3359 (1988).

93. As this paper was being written, a paper by Mosberg [Mosberg, H. I., ^{1}H n.m.r. investigation of conformational features of cyclic, penicillamine-containing enkephalin analogs, *Int. J. Peptide Protein Res. 29*:282–288 (1987)] appeared, which gave ^{1}H NMR data for several penicillamine-containing enkephalin analogues. The assignments for DPDPE are completely consistent with those reported here.

94. Hruby, V. J., L.-F. Kao, L. D. Hirning, and T. F. Burks, Conformation–biological activity relationships of conformationally constrained delta specific cyclic enkephalin. In *Peptides: Structure and Function*, C. M. Deber, V. J. Hruby, and K. D. Kopple, eds. Pierce Chemical Co., Rockford, Ill., pp. 487–490 (1985).

95. Anteunis, M. J., C. Becu, A. K. Lala, G. Verhegge, and K. Narayan-Lala, Glycyl methylene chemical shift non-equivalence in small peptides. Diastereoisomers of Leu–Gly–Phe. *Bull. Soc. Chim. Belg. 86*:161–186 (1977).

96. Anteunis, M. J. O., Glycyl methylene chemical shift non-equivalence. A useful conformational probe. *Tetrahedron Lett. 18*:1535–1538 (1977).

97. De Leeuw, F. A. A. M., and C. Altona, Component vicinal coupling constants for calculating side-chain conformations on amino acids. *Int. J. Peptide Protein Res. 20*:120–125 (1982).

98. Lewis, P. N., F. A. Momany, and H. A. Scheraga, Chain reversals in proteins. *Biochim. Biophys. Acta 303*:211–229 (1973).

99. Buccoleri, R. E., and M. Karplus, Prediction of the folding of short polypeptide segments by uniform conformational sampling. *Biopolymers 26*:137–168 (1987).

100. McCammon, J. A., and M. Karplus, Simulation of protein dynamics. *Annu. Rev. Phys. Chem. 31*:29–45 (1980).

101. Paine, G. H., and H. A. Scheraga, Prediction of the native conformation of a polypeptide by a statistical-mechanical procedure. I. Backbone structure of enkephalin. *Biopolymers 24*:1391–1436 (1985).

102. Paine, G. H., and H. A. Scheraga, Prediction of the native conformation of a polypeptide by a statistical-mechanical procedure. III. Probable and average conformations of enkephalin. *Biopolymers 26*:1125–1140 (1987).

103. Stillinger, F. H., and T. A. Weber, Hidden structure in liquids. *Physiol. Rev. A25*:978 989 (1982).

104. Hruby, V. J., L.-F. Kao, J. E. Shook, K. Gulya, H. I. Yamamura, and T. F. Burks, Design and synthesis of receptor selective peptide neurotransmitters. In *Peptides 1986: Proceedings of the 19th European Peptide Symposium*, D. Theodoropoulas, ed. W. de Gruyter, Berlin, pp. 385–388 (1987).

105. Vale, W., C. Rivier, and M. Brown, Regulatory peptides of the hypothalamus. *Annu. Rev. Physiol. 39*:473–527 (1977).

106. Terenuis, L., Somatostatin and ACTH are peptides with partial antagonist-like selectivity for opiate receptors. *Eur. J. Pharmacol. 38*:211–213 (1976).

107. Rezek, M., V. Havlecek, L. Leybin, F. S. LaBella, and H. G. Frieser, Opiate-like naloxone-reversible actions of somatostatin given intracerebrally. *Can. J. Physiol. Pharmacol. 56*:277–231 (1978).

108. Maurer, R. B., B. H. Gachiwiler, H. H. Buescher, R. C. Hill, and D. Roemer, Opiate antagonist properties of an octapeptide somatostatin analog. *Proc. Natl. Acad. Sci. USA 79*:4815–4817 (1982).

109. Pelton, J. T., K. Gulya, V. J. Hruby, S. Duckles, and H. I. Yamamura, Somatostatin analogs with affinity for opiate receptors in rat brain binding assay. *Peptides 6* (Suppl. 1):159–163 (1985).

110. Pelton, J. T., K. Gulya, V. J. Hruby, S. P. Duckles, and H. I. Yamamura, Conformationally restricted analogues of somatostatin with high μ-opiate receptor specificity. *Proc. Natl. Acad. Sci. USA 82*:236–239 (1985).

111. Nutt, R. F., D. F. Veber, P. E. Curley, R. Saperstein, and R. Hirschmann, Somatostatin analogs which define the role of the lysine-9 amino group. *Int. J Peptide Protein Res. 21*:66–73 (1983).

112. Pelton, J. T., W. Kazmierski, K. Gulya, H. I. Yamamura, and V. J. Hruby, Design and synthesis of conformationally constrained somatostatin analogues with high potency and specificity for μ opioid receptors. *J. Med. Chem. 29*:2370–2375 (1986).

113. Gulya, K., J. T. Pelton, V. J. Hruby, and H. I. Yamamura, Cyclic somatostatin octapeptide analogues with high affinity and selectivity toward mu opioid receptors. *Life Sci. 38*:2221–2230 (1986).

114. Shook, J. E., J. T. Pelton, W. S. Wire, L. D. Hirning, V. J. Hruby, and T. F. Burks, Pharmacological evaluation of a cyclic somatostatin octapeptide with antagonist activity at mu-opioid receptor in vitro. *J. Pharmacol. Exp. Ther. 240*:1–6 (1987).

115. Shook, J. E., J. T. Pelton, W. Kazmierski, P. K. Lemcke, W. S. Wire, V. J. Hruby, and T. F. Burks, Comparison of opioid antagonist properties of a cyclic somatostatin analog in vitro and in vitro. In *Progress in Opioid Research: Proceeding of the 1986 INRC*, NIDA Research Monograph 75. Rockville, Md., pp. 205–208 (1987).

116. Shook, J. E., J. T. Pelton, W. Kazmierski, P. K. Lemcke, R. G. Villar, V. J.

Hruby, and T. F. Burks, A cyclic somatostatin analog that precipitates withdrawal in morphine dependent mice. In *Proceedings of the 48th Annual Scientific Meeting of the Committee on Problems of Drug Dependence*, NIDA Research Monograph 76. Rockville, Md., pp. 295–301 (1987).

117. Shook, J. E., J. T. Pelton, P. K. Lemcke, F. Porreca, V. J. Hruby, and T. F. Burks, Mu opioid antagonist properties of a cyclic somatostatin octapeptide in vivo: Identification of mu receptor related functions. *J. Pharmacol. Exp. Ther. 242*:1–7 (1987).

118. Shook, J. E., J. T. Pelton, V. J. Hruby, and T. F. Burks, Peptide opioid antagonist separates peripheral and central opioid antitransit effects. *J. Pharmacol. Exp. Ther 243*:492–500 (1987).

119. Wynants, C., G. Van Binst, and H. R. Loosli, SMS 201-995, an octapeptide somatostatin analogue. Assignment of the ^{1}H 500 MHz n.m.r. spectra and conformational analysis of SMS-995 in dimethylsulfoxide. *Int. J. Peptide Protein Res. 25*:615–621 (1985).

120. Pelton, J. T., M. Whalon, W. Cody, and V. J. Hruby, Conformation of CTP-NH$_2$, a highly selective mu-opiate antagonist peptide by ^{1}H and ^{13}C NMR. *Int. J. Peptide Protein Res. 31*:109–115 (1988).

121. Wynants, C., E. Sugg, V. J. Hruby, and G. Van Binst, Conformational study of somatostatin analogue by high field N.M.R. spectroscopy in aqueous solution. *Int. J. Peptide Protein Res. 30*:541–547 (1987).

122. Sugg, E. E., D. Tourwe, W. Kazmierski, V. J. Hruby, and G. Van Binst, Proton N.M.R. investigation of the conformational influence of penicillamine residues on the disulfide ring system of opioid receptor selective somatostatin analogues. *Int. J. Peptide Protein Res. 31*:192–200 (1988).

12

Design of Conformationally Restricted Cyclopeptides for the Inhibition of Cholate Uptake of Hepatocytes

Horst Kessler, Andreas Haupt, and Martin Will
J. W. Goethe University, Frankfurt, Federal Republic of Germany

I. GENERAL REMARKS

Molecular recognition is not only important in understanding the selectivity of organic molecules; it is an essential concept for life processes. Most of the biological communication within living systems is based on molecular recognition. Often peptides are used as transmitting media for the following reasons:

1. A controlled synthesis of peptides and proteins at the ribosome guarantees easy accessibility.
2. The 25 natural amino acids allow a great variability in protein structure. Charges, steric hindrance, and lipophilic characters can be varied easily.

461

3. The high polarity and the ability to donate and accept hydrogen bonds induce sensitivity of the global structure to minor changes of the constituent amino acids or environmental effects.
4. The easy enzymatic degradation of peptides guarantees fast removal after the signal is induced. This allows a quick switching on and off of function.

The basic model in understanding molecular recognition was given by the "grandfather of bioorganic chemistry," Emil Fischer (1,2): the substrate is recognized by the receptor in forming a complex [called "supramolecule" by J. M. Lehn (3)]. We now believe that the conformational change of the receptor induced by the binding of a peptidic messenger results in the specific effect. Peptidic hormones, in general, however, have a high degree of flexibility. Hence, conformational changes of the substrate during binding also have to be considered for the "induced fit." It is known, for example, from the enkephalins (4) that different receptors can bind the same molecule in different conformations (Fig. 1).

In designing drugs for receptor-specific modulation, it is essential to know the receptor-bound conformation. As long as the complex is not experiment-

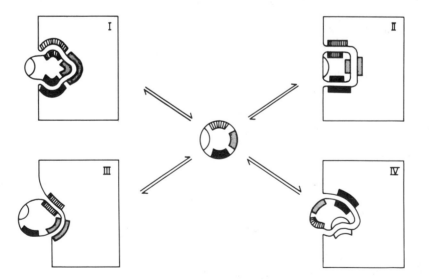

Figure 1 Different conformations of the same molecule can bind to different receptor types.

ally accessible, the introduction of rigidity into the substrate, followed by monitoring the biological activity, seems to be the best way toward an indirect determination of the bioactive conformation (5). Rigidity is mainly achieved by cyclization, but introduction of steric hindrance or peptidomimetics may also be used for this purpose. The possibilities for cyclization can be summarized as follows (6): head-to-tail cyclization of the backbone; side-chain to side-chain cyclization; side-chain to backbone cyclization; fixation of side chains; or combinations of those.

Under these circumstances, structure-activity studies can be performed in a conformationally controlled manner. In structure-activity relationships of peptides, variation of the side chains, variation of the chirality of certain residues, and the use of unnatural amino acids are commonly applied. As those changes are structural changes in constitution which may induce changes in the conformation as well, it is difficult to sort out the different influences. On the other hand, introduction of rigidity by cyclization can circumvent these problems by reducing the conformational flexibility of the peptidic drugs. The conformation of a biologically active peptide is determined by NMR spectroscopy, computer calculations [e.g., molecular dynamics (MD) calculations], and x-ray analysis (7). If the so determined conformations are identical in different environments (crystal, solvents of different polarity), we may consider it as "rigid," and conformational changes induced by binding to the receptor are unlikely because of energy consumption. A high biological activity, then, indicates a conformation close to the receptor-bound one of the flexible noncyclic precursor. A rigid cyclic peptide, having no biological activity, then expresses in that sense that the bioactive conformation cannot be realized at all because of the wrong spatial arrangement of important residues.

II. UPTAKE OF ORGANIC SUBSTRATES BY HEPATOCYTES

Organoprotection and cytoprotection by chemical substances are well-known phenomena and in some cases are already used clinically (8). The biochemical origin of these processes, however, is often not understood. In this work the cytoprotective activity of cyclic peptides against intoxication of rat liver cells by toxic agents is described (9). The prevention of phalloidin poisoning by antamanide [2], a cyclic decapeptide, is well known and has been reported in numerous publications by Wieland and co-workers (10). That both cyclic peptides, the poison and the antidote, are found in the same mushroom, *Amanita phalloides*, has attracted much interest. Later on it was found that somatostatin [1], a cyclic heterodetic peptide hormone, exhibits a similar effect (11,12). It was the aim of our study to determine if the

H—Ala—Gly—Cys—Lys—Asn—Phe—Phe—Trp   Pro—Phe—Phe—Val—Pro
　　　　　|　　　　　　　　　　　|　　　　　　　　　|　　　　　　　　　|
　　HO—Cys—Ser—Thr—Phe—Thr—Lys   Pro—Phe—Phe—Ala—Pro

1   **2**

Figure 2 Primary structure of somatostatin 1 and antamanide 2.

cytoprotection is related to the endocrine effects of this hormone. We also wanted to increase the activity by changing structures and to find out if a common structural element exists that is responsible for the cytoprotective effect.

The latter is not obvious at all from the constitution of both peptides, somatostatin and antamanide (Fig. 2). The solution of this problem will be given in Section III.A.2. In the course of our studies it has been shown that cytoprotection results from hepatocellular uptake inhibition of substances with liver toxicity (13,14). A directed transporter system in the liver cell membrane usually is responsible for the transport of cholate from blood via hepatocytes into the bile (15), a process of great importance for digestion. But other substances (16,17), mostly lipophilic ones, can be transported the same way, ephasizing the importance of this pathway for detoxification in animals. The problem arises when these substrates, which are transported, show inherent toxicity for the liver cell itself such as phalloidin, DMSO, ethanol, and others. Phalloidin, for instance (18,19), once having reached the interior of the hepatocyte, binds to actin and thus destabilizes the membrane (20). The typical formation of blisters in isolated hepatocytes induced by phalloidin is therefore a convenient way to test the inhibition of the transport in vitro (21). Another test is based on the direct measurement of the uptake inhibition of radioactive cholate or phalloidin (22) by cytoprotective agents.

The membrane proteins involved in the transport of all these different substrates were characterized by photoaffinity labeling techniques (23–25). It became evident that the same protein components were labeled by various radioactive and photoreactive analogs derived from cholic acid (26) as well as from antamanide, phalloidin (27), and one of the most active inhibitor peptides ("008") prepared by us in the course of this work (28,29), strongly supporting the hypothesis that all these substrates are transported into hepatocytes by the same system.

Table 1 Cytoprotection and Endocrine Activity of Somatostatin and Analogues

No.	Compound	Phalloidin uptake CD$_{50}$ (μM)[a]	Hormone activity[b]	Cholate uptake (%)[c]
1	Somatostatin	109.0	1	23 ± 7
3	H–D–Phe–Cys–Phe–T–P ol–Thr–Cys–Thr–Lys	50.0	0.33	—[d]
4	cyclo(–Pro–Phe–D–Trp–Lys–Thr–Phe–)	28.0	0.59	59.6
6	cyclo(–Phe–Phe–Trp–Lys–Thr–D–Phe–)	14.0	No effect	—
7	cyclo(–Phe–Phe–D–Trp–Lys–Thr–Phe–)	5.7	3.7	—
8	cyclo(–Gly–Phe–D–Trp–Lys–Thr–Pro–)	—	—	28 ± 1
9	cyclo(–Pro–Phe–D–Trp–Lys–Thr–)	—	—	29 ± 3
10	cyclo(–Pro–Phe–D–Trp–Lys–D–Thr–)	—	—	53 ± 2
11	cyclo(–Aib–Phe–D–Trp–Lys–Thr–)	—	—	37 ± 5

[a]Concentration of substance needed for a 50% inhibition of phalloidin uptake in isolated hepatocytes as described in Ref. 13.
[b]Measured as GH release inhibition (34).
[c]Effect of pretreatment of freshly isolated hepatocytes with somatostatin and its analogs on the prevention of plebs induced by phalloidin. Cytoprotection obtained from a single concentration of 50 μM (21).
[d]No biological testing was performed

III. STRUCTURE–ACTIVITY RELATIONSHIPS FOR HEPATOCELLULAR CHOLATE UPTAKE INHIBITION

A. Inhibitors Derived from Somatostatin

1. Active Sequence for Endocrine Activity and Cytoprotection

The active sequence of somatostatin—i.e., the region within the molecule responsible for the endocrine effects (inhibition of hormone release)—was localized only a short time after the isolation of the peptide hormone in 1972 (30). It was shown that the amino acid residues 6–11 of natural somatostatin represent the recognition area for the inhibition of glucagon, growth hormone (GH), and insulin secretion (31,32) (Fig. 3).

On the assumption that the rest of the molecule only functions to bring the important region into the right conformation, a large number of so-called "minisomatostatins" were developed (33). Those analogs possess a reduced conformational freedom owing to cyclization. If the active conformation at the receptor can still be realized under this reduced flexibility, the compound necessarily retains, at least partially, its biological activity. Moreover, there is hope that those constrained molecules may exhibit higher receptor selectivity which may culminate in a separation of insulin and glucagon release. Although this goal has not been reached, superpotent analogs with high in vivo stability have been synthesized (Fig. 4).

These results were achieved after extensive research mainly performed by Veber et al. at Merck, Sharpe & Dohme (MSD) (34) and Bauer et al. at SANDOZ (35). Compound 5 (in Fig. 4), for example, is about 100 times more active than natural somatostatin in the inhibition of insulin and glucagon secretion (36). All analogs exhibit increased enzymatic stability. We will concentrate here, however, on the cytoprotective effects.

The SANDOZ peptide (3 in Fig. 4) and the MSD peptide (4 in Fig. 4) were also tested for cytoprotection of rat liver cells against phalloidin poisoning (Table 1). As phalloidin uptake inhibition and GH release inhibition can be correlated for the examples 1, 3, and 4, our first working hypothesis was that the active regions responsible for the hormonal effect and cytoprotective

H—Ala—Gly—Cys—Lys—Asn—Phe —Phe—Trp
          | |
     HO—Cys—Ser—Thr—Phe —Thr—Lys

Figure 3 Active region of somatostatin for endocrine activity.

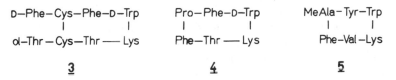

Figure 4 Minisomatostatins with superpotent endocrine activity by SANDOZ [3] and MSD [4, 5].

effect were identical. Therefore, we started from the very active MSD peptide 4, representing the sequence 7–11 of natural somatostatin, bridged by a proline residue and having the tryptophan in D configuration. We then took the normal sequence 6–11 of somatostatin and changed the chirality of amino acids in positions 6, 8, and 11, respectively. Our intention was to obtain a correlation between biological activities and conformation in solution. In all of the studied cyclic hexapeptides, a conformation with two β turns is

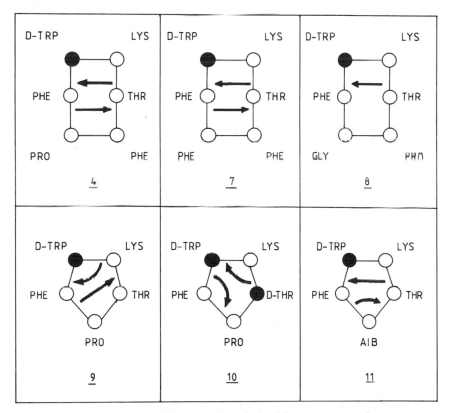

Figure 5 Cyclic penta- and hexapeptides derived from somatostatin.

observed in which a D amino acid tends to prefer the i + 1 position of a βII′ turn (Fig. 5) (37,38). In cyclic pentapeptides βII′γ or $\gamma\gamma$ conformations have been found (39,40) (Fig. 5), but it turned out that the βII′ turn in the Phe–D–Trp–Lys–Thr region is not sufficient for cytoprotection activity (8).

In addition, we found that high endocrine activity does not correlate directly with high cytoprotection activity (Table 1) (9). This gave us the first hint that the two effects, cytoprotection and GH release inhibition, were independent from each other. The inclusion of conformational arguments at this stage did not contribute to the clarification of these results.

2. Complete Decoupling of Endocrine Activity and Cytoprotection

In addition to variation in chirality, we also altered the direction of the peptide bonds. This can easily be achieved by cyclization of the reversed amino acid sequence ("retro-peptides"). This is unusual. There are many reports in the literature about "retro-inverso-peptides," in which the chirality of each amino acid residue is inverted and the sequence is reversed (41). In such retro-inverso-peptides the side chains may adopt similar spatial arrangements as the stem peptide. However, this cannot be achieved in retro-peptides (9) (Fig. 6). In fact, it has been found that modified cyclic "retro-inverso" somatostatins exhibit similar biological activities to the unchanged sequence (42). To our surprise, the cyclic hexapeptide cyclo(–D–Trp–Phe–Phe–Phe–Thr–Lys–) [12], which is the retro-sequence of cyclo(–D–Trp–Lys–Thr–Phe–Phe–Phe–) [7], still exhibits the high activity in phalloidin

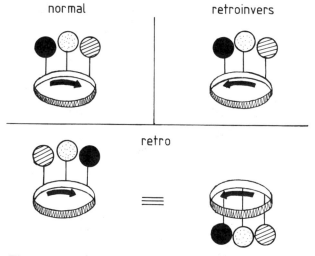

Figure 6   Schematic drawing of a stem peptide, its "retro," and "retroinverso" structure.

uptake inhibition. Moreover, no effect was found for GH release inhibition (43) (Table 2).

These results support the above-mentioned lack of correlation between the two effects. To account for the effect that peptides and their "retro" analogs are both active, we assume a small recognition area responsible for cytoprotective activity. This is emphasized by a comparison of the amount of substance required for efficient cytoprotection: although hormonal activities require nanomolar quantities, the discussed effect is observed only in the micromolar order. Only a small recognition area of relatively low selectivity can be met by both structures, a stem peptide and its retroanalog. The different specifity compared to hormonal effects is further expressed by the fact that the peptides in all cases were significantly more active when the lysine side chain was protected by a Z group than in the case of unprotected compounds (e.g., compounds 13 and 14 in Table 2) (28). The accumulation of aromatic amino acids within these peptides gives the impression that those residues are important in the binding process. In any case, each of the amino acids has to be checked for its contribution to the binding (see next section).

At this stage of our investigations, the retro-peptide cyclo(–D–Pro^1–Phe^2–Thr^3–Lys^4(Z)–Trp^5–Phe^6–) (13 "008(Z)") happened to be the most active one found so far (44), exceeding the activity of antamanide by a factor of 3. Therefore, its three-dimensional structure was investigated in detail by state-of-the-art NMR techniques and subsequent structural refinement by MD calculations (45). Homo- and heteronuclear 1-D and 2-D NMR techniques have been used to assign all proton and carbon resonances (46). Conformational analysis of the backbone is based on the temperature dependency of NH chemical shifts, the $^3J(HN-C\alpha H)$ coupling constants and NOE effects. Because of the small NOEs of a molecule of this size, NOEs were determined in the rotating frame (ROE) (47) by using a pulsed ROESY experiment. To suppress contributions from TOCSY transfer (J-coupling), small flip angles ($\beta = 18°$) were used (48). As the lock field depends strongly on the offset frequency, an offset correction was performed to get reliable volume integrals of the ROE cross peaks (49). The ROEs thus obtained were transformed into distances r_{ij} ($r_{ij}^6 \times ROE_{ij} = const.$) and then used as constraints in the molecular dynamics calculation via the GROMOS program package (50,51).

The resulting averaged backbone conformation is shown in Figure 7. The resulting averaged backbone conformation is shown in Figure 7. The hydrogen-bonding pattern is a result of the restrained dynamics and is not used as a restriction when the calculation starts. The thus calculated hydrogen bondings are in good agreement to the temperature dependency of the NH proton chemical shifts. Interesting features of this structure are the bifurcated hydrogen bonding of the Thr^3 NH and a weak βI turn (unfavorable distance and angle) between the Phe^6–NH and the Thr^3–CO. In

Table 2 Cytoprotective and Endocrine Activity of Cyclic Hexapeptides Derived from Somatostatin

No.	Compound	Cholate uptake CD_{50} (μE)[a]	Phalloidin uptake CD_{50} (kM)[b]	Hormone effect[c]
<u>7</u>	cyclo(–Phe–Phe–D–Trp–Lys–Thr–Phe–)	—[d]	5.7	3.7
<u>12</u>	cyclo(–Phe–Thr–Lys–D–Trp–Phe–Phe–)	10.0	5.1	—
<u>13</u>	cyclo(–Phe–Thr–Lys(Z)–Trp–Phe–D–Pro–)	1.5	1.0	—
<u>14</u>	cyclo(–Phe–Thr–Lys–Trp–Phe–D–Pro–)	3.0	1.5	—
<u>15</u>	cyclo(–D–Pro–Thr–Lys(Z)–D–Trp–Phe–D–Pro–)	2.0	3.3	—
<u>16</u>	cyclo(–/–Pro–Phe–Thr–Phe–Trp–Phe–)	2.0	—	—

[a]Concentration of substance needed for a 50% inhibition of phalloidin uptake in isolated hepatocytes.
[b]Measured as GH release inhibition (33).
[c]Effect of pretreatment of freshly isolated hepatocytes with somatostatin and its analogs on the prevention of plebs induced by phalloidin. Cytoprotection obtained from a single concentration of 50 μM (21).
[d]No biological testing was performed.

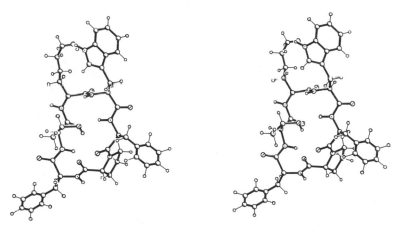

Figure 7 Averaged conformation of "008" obtained from MD calculations using NMR information. The side-chain conformation of Phe^2 does not show the most stable conformation in solution, because insufficient NOE restraints to the side-chain protons were available.

addition, it turned out that the Thr OH group is involved in hydrogen bonding as a donor (to CO of Phe^6) as well as an acceptor (to the NHs of Trp^5 and Phe^6). Furthermore, the Trp^5–NH forms a weak γ-turn in bonding to the Thr^3–CO.

The population of the three staggered rotamers of the side chains (except for Lys) was determined from homo and heteronuclear coupling constants. $^3J(HC\alpha$–$C\beta H)$ couplings obtained via the DISCO (52) and E.COSY technique (53) yield the population ratios of the three rotamers (54), whereas the heteronuclear coupling $^3J(^{13}CO$–$C\alpha C\beta H)$ can be used to assign the diastereotopic β protons unambiguously (54,55). The heteronuclear coupling information is most easily obtained from a routine COLOC spectrum (55,56). The dominant conformation of the side chains is given in Figure 8.

Unfortunately, this compound could not be crystallized, but an x-ray structure was obtained from a derivative where the Lys residue is substituted by Phe (compound 16, $CD_{50} = 2.0\ \mu M$) (45). Comparison of the NMR spectra provides evidence for identical solution conformations for the two compounds. The crystal structure of the Phe^4 analog 16 and the solution structure of 008 are presented in Figure 8.

Whereas the backbone conformation and the orientation of the aromatic side chains are nearly identical in the two peptides, the Thr side chain exhibits remarkable differences. The orientation of the Thr hydroxyl group in the crystalline state reveals the existence of an intermolecular hydrogen bond to a

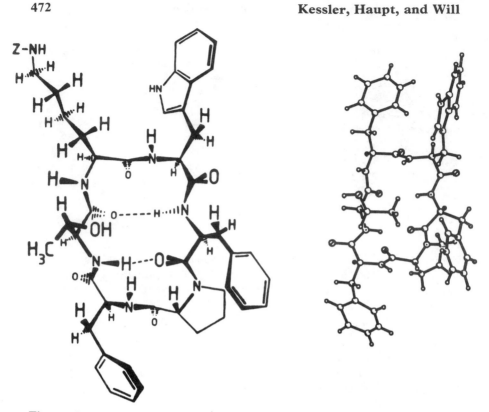

Figure 8 X-ray structure of (Phe⁴) "008" (right) and solution structure of "008" (left).

neighbored molecule in contrast to the intramolecular hydrogen bonding as present in solution (45). Such a remarkable difference in the side chain seems to be typical of dissolution of a crystal: intermolecular hydrogen bridges are broken, and, in solution, intramolecular bonding is preferred (57). A very similar difference was observed for the methyl-butenyl-threonine side chain (MeBmt) in cyclosporin A (58). For further elucidation of the recognition area, 008 was taken as the starting point for conformationally controlled structure activity studies.

3. New Search for the "Active Sequence"

To define the importance of the side chains of each amino acid for biological activity within the above-mentioned peptide, we synthesized analogs of this compound where all residues were replaced one by one by an alanine residue, and D-alanine for D-proline. The conformation of all Z-protected cyclic peptides was determined by NMR spectroscopy in d_6-DMSO solution (59). It turned out that five of the six analogs adopt a backbone conformation very similar to that of the parent compound. Hence, for these peptides the change in biological activity directly reflects the importance of the side chains.

Only the (Ala3)–008 [18], in which the Thr residue is substituted, exhibits a switching of the Lys–Trp amide bond, resulting in a different kind of β loop (βII) in this region of the molecule (59). The conformational change in 18 is an independent proof for the influence of the Thr 10 OH group on the backbone conformation: without the hydrogen acceptor ability of the hydroxyl group, the Trp^5–NH is not locked into the specific arrangement shown in Figure 7, and the Lys–Trp peptide bond is free to flip (60). However, we have to point out that the resulting βII turn does not agree with the rules derived from protein x-ray structures, which would suggest a βI turn for two L-amino acids in the i + 1 and i + 2 positions (61,62). Up to now, we have found several exceptions to these rules in cyclic peptides.

Determination of the side-chain rotamers of the aromatic amino acids indicates that their spatial arrangement is identical in all compounds including 18. Such identical conformations for all these peptides represents an ideal condition to determine the influence of each amino acid side chain on biological activity in terms of steric and lipophilic effects. The results are summarized in Table 3, and the following conclusions may be drawn:

1. All alanine-containing peptides exhibit cytoprotection activity.
2. Substitution of each of the aromatic amino acid residues by alanine leads to a decrease of biological activity. This emphasizes the importance of these amino acids for recognition.
3. D-Ala¹ instead of D–Pro¹ and Ala³ instead of Thr³ yield slightly enhanced biological activity.

Table 3 Inhibition of Cholate Uptake by Alanine Derivatives of "008"

No.	Compound	$CD_{50} (\mu M)^a$
13	cyclo(–Phe–Thr–Lys(Z)–Trp–Phe–D–Pro–)	1.5
17	cyclo(–Ala–Thr–Lys(Z)–Trp–Phe–D–Pro–)	5.0
18	cyclo(–Phe–Ala–Lys(Z)–Trp–Phe–D–Pro–)	0.5
19	cyclo(–Phe–Thr–Ala–Trp–Phe–D–Pro–)	4.0
20	cyclo(–Phe–Thr–Lys(Z)–Ala–Phe–D–Pro–)	7.0
21	cyclo(–Phe–Thr–Lys(Z)–Trp–Ala–D–Pro–)	3.7
22	cyclo(–Phe–Thr–Lys(Z)–Trp–Phe–D–Ala–)	1.0

[a]Concentration of substance needed for a 50% inhibition of phalloidin uptake in isolated hepatocytes as described in Ref. 13.

4. Substitution of Lys⁴(Z) by Ala⁴ reduces the activity to a similar level as
    the Lys-deprotected stem peptide 14 (Table 2).

These facts indicate that the cytoprotection activity is highly dependent on
lipophilic effects. Nevertheless, lipophilicity per se cannot guarantee high
cytoprotection (e.g., modification of the Lys side-chain amino group by
various carboxylic residues gave the best results with lipophilic aromatic
groups in contrast to lipophilic aliphatic residues such as oleic acid and
palmitic acid) (63).

B. Inhibitors Derived from Antamanide

To get more details about the recognition area, we compared the conformation and chemical structure of our stem peptide cyclo(–D–Pro¹–Phe²–
Thr³–Lys⁴(Z)–Trp⁵–Phe⁶–), [13], with other cytoprotective cyclic peptides
like antamanide [2] and cyclolinopeptide A [23]. The latter peptides exhibit
partial sequence homology (Pro–Pro–Phe–Phe–Xaa; Xaa = Val for 2,
Xaa = Leu for 23), and for both a high activity has been found in our test
system (Table 4). At first look, the important structural elements common to
all active peptides seem to be two adjacent aromatic amino acids like Phe,
Phe or Phe, Trp and a neighboring Pro or D-Pro residue. In addition to
sequential requirements, the backbone conformation and the spatial arrangement of the side chains are of great importance.

For example, the synthetic cyclic pentapeptide cyclo(–Pro–Pro–Phe–Phe–
Gly–) [25] (64) does not exhibit any biological activity, although sequence
homology is realized (Table 4). A look at the conformation of this peptide
helps to elucidate the origin of this contradiction: the spatial structure of the
Pro–Phe–Phe region is completely different from the one determined for
antamanide in crystal (65) and in solution (66) (Fig. 9).

Antamanide itself exhibits an equilibrium of up to four different conformations in solution (67). To a large extent, the solution conformation is
similar to the crystal structure. Because of slight differences it is difficult to
use these conformations for the discussion of the bioactive structure. We
therefore synthesized the more rigid cyclic hexapeptide cyclo(–D–Pro–Phe–
Phe–Pro–Phe–Phe) [24, "PFF"] combining the structural elements of the
somatostatin-derived 13 and antamanide and containing the suggested
structural elements required for a cytoprotective effect (68). Indeed, the
concentration needed for a 50% inhibition of cholate uptake was 3 μM, thus
being only slightly less active than cyclo(–D–Pro¹–Phe²–Thr³–Lys⁴(Z)–
Trp⁵–Phe⁶–) [13]. We were able to put this result on a molecular basis by
comparing the NMR-derived conformation of 008(Z) [13] in DMSO with
the x-ray structure of PFF [24]: the Phe–Phe–D–Pro–Phe region of PFF

Table 4 Hepatocellular Cholate Uptake Inhibition for Cyclolinopeptide A, Antamanide, and Model Compounds

No.	Structure	Compound	$CD_{50}(\mu M)$[a]
2	cyclo(–Phe–Pro–Pro–Phe–Phe–Val–Pro–Pro–Ala–Phe–)	Antamanide	8.0
23	cyclo(–Val–Pro–Pro–Phe–Phe–Leu–Ile–Ile–Leu–)	Cyclolinopeptide A	3.0
24	cyclo(–D–Pro–Phe–Phe–Pro–Phe–Phe–)	("PFF")	3.0
25	cyclo(–Pro–Pro–Phe–Phe–Gly–)		Inactive

[a]Concentration of substance needed for a 50% inhibition of phalloidin uptake in isolated hepatocytes as described in Ref. 13.

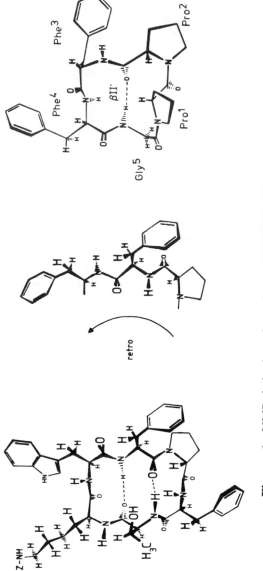

Figure 9 NMR-derived conformations of "008(Z)" (left), partial structure of antamanide (2, in the middle), and cyclo(–Pro–Pro–Phe–Gly–) (25, on the right).

[24] and the Trp–Phe–D–Pro–Phe region of 008(Z) [13] can be superimposed accurately (68) (Fig. 10).

This is most important, as the side chains of 008 in solution populate several rotamers with their dominating orientation equivalent to the one for PFF [24] in the crystalline state. The aromatic side chains of 008(Z) adopt the conformation shown in Figure 10 to the following percentages: Phe^2 = 80%, Trp^5 = 75%, Phe^6 = 58% (55). In addition, on dissolving crystals of PFF [24], the NMR spectrum obtained exhibits two conformations differing by cis/trans isomerism about the one Pro–Phe bond in slow exchange. The amount of the conformation that corresponds to the crystal structure varies from about 40% to 70% depending strongly on the solvent polarity (69). This demonstrates the difficulty in obtaining conformation activity relationships by comparing only two compounds under one condition. When, however, cytoprotective activity is observed, almost identical spatial structures have been found for all cyclic hexapeptides (44) including the conformation of the aromatic side chains. Preliminary results in other solvents like CDCl$_3$ and H$_2$O (with unprotected Lys side chain) support these findings (52). The structures of antamanide (66,67) and cyclolinopeptide A (70) in solution are more complicated. These peptides can

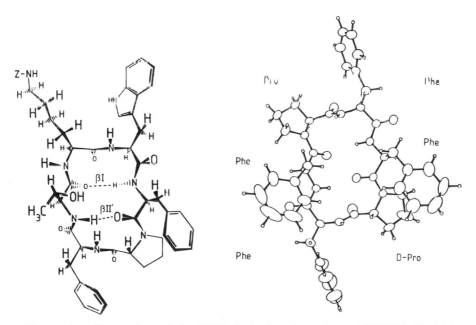

Figure 10 Comparison of the NMR-derived conformation of "008(Z)" (13, left) with the x-ray structure of "PFF" (24, right).

adopt, at least in the Pro–Phe region, a similar global structure. For this it is necessary to arrange the molecule in a way that the Pro^8–Phe^9 of antamanide corresponds to the partial "retro-inverso" structure Phe^6–D–Pro^1 in 008(Z). These statements need further investigations, which are currently under way.

When the spatial structures are not available, it is impossible to determine the necessity of molecular substructures for biological activity by constitution-activity relationships in flexible molecules. Wieland's group has performed extensive structure-activity studies on antamanide and has synthesized about 80 derivatives (10). At that time an elucidation of the conformation was not possible, and the results gave the impression that almost all parts of the molecule would be necessary for biological activity. However, changes in the spatial structure of the binding site of antamanide may also be induced by constitutional variations far from the bioactive site of the substrate molecule. Therefore, without conformational control, it is difficult to draw definite conclusions about the recognition area.

IV. POSSIBLE APPLICATIONS

Although the biological assay to optimize activity was the competitive inhibition of cholate or phalloidin uptake by isolated hepatocytes, in vivo testing of liver cytoprotection has been performed as well (11,12). The results show the potential usefulness of these compounds. The high lipophilicity of our analogs prevented further studies in other test systems. Therefore, it was important to improve the water solubility. This was achieved either by deprotection of the Lys side chain or by attaching polar groups (e.g., sulfate, polyethyleneglycol) to the Thr and/or a Tyr hydroxyl group (71) without considerable loss of biological activity. These compounds exhibit high potency in the protection against taurocholate- and cerulein-induced pancreatitis (72) and against alcohol-induced ulceration of the stomach mucosa (73). Furthermore, significant protection of the liver against ischemia was observed (74). Although the origins of these biological effects are unknown at this time, there is no doubt that they open new areas for possible applications. They also leave substantial work for the future to elucidate the mechanisms of the effects.

V. CONCLUSIONS

In the search for superpotent cytoprotective peptides, we synthesized a large number of conformationally restricted cyclic penta- and hexapeptides. Their conformations were determined by NMR spectroscopy, by restrained molecular dynamics calculations, and partially by x-ray analysis. The following results were obtained:

1. It was shown that endocrine activity and cytoprotection of somatostatins have different structural requirements.
2. It was possible to find compounds that exhibit an enhanced cytoprotective effect but no longer show endocrine activity.
3. By structure-activity studies we found compounds that were 2 orders of magnitude more potent in cytoprotection than somatostatin.
4. It was possible to localize the common structural features (including the spatial arrangement) of the "somatostatins and antamanides" structure responsible for the cytoprotective activity.

The topic presented in this chapter is an example of molecular modeling of bioactive molecules without knowledge of the receptor. This approach certainly requires the synthesis and conformational studies of more compounds than in cases where the structure of the target is known. In addition, rigidization is an important requirement to draw structural conclusions. Such studies follow a narrow path between the loss of activity by fixation of the wrong conformation and compounds with too high a flexibility to allow definite conclusions. Even our cyclic peptides exhibit partial flexibilities, mainly in the side chains. Our conclusions are based on the simplifying assumption that the most stable conformation is close to that bound to the receptor. If rigidity is accompanied by high biological activity, it seems to be proper to assume that a change in the conformation would consume extra energy in the binding process and is therefore unlikely.

The studies shown here are certainly an example of the combined use of synthesis and conformational analysis being used to design compounds of higher biological activities. It is obvious that the next target is the isolation of the hepatic receptor by affinity chromatography. The structure of the receptor will certainly help to find more active molecules and to understand the biochemical mechanism of the cytoprotection process in a more rational way.

ACKNOWLEDGMENTS

The article presented here is based on the work of a number of co-workers for the synthesis and conformational analysis of the cyclic peptides: M. Bernd, I. Damm, V. Eiermann, G. Gemmecker, C. Griesinger, A. Müller, K. Wagner, and J. Zarbock.

The biological assays were done by Professor Frimmer, Dr. Ziegler in Giessen, Professor Rao in Bonn, Professor Usadel in Heidelberg/Mannheim, Professor Szabo at Harvard Medical School, Dr. Sandow at Hoechst Company, and others. Discussions with these colleagues and with the late Professors T. Wieland and R. Geiger were stimulating. We are indebted to all of them.

Financial support was given by the Fonds der Chemischen Industrie, the Deutsche Forschungsgemeinschaft, and the Bundesminister für Forschung und Technologie.

REFERENCES

1. Fischer, E., Einflüsse der Konfiguration auf die Wirkung der Enzyme. *Berichte Chem. Gesellschaft 27*:2985–2993 (1894).
2. Hruby, V. J., Structure and conformation related to the activity of peptide hormones. In *Perspectives in Peptide Chemistry*, A. Eberle, R. Geiger, T. Wieland, eds. Karger, Basel, New York, pp. 207–221 (1981).
3. Lehn, J. M., Supramolecular chemistry: Receptors, catalysts and carriers. *Science 227*:849–856 (1985).
4. Schiller, P. W., Conformational analysis of enkephalins and conformation activity relationship. In *The Peptides*, S. Udenfried, J. Meienhofer, eds. Academic Press, Orlando, Fla., pp. 219–268 (1984) and references cited therein.
5. Kessler, H., Conformation and biological activity of cyclic peptides. *Angew. Chem. 94*:509–520; *Int. Ed. Engl. 21*:512–523 (1982).
6. Hruby, V. J., Conformational restrictions of biologically active peptides via amino acid side chain groups. *Life Sci. 31*:189–199 (1982).
7. Kessler, H., K. Wagner, and M. Will, Analysis of peptide conformations by NMR spectroscopy. In *Proceedings of the IXth International Symposium on Medicinal Chemistry*, E. Winterfeld, ed. E. Mutschler, Berlin, pp. 143–157 (1987).
8. *International Symposium on Mechanisms of Cell Injury, Cytoprotection-Organoprotection*, Heidelberg, June 9–11, 1986. *Klin. Wochenschr.*, K. H. Usadel, ed. Suppl. VII, *64*:1–155 (1986).
9. Kessler, H., M. Gehrke, A. Haupt, M. Klein, A. Müller, and K. Wagner, Common structural features for cytoprotection activities of somatostatin, antamanide and related peptides. *Klin. Wochenschr. 64* (Suppl. VII):74–78 (1986).
10. Wieland, T., *Peptides of Poisonous Amanita Mushrooms*. Springer-Verlag, New York (1986).
11. Szabo, S., and K. H. Usadel, Cytoprotection-organoprotection by somatostatin: Gastric and hepatic lessions. *Experientia 38*:245 (1982).
12. Usadel, K. H., H. Kessler, G. Rohr, K. Kusterer, K. D. Palitzsch, and U. Schwedes, Cytoprotective properties of somatostatin. *Klin. Wochenschr. 64* (Suppl. VII):59–63 (1986).
13. Ziegler, K., M. Frimmer, H. Kessler, I. Damm, V. Eiermann, S. Koll, and J. Zarbock, Modified somatostatins as inhibitors of a multispecific transport system for bile acids and phallotoxins in isolated hepatocytes. *Biochim. Biophys. Acta 845*:86–93 (1985).
14. Petzinger, E., Competitive inhibition of the uptake of demethylphalloin by cholic acid in isolated hepatocytes. *Naunyn-Schmiedeberg's Arch. Pharmacol. 316*:345–349 (1981).
15. Petzinger, E., and M. Frimmer, Energy linked uptake of demethylphalloin by isolated rat liver cells. *Arch Pharmacol. 319*:87–92 (1982).

16. Frimmer, M., and R. Kroker, Phalloidin-antagonisten. *Drug Res.* 25:394–396 (1975).

17. Frimmer, M., E. Petzinger, and K. Ziegler, Protective effect of anionic cholecystographic agents against phalloidin on isolated hepatocytes by competitive inhibition of the phallotoxin uptake *Naunyn-Schmiedeberg's Arch. Pharmacol.* 313:85–89 (1980).

18. Frimmer, M., Phalloidin—Ein leberspezifisches Pilzgift. *Biol. Unserer Zeit* 5:147–152 (1979).

19. Frimmer, M., What we have learned from phalloidin. *Toxicol. Lett.* 35:169–182 (1987).

20. Lengsfeld, A. M., I. Löw, T. Wieland, P. Dancker, and W. Hasselbach, Interaction of phalloidin with actin. *Proc. Natl. Acad. Sci. USA* 71:2803–2807 (1974).

21. Rao, G. S., H. Lemoch, H. Kessler, I. Damm, V. Eiermann, S. Koll, J. Zarbock, and K. H. Usadel, Prevention of phalloidin induced lesions on isolated rat hepatocytes. *Klin. Wochenschr.* 64 (Suppl. VII):79–86 (1986).

22. Ziegler, K., E. Petzinger, E. Grundmann, and M. Frimmer, Decreased sensitivity of isolated hepatocytes from baby rats, from regenerating and from poisoned livers to phalloidin. *Naunyn-Schmiedeberg's Arch. Pharmacol.* 306:295–300 (1979).

23. Eberle, A. N., Photoaffinity labelling of peptide hormone receptors. *J. Receptor Res.* 3:313–326 (1983).

24. Chowdry, V., and F. H. Westheimer, Photoaffinity labelling of biological systems. *Annu. Rev. Biochem.* 48:293–325 (1979).

25. Ziegler, K., and M. Frimmer, Photoaffinity labelling of whole cells by flashed light: A simple apparatus for high energy ultraviolet flashes. *Biochim. Biophys. Acta* 855:143–146 (1986).

26. Ziegler, K., M. Frimmer, and H. Fasold, Further characterization of membrane proteins involved in the transport of organic anions in hepatocytes. *Biochim. Biophys. Acta* 769:117–129 (1984).

27. Wieland, T., M. Nassal, W. Kramer, G. Fricker, U. Bickel, and G. Kurz, Identity of hepatic membrane transport system for bile salts, phalloidin, and antamanide by photoaffinity labelling. *Proc. Natl. Acad. Sci. USA* 78:5232–5234 (1981).

28. Kessler, H., A. Haupt, M. Frimmer, and K. Ziegler, Synthesis of a cyclic retro analogue of somatostatin suitable for photoaffinity labelling. *Int. J. Peptide Protein Res.* 621–628 (1987).

29. Ziegler, K., and M. Frimmer, Molecular aspects of cytoprotection by modified somatostatins. *Klin Wochenschr.* 64 (Suppl. VII):87–89 (1986).

30. Brazeau, P., W. Vale, R. Burgus, N. Ling, M. Butcher, J. Rivier, and R. Guillemin, Hypothalamic polypeptide that inhibits the secretion of immunoreactive pituitary growth hormone. *Science* 179:77–79 (1973).

31. Arison, B. H., R. Hirschmann, and D. F. Veber, Inferences about the conformation of somatostatin at a biological receptor based on NMR studies. *Bioorg. Chem.* 7:447–451 (1978).

32. Hallenga, K., G. van Binst, M. Knappenberg, J. Brison, A. Michel, and J. Dirkx, The conformational properties of some fragments of the peptide hormone somatostatin. *Biochim. Biophys. Acta* 577:82–101 (1979).

33. Veber, D. F., Conformational considerations in the design of somatostatin analogs showing increased metabolic stability. In *Peptides, Proceedings of the Sixth American Peptide Symposium*, E. Gross, J. Meienhofer, eds. Pierce Chemical Co., Rockford, Ill., pp. 409–419 (1979).

34. Veber, D. F., R. M. Freidinger, D. Schwenk-Perlow, W. J. Paleveda, F. W. Holly, R. G. Strachnan, R. F. Nutt, B. H. Arison, C. Homnick, W. C. Randall, M. S. Glitzer, R. Saperstein, and R. Hirschmann, A potent cyclic hexapeptide analogue of somatostatin. *Nature 292*:55–58 (1981).

35. Bauer, W., U. Briner, W. Doepfner, R. Haller, R. Huguenin, P. Marbach, T. J. Petcher, and J. Pless, A very potent and selective octapeptide analogue of somatostatin with prolonged action. *Life Sci. 31*:1133–1140 (1982).

36. Nutt, R. F., C. D. Colton, D. F. Veber, E. L. Slater, and R. Saperstein, Somatostatin analogs with improved oral bioavailability. *Klin. Wochenschr. 64* (Suppl. VII):71–73 (1986).

37. Kessler, H., M. Bernd, and I. Damm, Peptide conformations 23: NMR investigations of cyclic hexapeptides containing the active sequence of somatostatin. *Tetrahedron Lett., 23*:4685–4689 (1982).

38. Kessler, H., M. Bernd, H. Kogler, J. Zarbock, O. W. Sorensen, G. Bodenhausen, and R. R. Ernst, Peptide conformations 28: Relayed heteronuclear correlation spectroscopy and conformational analysis of cyclic hexapeptides containing the active sequence of somatostatin. *J. Am. Chem. Soc. 105*:6944–6952 (1983).

39. Kessler, H., and V. Eiermann, Peptide conformations 24: Homo- and heteronuclear 2D NMR spectroscopy of cyclic pentapeptides containing the active sequence of somatostatin. *Tetrahedron Lett. 23*:4689–4692 (1982).

40. Eiermann, V., Dissertation: Cyclische Somatostatinanaloge—Synthese und Konformationsstudien. Frankfurt am Main (1983).

41. Goodman, M., and M. Chorev, On the concept of linear modified retro-peptide structures. *Acc. Chem. Res. 12*(1):1–7 (1979).

42. Freidinger, R. M., C. D. Colton, D. S. Perlow, W. L. Whitter, W. J. Paleveda, D. F. Veber, B. H. Arison, and R. Saperstein, Modified retro enantiomers are potent somatostatin analogues. In *Peptides, Proceedings of the Eighth American Peptide Symposium*, H. Hruby, D. H. Rich, eds. Pierce Chemical Company, Rockford, Ill., pp. 349–352 (1983).

43. Bickel, M., H. Kessler, W. König, V. Teetz, and W. Stoll, Long-term inhibition of gastric acid and secretion by somatostatin and analogues in rats. *Acta Endocrinol. 253* (Suppl.):106–107 (1983).

44. Kessler, H., A. Haupt, M. Klein, and K. Wagner, Common structural features for cytoprotection activity of cyclic retro-analogues of somatostatin. In *Peptides, Proceedings of the 19th European Peptide Symposium*, K. Theodoropoulos ed. W. de Gruyter, Berlin, pp. 327–330 (1987).

45. Kessler, H., J. W. Bats, C. Griesinger, S. Koll, K. Wagner, and M. Will, Conformational analysis of a superpotent cytoprotective cyclic somatostatin analogue. *J. Am. Chem. Soc. 110*:1033–1049 (1988).

46. Kessler, H., W. Bermel, A. Müller, and K. H. Pook, Modern nuclear magnetic resonance spectroscopy of peptides. In *The Peptides*, Vol. 7, S. Udenfriend, J. Meienhofer, V. J. Hruby, eds., Academic Press, New York, pp. 438–473 (1985).

47. Bothner-By, A. A., R. L. Stephans, J. Lee, C. D. Warren, and R. W. Jeanloz, Structure determination of a tetrasaccharide: Transient nuclear overhauser effects in the rotating frame. *J. Am. Chem. Soc. 106*:811–813 (1984).

48. Kessler, H., C. Griesinger, R. Kerssebaum, K. Wagner, and R. R. Ernst, Separation of cross relaxation and J cross-peaks in 2D rotating frame NMR spectroscopy. *J. Am. Chem. Soc. 109*:607–609 (1987).

49. Griesinger, C., and R. R. Ernst, Frequency offset effects and their elimination in NMR rotating frame cross-relaxation spectroscopy. *J. Magn. Reson. 75*:261–271 (1987).

50. Van Gunsteren, W. F., GROMOS—Groningen molecular simulation system. *J. Mol. Biol. 183*:461–477 (1985).

51. Hermans, J. (ed.), *Molecular Dynamics and Protein Structure.* Polycrystal Book Service, Western Springs, Ill. (1985).

52. Kessler, H., A. Müller, and H. Oschkinat, Differences and sums of traces within (OSY spectra (DISCO) for the extraction of coupling constants. *Magn. Reson. Chem. 23*:844–852 (1985).

53. Griesinger, C., O. W. Soerensen, and R. R. Ernst, Two-dimensional correlation of connected NMR-transitions. *J. Am. Chem. Soc. 107*:6394–6396 (1985).

54. Bystrov, V. F., Progress in NMR spectroscopy. *10*:41–81 (1976).

55. Kessler, H., C. Griesinger, and K. Wagner, Peptide conformations 42: Conformation of side chains in peptides using heteronuclear coupling constants obtained by two-dimensional NMR spectroscopy. *J. Am. Chem. Soc. 109*:6927–6933 (1987).

56. Kessler, H., C. Griesinger, J. Zarbock, and H. R. Loosly, Assignment of carbonyl carbons and sequence analysis in peptides by heteronuclear shift correlation via small coupling constants with broadband decoupling in t1 (COLOC). *J. Magn. Reson. 57*:331–337 (1984).

57. Kessler, H., G. Zimmermann, H. Forster, J. Engel, G. Oepen, and W. S. Sheldrick, Does a molecule have the same conformation in the crystalline state and in solution? *Angew. Chem. Int. Ed. Engl. 20*:1053–1055 (1981).

58. Loosli, H. R., H. Kessler, H. Oschkinat, H. P. Weber, T. J. Petcher, and A. Widmer, Peptide conformations 31: The conformation of cyclosporin A in crystal and in solution. *Helv. Chim. Acta 68*:682–704 (1985).

59. Kessler, H., G. Gemmecker, A. Haupt, M. Klein, K. Wagner, and M. Will, Alanine containing analogues of cyclo(–D–Pro–Phe–Thr–Lys(Z)–Trp–Phe)— conformationally controlled structure-activity-relationships, *Tetrahedron 44*:745–759 (1988).

60. Kessler, H., K. Wagner, and M. Will, Conformational analysis of a cyclic hexapeptide by rotating frame NOE evaluation and molecular dynamics calculation. In *Peptides 1987, Proceedings of the 10th American Peptide Symposium* (in press).

61. Smith, J. A., and L. G. Pease, Reverse turns in peptides and proteins. *Crit. Rev. Biochem. 8*:315–399 (1980).

62. Rose, G. D., L. M. Gierasch, and J. Smith, Turns in peptides and proteins. *Adv. Protein Chem. 37*:1–107 (1985).

63. Kessler, H., A. Haupt, and M. Schudok (to be published).

64. Kessler, H., and A. Müller, Eine ungewöhnliche Konformation in dem cyclischen Pentapeptid cyclo(-Pro-Pro-Phe-Phe-Gly-) in DMSO. *Liebigs Ann. Chem.* 1687-1704 (1986).

65. Karle, I. L., J. Karle, T. Wieland, W. Burgermeister, H. Faulstich, and B. Witkop, Conformation of the lithium-antamanide complex and sodium-(Phe4, Val6)antamanide complex in the crystalline state. *Proc. Natl. Acad. Sci. USA* 70:1836-1840 (1973).

66. Kessler, H., and A. Müller (to be published).

67. Kessler, H., C. Griesinger, J. Lautz, A. Müller, W. F. van Gunsteren, and H. J. C. Berendsen, Conformational dynamics detected by nuclear magnetic resonance NOE values and J coupling constants, *J. Am. Chem. Soc.* 110:3393-3396 (1988).

68. Kessler, H., M. Klein, A. Müller, K. Wagner, J. W. Bats, M. Frimmer, and K. Ziegler, Conformational prerequisites for the in vitro inhibition of cholate uptake in hepatocytes by cyclic analogues of antamanide and somatostatin. *Angew. Chem. 98*: 1030-1031; *Int. Ed. Engl. 25*:997-999 (1986).

69. Kessler, H., and K. Wagner, Unpublished results.

70. Benedetti, E., V. Pavone, et al., First Capri Conference on Conformation and Biological Activity on Peptides, May 23-26, 1988, Capri, Italy. *1986*, D. Theodoropoulos, ed. W. de Gruyter, Berlin, pp. 327-330 (1987).

71. Kessler, H., A. Haupt, and M. Schudok, Cyclische Peptide mit Cytoprotektiver Wirkung. Deutsches Patent P 36 14 904.7 (HOE 86/F 096) und P 37 03 159.7 (HOE 87/F 026) (3.2.1987).

72. Rohr, G., V. Keim, and K. H. Usadel, Prevention of experimental pancreatitis by somatostatin. *Klin. Wochenschr. 64* (Suppl. VII):93-96 (1986).

73. Kusterer, K., G. Rohr, U. Schwedes, K. H. Usadel, and S. Szabo, Gastric mucosal protection by somatostatins. *Klin. Wochenschr. 64* (Suppl. VII):97-99 (1986).

74. Kusterer, K., K. D. Palitzsch, C. Bloechle, T. Konrad, G. Brendenscheg, G. Rohr, U. Schwedes, H. Kessler, and K. H. Usadel, Iloprost und Somatostatinanaloge besitzen einen protektiven Effekt bei der ischämischen Leberschädigung der Ratte. 42. Tagung der Deutschen Gesellschaft für Verdauungs- und Stoffwechselkrankheiten, Sept. 9-12, 1987, Salzburg.

Index